T0131005

Pediatric Gastroenterology

Editor

HARPREET PALL

PEDIATRIC CLINICS
OF NORTH AMERICA

www.pediatric.theclinics.com

Consulting Editor
BONITA F. STANTON

December 2021 • Volume 68 • Number 6

ELSEVIER

1600 John F. Kennedy Boulevard • Suite 1800 • Philadelphia, Pennsylvania, 19103-2899

http://www.theclinics.com

THE PEDIATRIC CLINICS OF NORTH AMERICA Volume 68, Number 6
December 2021 ISSN 0031-3955, ISBN-13: 978-0-323-92004-9

Editor: Kerry Holland
Developmental Editor: Axell Ivan Jade M. Purificacion

The Pediatric Clinics of North America (ISSN 0031-3955) is published bimonthly by Elsevier Inc., 360 Park Avenue South, New York, NY 10010-1710. Months of issue are February, April, June, August, October, and December. Periodicals postage paid at New York, NY and additional mailing offices. Subscription prices are $250.00 per year (US individuals), $984.00 per year (US institutions), $315.00 per year (Canadian individuals), $1048.00 per year (Canadian institutions), $376.00 per year (international individuals), $1048.00 per year (international institutions), $100.00 per year (US students and residents), $100.00 per year (Canadian students and residents), and $165.00 per year (international residents and students). To receive students/resident rare, orders must be accompanied by name of affiliated institution, date of term, and the signature of program/residency coordinator on institution letterhead. Orders will be billed at individual rate until proof of status is received. Foreign air speed delivery is included in all *Clinics* subscription prices. All prices are subject to change without notice. **POSTMASTER:** Send address changes to *The Pediatric Clinics of North America*, Elsevier Health Sciences Division, Subscription Customer Service, 3251 Riverport Lane, Maryland Heights, MO 63043. **Customer Service: 1-800-654-2452 (US and Canada). From outside of the US and Canada: 1-314-447-8871. Fax: 1-314-447-8029. For print support, E-mail: JournalsCustomerService-usa@elsevier.com. For online support, E-mail: JournalsOnlineSupport-usa@elsevier.com.**

Reprints. For copies of 100 or more, of articles in this publication, please contact the Commercial Reprints Department, Elsevier Inc., 360 Park Avenue South, New York, NY 10010-1710. Tel.: 212-633-3874; Fax: 212-633-3820; E-mail: reprints@elsevier.com.

The Pediatric Clinics of North America is also published in Spanish by McGraw-Hill Inter-americana Editores S.A., Mexico City, Mexico; in Portuguese by Riechmann and Affonso Editores, Rua Comandante Coelho 1085, CEP 21250, Rio de Janeiro, Brazil; and in Greek by Althayia SA, Athens, Greece.

The Pediatric Clinics of North America is covered in *MEDLINE/PubMed (Index Medicus)*, *Excerpta Medica*, *Current Contents*, *Current Contents/Clinical Medicine*, *Science Citation Index*, *ASCA*, *ISI/BIOMED*, and *BIOSIS*.

PROGRAM OBJECTIVE

The goal of the *Pediatric Clinics of North America* is to keep practicing physicians and residents up to date with current clinical practice in pediatrics by providing timely articles reviewing the state-of-the-art in patient care.

TARGET AUDIENCE

All practicing pediatricians, physicians and healthcare professionals who provide patient care to pediatric patients.

LEARNING OBJECTIVES

Upon completion of this activity, participants will be able to:

1. Review health equity, social determinants of health, and the impact of the COVID-19 pandemic on pediatric gastroenterology.
2. Discuss the pathogenesis and medical management of inflammatory bowel disease, esophagitis, and celiac disease.
3. Recognize advances in pediatric endoscopic procedures.

ACCREDITATIONS
Physician Credit

The Elsevier Office of Continuing Medical Education (EOCME) is accredited by the Accreditation Council for Continuing Medical Education (ACCME) to provide continuing medical education for physicians.

The EOCME designates this journal-based activity for a maximum of 13 *AMA PRA Category 1 Credit*(s)™. Physicians should claim only the credit commensurate with the extent of their participation in the activity.

All other healthcare professionals requesting continuing education credit for this this journal-based activity will be issued a certificate of participation.

ABP MAINTENANCE OF CERTIFICATION CREDIT

Successful completion of this CME activity, which includes participation in the activity and individual assessment of and feedback to the learner, enables the learner to earn up to 13 MOC points in the American Board of Pediatrics' (ABP)

Maintenance of Certification (MOC) program. It is the CME activity provider's responsibility to submit learner completion information to ACCME for the purpose of granting ABP MOC credit.

DISCLOSURE OF CONFLICTS OF INTEREST

The EOCME assesses conflict of interest with its instructors, faculty, planners, and other individuals who are in a position to control the content of CME activities. All relevant conflicts of interest that are identified are thoroughly vetted by EOCME for fair balance, scientific objectivity, and patient care recommendations. EOCME is committed to providing its learners with CME activities that promote improvements or quality in healthcare and not a specific proprietary business or a commercial interest.

The planning committee, staff, authors, and editors listed below have identified no financial relationships or relationships to products or devices they or their spouse/life partner have with commercial interest related to the content of this CME activity:

Ricardo Arbizu, MD, MS; Regina Chavous-Gibson, MSN, RN; Reuven Zev Cohen, MD; Rhea Daniel, MD; Udeme D. Ekong, MD, MPH; A. Jay Freeman, MD; Ben Freiberg, MD; Samuel Gnanakumar; Deborah A. Goldman, MD; Karoly Horvath, MD, PhD; Jennifer Jimenez, MD; Linola Juste, MPH; Sarah Kemme, MD; Julie Khlevner, MD; Amornluck Krasaelap, MD; Beth Loveridge-Lenza, MD; Daniel Mallon, MD, MSHPEd; Rajkumar Mayakrishnann; Jonathan Miller, MD; Tania Mitsinikos, MD; Paula Mrowczynski-Hernandez, RD; Amanda B. Muir, MD; Harpreet Pall, MD; Leonel Rodriguez, MD, MS; Melanie A. Ruffner, MD, PhD; Elizabeth A. Spencer, MD; Richard Taylor, III, MD; Sanu R. Yadav, MD; Sara E. Yerina, BSN, RN

The planning committee, staff, authors and editors listed below have identified financial relationships or relationships to products or devices they or their spouse/life partner have with commercial interest related to the content of this CME activity:

Marla C. Dubinsky, MD: Consultant: Abbvie, Celgene, Genentech, Janssen, Pfizer, Prometheus Labs, Salix, Takeda, UCB; Research: Janssen, Pfizer, Takeda; Co-Founder and shareholder: Trellus Health

Rohit Kohli, MBBS, MS: Research: Albireo Pharma, Epigen Biosciences, Mirum Pharmaceuticals, Takeda, Vision Pharmaceuticals; Consultant/Speaker: Alexion, Intercept Pharmaceuticals, Sanofi-Genzyme

Diana G. Lerner, MD: Founder: Lerner Media Inc.

Cara Mack, MD: Consultant: Albireo Pharma

Karen F. Murray, MD: Consultant: Gilead, Albireo Pharma

UNAPPROVED/OFF-LABEL USE DISCLOSURE
The EOCME requires CME faculty to disclose to the participants:
1. When products or procedures being discussed are off-label, unlabelled, experimental, and/or investigational (not US Food and Drug Administration [FDA] approved); and
2. Any limitations on the information presented, such as data that are preliminary or that represent ongoing research, interim analyses, and/or unsupported opinions. Faculty may discuss information about pharmaceutical agents that is outside of FDA-approved labelling. This information is intended solely for CME and is not intended to promote off-label use of these medications. If you have any questions, contact the medical affairs department of the manufacturer for the most recent prescribing information.

TO ENROLL
To enroll in the *Pediatric Clinics of North America* Continuing Medical Education program, call customer service at 1-800-654-2452 or sign up online at http://www.theclinics.com/home/cme. The CME program is available to subscribers for an additional annual fee of USD 324.00.

METHOD OF PARTICIPATION
In order to claim credit, participants must complete the following:
1. Complete enrolment as indicated above.
2. Read the activity.
3. Complete the CME Test and Evaluation. Participants must achieve a score of 70% on the test. All CME Tests and Evaluations must be completed online.

In order to claim MOC points, participants must complete the following:
1. Complete steps listed above for claiming CME credit
2. Provide your specialty board ID#, birth date (MM/DD), and attestation.
3. Online MOC submission is only available for the American Board of pediatrics' (ABP) Maintenance of Certification (MOC) program

CME INQUIRIES/SPECIAL NEEDS
For all CME inquiries or special needs, please contact elsevierCME@elsevier.com

Contributors

CONSULTING EDITOR

BONITA F. STANTON, MD
Professor of Pediatrics and Founding Dean, Robert C. and Laura C. Garrett Endowed Chair, Hackensack Meridian School of Medicine, President, Academic Enterprise, Hackensack Meridian Health, Nutley, New Jersey

EDITOR

HARPREET PALL, MD, MBA, CPE
Chair and Professor, Department of Pediatrics, Hackensack Meridian School of Medicine, Nutley, New Jersey; Department of Pediatrics, K. Hovnanian Children's Hospital, Jersey Shore University Medical Center, Neptune, New Jersey

AUTHORS

RICARDO ARBIZU, MD, MS
Section of Pediatric Gastroenterology, Hepatology and Nutrition, Associate Director, Neurogastroenterology and Motility Center, Assistant Professor, Yale School of Medicine, Yale New Haven Children's Hospital, New Haven, Connecticut

REUVEN ZEV COHEN, MD
Division of Pediatric Gastroenterology, Hepatology, and Nutrition, Emory University School of Medicine, Children's Healthcare of Atlanta, Atlanta, Georgia

RHEA DANIEL, MD
Department of Pediatric Gastroenterology, Hepatology, and Nutrition, McGovern Medical School, The University of Texas Health Science Center at Houston, Children's Memorial Hermann Hospital, Houston, Texas

MARLA C. DUBINSKY, MD
Professor of Pediatrics and Medicine, Chief of the Division of Pediatric Gastroenterology, Department of Pediatrics, Mount Sinai Kravis Children's Hospital, Co-Director, Susan and Leonard Feinstein Inflammatory Bowel Disease Clinical Center, Mount Sinai Hospital, Icahn School of Medicine, New York, New York

UDEME D. EKONG, MD, MPH
MedStar Georgetown Transplant Institute, MedStar Georgetown University Hospital, Associate Professor of Pediatrics and Surgery, Department of Pediatrics, Georgetown University School of Medicine, Washington, DC

A. JAY FREEMAN, MD
Division of Pediatric Gastroenterology, Hepatology, and Nutrition, Emory University School of Medicine, Children's Healthcare of Atlanta, Atlanta, Georgia

BEN FREIBERG, MD
Section of Pediatric Gastroenterology, Hepatology and Nutrition, Advanced Fellow, Pediatric Neurogastroenterology and Motility, Yale School of Medicine, Yale New Haven Children's Hospital, New Haven, Connecticut

DEBORAH A. GOLDMAN, MD
Department of Pediatric Gastroenterology, Hepatology and Nutrition, Cleveland Clinic Children's Hospital, Clinical Assistant Professor of Pediatrics, Cleveland Clinic Lerner College of Medicine of Case Western Reserve University, Cleveland, Ohio

KAROLY HORVATH, MD, PhD
Professor of Pediatrics, Florida State University, Center for Digestive Health and Nutrition, Arnold Palmer Hospital for Children, Orlando Health, Orlando, Florida

JENNIFER JIMENEZ, MD
Department of Pediatrics, Hackensack Meridian School of Medicine, Nutley, New Jersey; Pediatric Gastroenterologist, Division of Pediatric Gastroenterology and Nutrition, Department of Pediatrics, K. Hovnanian Children's Hospital, Jersey Shore University Medical Center, Neptune, New Jersey

LINOLA JUSTE, BS
Division of Gastroenterology, Hepatology and Nutrition, Children's Hospital of Philadelphia, Philadelphia, Pennsylvania

SARAH KEMME, MD
Section of Gastroenterology, Hepatology, and Nutrition, Digestive Health Institute, University of Colorado Denver School of Medicine, Children's Hospital Colorado, Aurora, Colorado

JULIE KHLEVNER, MD
Associate Professor of Pediatrics, Director, Gastrointestinal Motility Center, Division of Pediatric Gastroenterology, Hepatology and Nutrition, Morgan Stanley Children's Hospital, Columbia University Irving Medical Center, New York, New York

ROHIT KOHLI, MBBS, MS
Division Chief, Gastroenterology, Children's Hospital Los Angeles, Los Angeles, California

AMORNLUCK KRASAELAP, MD
Assistant Professor of Pediatrics, University of Missouri School of Medicine, University of Kansas, Children's Mercy Hospital, Kansas City, Missouri

DIANA G. LERNER, MD
Associate Professor of Pediatrics, Division of Pediatric Gastroenterology, Hepatology and Nutrition, Department of Pediatrics, Medical College of Wisconsin, Milwaukee, Wisconsin

BETH LOVERIDGE-LENZA, MD
Pediatric Gastroenterologist, Jersey Shore University Medical Center, Division of Pediatric Gastroenterology and Nutrition, K. Hovnanian Children's Hospital, Hackensack Meridian Health, Neptune, New Jersey

CARA L. MACK, MD
Section of Gastroenterology, Hepatology, and Nutrition, Professor of Pediatrics, Hewit, Andrew Chair in Pediatric Liver Disease, Digestive Health Institute, University of Colorado Denver School of Medicine, Children's Hospital Colorado, Aurora, Colorado

DANIEL MALLON, MD, MSHPEd
Department of Pediatrics, Assistant Professor, Division of Gastroenterology, Hepatology and Nutrition, Cincinnati Children's Hospital Medical Center, University of Cincinnati College of Medicine, Cincinnati, Ohio

JONATHAN MILLER, MD
Fellow, Division of Pediatric Gastroenterology, Hepatology and Nutrition, Morgan Stanley Children's Hospital, Columbia University Irving Medical Center, New York, New York

TANIA MITSINIKOS, MD
Director, Fatty Liver Clinic, Children's Hospital Los Angeles, Los Angeles, California

PAULA MROWCZYNSKI-HERNANDEZ, RD
Dietitian, Fatty Liver Clinic, Children's Hospital Los Angeles, Los Angeles, California

AMANDA B. MUIR, MD
Assistant Professor of Pediatrics, Division of Gastroenterology, Hepatology and Nutrition, Department of Pediatrics, Children's Hospital of Philadelphia, University of Pennsylvania Perelman School of Medicine, Philadelphia, Pennsylvania

KAREN F. MURRAY, MD
Professor and Chair, Department of Pediatrics, Cleveland Clinic Lerner College of Medicine, Physician-in-Chief, Cleveland Clinic Children's Hospital, Cleveland, Ohio

HARPREET PALL, MD, MBA, CPE
Chair and Professor, Department of Pediatrics, Hackensack Meridian School of Medicine, Nutley, New Jersey; Department of Pediatrics, K. Hovnanian Children's Hospital, Jersey Shore University Medical Center, Neptune, New Jersey

LEONEL RODRIGUEZ, MD, MS
Section of Pediatric Gastroenterology, Hepatology and Nutrition, Chief, Pediatric Gastroenterology and Hepatology, Director, Neurogastroenterology and Motility Center, Associate Professor of Pediatrics, Yale School of Medicine, Yale New Haven Children's Hospital, New Haven, Connecticut

MELANIE A. RUFFNER, MD, PhD
Assistant Professor of Pediatrics, Division of Allergy and Immunology, Department of Pediatrics, Children's Hospital of Philadelphia, University of Pennsylvania Perelman School of Medicine, Philadelphia, Pennsylvania

ELIZABETH A. SPENCER, MD
Assistant Professor, Department of Pediatrics, Mount Sinai Kravis Children's Hospital, Susan and Leonard Feinstein Inflammatory Bowel Disease Clinical Center, Mount Sinai Hospital, Icahn School of Medicine, New York, New York

RICHARD TAYLOR, III, MD
Pediatric Residency Program, Department of Pediatrics, Pediatric Chief Resident, Cincinnati Children's Hospital Medical Center, University of Cincinnati College of Medicine, Cincinnati, Ohio

SANU R. YADAV, MD
Department of Pediatric Gastroenterology, Hepatology and Nutrition, Cleveland Clinic Children's Hospital, Cleveland, Ohio

SARA E. YERINA, BSN, RN
MedStar Georgetown Transplant Institute, MedStar Georgetown University Hospital, Washington, DC

Contents

Social determinants of health (SDH) as outlined by Healthy People 2020 encompasses 5 key domains: economic, education, social and community context, health and health care, and neighborhood and built environment. This article emphasizes pediatric populations and some of the existing SDH and health care disparities seen in pediatric gastroenterology. We specifically review inflammatory bowel disease, endoscopy, bariatric surgery, and liver transplantation. We also examine the burgeoning role of telehealth that has become commonplace since the coronavirus disease 2019 era.

Pediatric gastroenterologists took on a variety of challenges during the coronavirus disease 2019 pandemic, including learning about a new disease and how to recognize and manage it, prevent its spread among their patients and health professions colleagues, and make decisions about managing patients with chronic gastrointestinal and liver problems in light of the threat. They adapted their practice to accommodate drastically decreased numbers of in-person visits, adopting telehealth technologies, and instituting new protocols to perform endoscopies safely. The workforce pipeline was also affected by the impact of the pandemic on trainee education, clinical experience, research, and job searches.

Inflammatory bowel disease (IBD) describes a heterogenous group of diseases characterized by chronic inflammation of the intestinal tract. The IBD subtypes, Crohn's disease, ulcerative colitis, and IBD-Unspecified, each have characteristic features, but heterogeneity remains even among the subtypes. There has been an explosion of new knowledge on the possible pathogenesis of IBD over the last 2 decades mirroring innovation and refinement in technology, particularly the generation of large scale – "-omic" data. This knowledge has fostered a veritable renaissance of novel diagnostics, prognostics, and therapeutics, with patients with IBD seeing hope bloom in the increasingly large armamentarium of IBD therapies.

However, while there are increased numbers of therapies and more pathways being targeted, the number of medications for IBD is still finite and the efficacy has reached a plateau. Precision medicine (PM) is much needed to rationally select and optimize IBD therapies in the new reality of wider but still limited choice with a concurrent, increasingly fine resolution on the significance and utility of clinical, genetic, microbial, and proteomic characteristics that define individual patients. PM is a rapidly changing art, but this review will strive to detail the current state and future directions of PM in pediatric IBD.

technology have increased our understanding of gastrointestinal physiology and that knowledge has been applied to develop new diagnostic studies and therapeutic interventions. We present an overview of the clinical presentation, diagnosis, and treatment of common primary and secondary functional and motility disorders affecting the upper gastrointestinal tract in children.

Functional and motility gastrointestinal disorders are the most common complaints to the pediatric gastroenterologist. Disorders affecting the small intestine carry a significant morbidity and mortality due to the severe limitation of therapeutic interventions available and the complications associated with such interventions. Congenital colorectal disorders are rare but also carry significant morbidity and poor quality of life plus the social stigma associated with its complications. In this review, we summarize the clinical presentation, diagnostic evaluations, and the therapeutic interventions available for the most common and severe gastrointestinal functional and motility disorders of the small bowel, colon, and anorectum.

Pediatric pancreatitis describes a spectrum covering acute pancreatitis, acute recurrent pancreatitis, and chronic pancreatitis, each with varying clinical manifestations and risk factors requiring a tailored diagnostic approach. We emphasize management strategies based on age, risk factors, recurrence, and complications. A discussion of the role of therapeutic endoscopy is reviewed and highlights the growing role of endoscopic ultrasound and endoscopic retrograde cholangiopancreatography in children with pancreatitis. Particular diagnostic challenges in autoimmune pancreatitis are reviewed with an emphasis on differentiating this entity from alternate pancreaticobiliary pathologies. Finally, we explore a multidisciplinary approach to acute recurrent and chronic pancreatitis.

In chronic hepatitis, a broad differential diagnosis should be considered to accurately identify the cause(s) of liver injury. Autoimmune liver diseases (autoimmune hepatitis, primary sclerosing cholangitis, overlap syndrome) can occur in the setting of limited symptoms; therefore, a high index of suspicion and appropriate diagnostic workup should be performed. Most children with autoimmune hepatitis achieve sustained remission with medical therapy; however, there are no equivalent therapies for primary sclerosing cholangitis that impact the progression of disease. Research should include biomarker studies to predict histologic remission in autoimmune hepatitis and mechanistic studies to define future treatment targets for primary sclerosing cholangitis.

Obesity has led fatty liver disease to become the most common chronic liver disease in children worldwide. Pediatric professional organizations have agreed that screening for fatty liver disease in children is the need of the hour. Once identified, prevention is key through appropriate dietary and activity prescriptions. Research continues to identify key pathways and genetic risk factors that predispose certain children to the more severe manifestations of this silent epidemic. We hope these novel observations lead to breakthrough treatments for these children that are severely impacted, such that they may no longer need liver transplantation as young adults.

Hepatitis C in children is on the rise due to perinatal transmission from infected mothers, and high-risk practices in adolescents and young adults. Prevalence remains underestimated because children at high risk are often not screened. Treatment has evolved over the past decade with the advent of new drugs, and global elimination is now possible. Direct-acting antiviral combinations are safe and effective, with sustained viral suppression rate >90%, and Food and Drug Administration–approved for children ≥3 years old. Although challenging, efficient screening and treatment of chronic hepatitis C virus early is cost-effective and reduces burden of disease and its complications.

Biliary atresia (BA) is a common cause of jaundice in infancy. There is increasing evidence that newborn screening with direct or conjugated bilirubin leads to earlier diagnosis. Although the Kasai portoenterostomy is the primary treatment, there are scientific advances in adjuvant therapies. As pediatric patients transition to adult care, multidisciplinary care is essential, given the complexity of this patient population.

PEDIATRIC CLINICS OF NORTH AMERICA

FORTHCOMING ISSUES

February 2022
International Aspects of Pediatric Infectious Diseases
Chokechai Rongkavilit and Fouzia Naeem, *Editors*

April 2022
Pediatric Otolaryngology
Huma Quraishi and Michael Chee, *Editors*

June 2022
Pediatric Critical Care
Mary Lieh-Lai and Katherine Cashen, *Editors*

RECENT ISSUES

October 2021
Covid-19 in Children
Elizabeth Secord and Eric John McGrath, *Editors*

August 2021
Pediatric Neurosurgery in Primary Care
Jonathan Martin and Greg Olavarria, *Editors*

June 2021
Integrated Behavioral Health in Pediatric Practice
Roger Apple, Cheryl Adele Dickson, Maria Demma I. Cabral, *Editors*

SERIES OF RELATED INTEREST

Gastroenterology Clinics of North America
www.gastro.theclinics.com

Foreword

New Clinical Responsibilities for All Physicians, Including Pediatricians

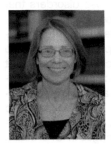

Bonita F. Stanton, MD
Consulting Editor

When the COVID-19 pandemic demonstrated the ability and speed to cause enormous confusion, pain, and mortality, the medical profession was stunned. The speed and efficiency of this virus and vast expanse of symptoms suggested that most if not all our organ systems could be involved in the infection. The fact that those patients surviving an acute infection could live on with significant long-term, minor to major sequalae covering a wide variety of unpredictable symptoms has been all the more concerning.[1–4]

Of interest (and offering considerable relief) to pediatricians across the globe, children appeared to be less likely to contract the disease or to suffer severe symptoms. In general, they seemed much less likely to develop severe illness compared with adults, especially adults over the age of 65 years.[5]

As the first year of the pandemic wore on, physicians in general, and perhaps pediatricians in particular, began to take solace from the facts that the medical profession was beginning to understand COVID-19 better and that progress with regard to effective vaccines was moving along quickly, leading to growing optimism that perhaps this would be a disease that could be stopped from spreading and ultimately eliminated. Earlier in 2021, there had been a growing sense that with the increased availability of effective vaccines not only among developed nations but also increasingly among middle-income nations that the pandemic might be soon coming to an end, or at least be "under control."

Sadly, this optimistic trajectory was derailed in late spring and summer of 2021 when the Delta variant spread across the globe and established itself as substantially more virulent than its predecessors. The Delta variant rapidly became the most prevalent COVID strain across the globe. The variant is noteworthy for several reasons, including

Pediatr Clin N Am 68 (2021) xv–xvii
https://doi.org/10.1016/j.pcl.2021.09.002
0031-3955/21/© 2021 Published by Elsevier Inc.

higher rates of breakthrough among the vaccinated and substantially higher concentrations of the Delta strain of the virus compared with other COVID-19 strains in the nasal passages of vaccinated.[6]

The trajectory of the disease over the past 4 to 8 weeks with the Delta variant has made it clear that this path is not becoming a reality. Of particular importance is the observation that an increasingly higher proportion of hospitalized COVID-19 patients are young adults and even children aged less than 20 years.[7]

Therefore it is timely that this issue of Pediatric Clinics of North America, edited by Harpreet Pall and his colleagues from across the globe, in focusing on a wide array of pediatric gastrointestinal (GI) disorders, has identified many of those disorders that may result from or be exacerbated by COVID-19. The authors also describe COVID-driven changes in clinical practice, such as dramatically increased use of telemedicine, more intensive sterilization practices before and after GI procedures, and so forth, and how these changes may impact the health care of children. Given that COVID-19 is likely to remain a global pandemic that is impacting children, it is important that we take this into consideration as we train our current and future pediatricians, including but not limited to those whose professional focus is pediatric gastroenterology. Dr Pall and the authors who worked with him on this issue have done an excellent job balancing the new COVID-necessitated changes in GI practice with other breakthroughs in pediatric GI to bring us this very timely issue of *Pediatric Clinics of North America*.

Bonita F. Stanton, MD
Hackensack Meridian School of Medicine
123 Metro Boulevard
Suite M-4110
Nutley, NJ 07110, USA

E-mail address:
bonita.stanton@hmhn.org

REFERENCES

1. Wu Z, McGppgan JM. Characteristics of and important lessons from the coronavirus disease 2019 (COVID-19) outbreak in China: summary of a report of 72 314 cases from the Chinese Center for Disease Control and Prevention. JAMA 2020; 323(13):1239–42.
2. Majumder J, Minko T. Recent developments on therapeutic and diagnostic approaches for COVID-19. AAPS J 2021;23(1):14. https://doi.org/10.1208/s12248-020-00532-2.
3. Ortiz-Prado E, Simbaña-Rivera K, Gómez- Barreno L, et al. Clinical, molecular, and epidemiological characterization of the SARS-CoV-2 virus and the coronavirus disease 2019 (COVID-19), a comprehensive literature review. Diagn Microbiol Infect Dis 2020;98(1):115094.
4. Al Samman M, Caggiula A, Ganguli S, et al. Non-respiratory presentations of COVID-19, a clinical review. Am J Emerg Med 2020;38(11):2444–54.
5. Vakili S, Savardashtaki A, Jamalnia S, et al. Laboratory findings of COVID-19 infection are conflicting in different age groups and pregnant women: a literature review. Arch Med Res 2020;51(7):603–7.
6. Pouwels KB, Pritchard E, Matthews PC, et al, the COVID-19 Infection Survey Team. Impact of Delta on viral burden and vaccine effectiveness against new SARS-CoV-2 infections in the UK. Preprint Oxford. Available at: https://www.ndm.ox.ac.uk/

files/coronavirus/covid-19-infection-survey/finalfinalcombinedve20210816.pdf. Accessed September 11, 2021.
7. Pola A, Murthy KS, Santhekadur PK. COVID-19 and gastrointestinal system: a brief review. Biomed J 2021;44(3):245–51. https://doi.org/10.1016/j.bj.2021.01.001.

Preface

Advances in Pediatric Gastroenterology

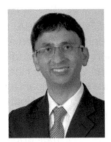

Harpreet Pall, MD, MBA, CPE
Editor

It is my pleasure to present this very special gastroenterology-focused issue of *Pediatric Clinics of North America*. As the editor of this issue, I have had the opportunity to collaborate with talented experts on a variety of topics important to the pediatric gastroenterology community.

The last few years have brought remarkable scientific advancements in the field of pediatric gastroenterology. In this issue, we highlight the topics that continue to be particularly relevant. Most recently, the COVID-19 pandemic has created new challenges worldwide in our specialty. Many aspects have been impacted, including exacerbation of health disparities, fellow training, and care delivery.

Included in this issue are articles relevant to the pandemic, such as health equity and social determinants of health (Rhea Daniel, MD, Jennifer Jimenez, MD, and Harpreet Pall, MD, MBA, CPE) and the impact of COVID-19 on pediatric gastroenterology (Richard Taylor III, MD and Daniel Mallon, MD, MSHPEd). There has been an explosion of new knowledge in the pathogenesis of inflammatory bowel disease, and an update on precision medicine is provided (Elizabeth Spencer, MD and Marla Dubinsky, MD). Medical management of eosinophilic esophagitis continues to be relevant (Melanie Ruffner, MD, PhD, Linola Juste, BS, and Amanda Muir, MD), and celiac disease (Jennifer Jimenez, MD, Beth Loveridge-Lenza, MD, and Karoly Horvath, MD, PhD) has promising therapeutic options on the horizon. Several advances in endoscopic procedures are discussed (Amornluck Krasaelap, MD and Diana Lerner, MD) as well as upper gastrointestinal functional and motility disorders (Jonathan Miller, MD, Julie Khlevner, MD, and Leonel Rodriguez, MD) and lower gastrointestinal functional and motility disorders (Ricardo Arbizu, MD, Ben Freiberg, MD, and Leonel Rodriguez, MD). Finally, important pancreatic and liver diseases are highlighted, with discussions on pancreatitis in children (Reuven Zev Cohen, MD and A. Jay Freeman, MD), autoimmune liver disease (Sarah Kemme, MD and Cara Mack, MD), nonalcoholic fatty liver

Pediatr Clin N Am 68 (2021) xix–xx
https://doi.org/10.1016/j.pcl.2021.09.001
0031-3955/21/© 2021 Published by Elsevier Inc.

disease (Tania Mitsinikos, MD, Paula Mrowczynski-Hernandez, RD, and Rohit Kohli, MBBS, MS), hepatitis C (Sanu Yadav, MD, Deborah A. Goldman, MD, and Karen F. Murray, MD), and biliary atresia/neonatal cholestasis (Sara E. Yerina, BSN, RN and Udeme D. Ekong, MD, MPH).

It has truly been a pleasure to edit the contributions of such a talented group of authors. I would like to thank them for preparing thoughtful, concise, and cutting-edge articles. I very much hope you enjoy this special gastroenterology issue of *Pediatric Clinics of North America*.

Harpreet Pall, MD, MBA, CPE
Department of Pediatrics
Hackensack Meridian School of Medicine
Hackensack Meridian K. Hovnanian Children's Hospital
Jersey Shore University Medical Center
1945 State Route 33
Neptune, NJ 07753, USA

E-mail address:
Harpreet.pall@hmhn.org

Health Equity and Social Determinants of Health in Pediatric Gastroenterology

Rhea Daniel, MD[a], Jennifer Jimenez, MD[b,c], Harpreet Pall, MD[b,c],*

KEYWORDS

- Social determinants of health • Pediatrics • Liver transplant
- Inflammatory bowel disease • Obesity • Endoscopy

KEY POINTS

- The current COVID-19 pandemic has brought existing health care disparities to the fore-front of national discussions and made it clear that healthy equity needs to be a priority in future research and health care implementation.
- As telehealth continues to advance, special care should be given to addressing the digital divide to provide care with an equitable lens.
- Considering social determinants of health when creating initial care plans for patients can help mitigate adverse events and increase efficiency in healthcare.

INTRODUCTION

Social determinants of health (SDH) as outlined by Healthy People 2020 encompasses 5 key domains: economic, education, social and community context, health and health care, and neighborhood and built environment.[1] The recognition that health starts in our homes and communities and is shaped by a myriad of factors has led to an explosion of research attempting to understand the interaction between medical interventions, outcomes, and SDH. The current coronavirus disease 2019 (COVID-19) pandemic has brought existing health care disparities to the forefront of national discussions and made it clear that healthy equity needs to be a priority in future research and health care implementation. A few months after the start of the pandemic the Centers for Disease Control and Prevention reported that 21.8% of COVID-19 cases in the United States (US) occurred in black patients and 33.8% occured in Latino patients

[a] Department of Pediatric Gastroenterology, Hepatology, and Nutrition, McGovern Medical School, University of Texas Health Science Center and Children's Memorial Hermann Hospital, Houston, TX 70007, USA; [b] Department of Pediatrics, Hackensack Meridian School of Medicine, Nutley, NJ, USA; [c] Department of Pediatrics, K. Hovnanian Children's Hospital at Jersey Shore University Medical Center, Neptune, NJ, USA
* Corresponding author. Department of Pediatrics, Hackensack Meridian School of Medicine, Nutley, NJ.
E-mail address: harpreet.pall@hmhn.org

Pediatr Clin N Am 68 (2021) 1147–1155
https://doi.org/10.1016/j.pcl.2021.07.004
0031-3955/21/© 2021 Elsevier Inc. All rights reserved.

despite these groups comprising only 13% and 18% of the population, respectively.[2] As the pandemic has progressed, the numbers have continued to change but the racial disproportion has remained with mortality rates among black patients more than 2 times greater than that among white patients.[2] Although the highest burden of morbidity and mortality related directly to COVID-19 infections falls upon adults, the effects of the pandemic are transmitted to children and young adults in a multitude of ways. For example, children of disproportionately affected communities are more likely to experience loss or disability of a primary parent or caregiver due to COVID-19 compared with white children. Similarly, they are more likely to experience financial hardships and economic unrest in their home from parental loss of income due to an overrepresentation of ethnic and minority populations in service industries.[3] The cumulative effect of these experiences and toxic stressors, whether created by the COVID-19 pandemic or exacerbated by it, add to the burden of adverse childhood experiences (ACEs) in these communities. Studies have shown that ACEs contribute to physiologic disruptions that persist into adulthood and are associated with multiple poor health outcomes, including cardiovascular disease, asthma, and depression even in the absence of health-threatening behaviors.[4] In this way, the COVID-19 pandemic has the potential to propagate health disparities currently highlighted by the pandemic itself. It is important to examine current health care inequities that exist in our country today and focus on mitigating these disparities in the future.

This article emphasizes pediatric populations and some of the existing SDH and health care disparities seen in pediatric gastroenterology. We look specifically at inflammatory bowel disease (IBD), endoscopy, bariatric surgery, and liver transplantation. We also examine the burgeoning role of telehealth that has become commonplace since the COVID-19 era.

LIVER TRANSPLANT

The only effective treatment of end-stage liver disease (ESLD) is liver transplantation. Owing to the limited availability of organs, there is a greater demand than available supply, leading to inequitable access across the country. Before receiving a liver transplant, patients are required to be evaluated by a physician and listed as an eligible candidate for transplant. As part of the initial evaluation national guidelines require a patient's social support system to be assessed and deemed adequate. The 2013 practice guidelines by the American Association for the Study of Liver Diseases and the American Society of Transplantation lists lack of adequate social support as a contraindication to liver transplant.[5] Unlike some of the other contraindications listed, such as acquired immunodeficiency syndrome, extrahepatic malignancy, hemangiosarcoma, and uncontrolled sepsis, the eligibility exclusion based on social support is subjective and the criterion used to determine what is "adequate" is ill-defined.[5] Despite the lack of evidence-based guidelines available to help direct the assessment of social support, a study by Ladin and colleagues[6] surveying 584 transplant providers found social support to be the second most influential factor in listing decisions. As Barry and colleagues[7] point out, using adequate social support as a requirement for organ transplant eligibility runs the risk of systematically excluding patients with limited socioeconomic means and minorities who may not be able to meet perceived requirements due to limitations on their available support systems, which are outside of their control and often stem from broader social inequities.

A study by Ross and colleagues[8] used community health scores (CHS) as a composite indicator of proxy variables for community health to investigate sociodemographic determinants of waitlist and posttransplant survival in ESLD. Higher CHS

scores indicate high-risk communities with less access to care.[8] The study found patients who reside in the highest CHS areas are more likely to be of Black race, live
further from their listing transplant center, have public insurance, and fewer candidates are listed for each person dying from liver disease in that area.[8] The death
rate from ESLD was two times higher than that of the lowest risk CHS communities.[8]
Notably, patients in the highest CHS communities derived equal benefit from transplant and postoperative survival was equivalent to that of lower risk areas.[8] As demonstrated in this study, geographic residence plays a significant role in transplantation
listing. Area of residence is a well-known factor in health and health care outcomes
with a large body of literature describing health and life expectancy disparities in rural
communities compared with urban areas.[9–11]

TELEHEALTH

The current COVID-19 pandemic has underscored the aforementioned disparities and
has led to an unprecedented and rapid advancement in the use of telehealth that has
been supported by increased Medicaid and Medicare reimbursement. A recent study
evaluating the role of telehealth in liver transplantation found that patients who underwent initial transplant evaluation remotely via telehealth experienced a significant 85%
reduction in time from referral to evaluation and 74% reduction in time to listing
compared with the usual care group.[12] Although there was no difference in pretransplant mortality or time to transplantation, the use of telehealth can help reduce the
financial burden and time associated with medical visits, which is especially beneficial
to caregivers and patients living far from transplant centers or experiencing low job
flexibility.

   Although telehealth has the ability to bridge gaps in health care by increasing access, concerns have been raised that telehealth may actually create or increase health
care inequities and deepen the digital divide. The digital divide refers to the inequalities
between individuals, households, and other groups of different demographic and socioeconomic levels to access information and communication technologies and have
the knowledge and skills needed to effectively use the information gained from con-
necting.[13,14] This digital divide occurs in the context of all domains of SDH and can
perpetuate inequities based on various social factors.[15]

   A study by Wegermann and colleagues[16] showcases how the digital divide is man-
ifested in clinical practice. The study evaluated how racial and socioeconomic disparities in patients with liver disease impact the use of telehealth services since the start
of the COVID-19 pandemic. The investigators found that telehealth visit attempts
among patients self-identifying race/ethnicity as Latino or other were less likely to
be completed and visits by patients self-identifying as black race/ethnicity were associated with an increased odds of completion of a telephone versus video visit
compared with white patients.[16] Similarly, patients with Medicaid or Medicare insurance had an increased odds of completing a telephone versus video visit compared
with patients with private insurance.[16] Although telehealth has the potential to increase
health care access, the aforementioned study highlights the fact that most telehealth
programs require patients to have access to broadband Internet services. However,
33% of rural Americans lack access to high-speed broadband Internet that supports
video-based telehealth visits.[17] In rural northern Michigan where 40% of residents lack
access to high-speed broadband Internet, hospitals are working to overcome this access issue by offering telephonic visits instead of video visits and providing the option
for patients to drive to designated locations with broadband Internet services to complete video visits in their car.[17] As telehealth continues to advance, special care should

be paid to addressing the digital divide to optimize access and knowledge regarding telehealth services to bolster health care equity.

INFLAMMATORY BOWEL DISEASE

IBD affects more than 600,000 adults and children in the US and Canada alone.[18] Emerging data highlights potential health care disparities among children with IBD from different racial groups and lower-income neighborhoods. For example, although black patients are suspected to have an overall lower prevalence of IBD, in the US studies demonstrate that they are more likely to experience IBD-related hospitalizations and higher IBD-related mortality when compared with white and Latino patients.[19] In a study by Dotson and colleagues[20] looking at pediatric patients with Crohn disease (CD) within the Improve Care Now registry, differences in 1-year remission rates were observed, suggesting that black patients may have an increase in disease activity during the first year of diagnosis, despite similar treatment and number of follow-up visits. Their data suggested that CD is more severe in black children and/or they respond less well or less quickly to existing medication options.[20] Differences in disease extent and severity have also been noted to be a factor for children of different races in several studies. Black children with ulcerative colitis (UC) were more likely to demonstrate proctitis or left-sided colitis and increased rates of perianal disease when compared with white patients with UC.[21,22] Among Latino patients with IBD in the US, an increased prevalence of UC has been reported, with Latino patients born outside of the US having an increased prevalence of UC compared with Latino patients born within the US and non-Latino white patients.[21] Barnes and colleagues[22] evaluated 295 hospitalized pediatric patients with IBD between 2000 and 2012. Their study demonstrated an increased length of stay (LOS) among black and Latino children when compared with white children.[22] In a later study, Barnes and colleagues[23] highlighted that the more severe presentations and increased LOS for black children may be in part due to the increase in stricturing and penetrating disease. One of the investigators' conclusions was to consider earlier initiation of biological therapy to potentially reduce CD-related complications.[23]

When looking at disparities among pediatric patients with IBD in the emergency department (ED) setting, there was an increase in repeat visits observed particularly in black children with IBD and patients with Medicaid insurance. ED visits of 2618 pediatric patients with a primary diagnosis of CD were analyzed between 2007 and 2013 by Dotson and colleagues.[24] The investigators observed that the proportion of patients with repeat visits to the ED were greater for black children (33%) than white children (22%) and greater for Medicaid-insured (27%) than privately insured patients (21%) with white children having a higher median neighborhood income and more likely to have private insurance (57% vs 30% respectively).[24] Their results suggest an opportunity to improve outpatient management of children with IBD particularly among black children and those with Medicaid so that nonemergent problems are more effectively handled in the office setting rather than ED. Their observations led to changes that included extending evening and weekend clinic hours, implementing electronic patient portals to increase communication between multiple providers, and fully integrating supportive multidisciplinary teams including case managers, social workers, and psychologists into their practice.[24]

When looking specifically at low socioeconomic status (SES), Benchimol and colleagues[25] highlighted disparities in health service use among Canadian children with IBD. The investigators compared 2 cohorts of pediatric patients with IBD from the Ontario Crohn's and Colitis Cohort, which includes patients with pediatric-onset

IBD between the ages of 6 months and 18 years.[25] Comparing 2 groups from this cohort (944 patients living in neighborhoods of the lowest income compared with 1286 patients living in neighborhoods of the highest income), they found that children from low-income neighborhoods had higher IBD-related physician visit rates, hospitalization rates, and ED usage than those from higher-income neighborhoods, which was consistent with previous Canadian studies.[25] Their study also highlighted higher rates of surgery in lower-income children with CD, especially those diagnosed after 2000.[25] The investigators theorized that this finding may be possibly related to access to biological agents, given that the landmark studies were published on the efficacy of these medications in CD in the early 2000s.[25]

PEDIATRIC OBESITY AND BARIATRIC SURGERY

Pediatric obesity is a national public health crisis involving more than 13 million children and adolescents in the US and affects patients of Latino background and black youth at a significantly higher rate than whites.[26,27] Despite this, use of metabolic bariatric surgery (MBS) is the lowest in black and Latino youth. The National Health and Nutrition Examination Survey cross-sectional data (N = 19,225) demonstrated that the US prevalence of youth severe obesity increased in Latino and non-Latino black children; however, non-Latino white children had higher rates of MBS use (45.8%) compared with Latinos (22.7%) and non-Latino blacks (14.2%).[28] There are some data that support MBS over medical therapy for pediatric patients with severe obesity. A study by Inge and colleagues[29] demonstrated that compared with medical therapy (metformin and a lifestyle intervention program focusing on weight loss through behavior modification), treatment with MBS in severely obese adolescents with type 2 diabetes was associated with better glycemic control, weight reduction, and improvement in comorbidities. In a later study, Inge and colleagues[30] also demonstrated that adolescents who undergo MBS experience remission in cardiovascular comorbidities compared with adults who undergo MBS. Regarding differences among male and female use of MBS, Perez and colleagues[31] demonstrated that female adolescents were significantly more likely than males to undergo MBS for the management of severe obesity. Among racial minorities, Medicaid insurance was associated with a further decreased likelihood of undergoing MBS when compared with privately insured patients, whereas the opposite effect was observed among white patients.[31]

There are opportunities to work toward overcoming these disparities, including increasing access to education on MBS for community pediatricians and pediatric gastroenterologists, particularly those providers who care for multiethnic populations in both community and clinic/hospital settings. When medical management to achieve weight loss is ineffective despite a multidisciplinary team approach, physicians should offer information regarding the risk versus benefits of surgical approaches to overcome obesity.[32]

PEDIATRIC ENDOSCOPY

The literature regarding how health disparities affect the use of pediatric gastroenterology procedures is limited. No-show rate in the endoscopy unit is a key barrier to high-quality services and efficiency. One recent study addressing the barriers to potential no-show (transportation, insurance, health literacy, etc.) was able to decrease the no-show rate from an average of 7% in the preintervention phase to 2% in the postintervention phase.[33]

A recent study identified various factors associated with higher use of emergent gastrointestinal (GI) procedures, including age less than 5 and greater than 18 years, black or non-Caucasian race, male gender, Medicaid insurance, and Spanish speaking language.[34] Although this study identified previously undescribed associations between health disparities and emergent GI procedures, the role of SES, specifically poverty, was not assessed.

In a follow-up study, the investigators expanded on this knowledge by stratifying SES by geocoding.[35] Geocoding or geospatial mapping enables us to not only identify trends at the population levels but also identify high-risk patient populations. Using census tracts enables us to gain valuable information about measures of markers of economic deprivation.[36–39] SES is a composite of many factors that make up a patient's health and wellness and encompasses far more than individual health disparity variables. This study is the first report using geospatial mapping to study health disparities within the realm of pediatric gastroenterology. The study aimed to characterize risk factors and determine the role of SES on emergent versus nonemergent GI procedures.[35] A retrospective chart review with 2556 patient records was performed. Demographic data and SES categories were determined. Most emergent procedures were performed on an inpatient basis. Health disparity factors analyzed included age, gender, insurance type, race, language, and SES using census tracts. Using geocoded data, the investigators found that as SES increases by 1, emergent risk for procedures decreased by 2.9% (odds ratio, 0.97; $P = .045$). These results show that SES was inversely correlated with the risk of having an emergent procedure and suggest that geospatial mapping can be used as a screening tool to evaluate health care disparities. Additional work is needed to identify and address the underlying causes of poverty and help improve access to outpatient care in disadvantaged and vulnerable groups.

SUMMARY

Disparities exist throughout health care. This article highlights examples of inequities that exist in pediatric gastroenterology, including liver transplant, IBD, obesity, and endoscopy.

We also discuss the increasing prevalence of telehealth services. Telehealth will potentially allow physicians to bridge gaps in health care and provide increased medical access to rural and disadvantaged populations. Special attention should be paid to minimizing the digital divide while developing and integrating these technologies into our health care delivery system.

CLINICS CARE POINTS

- As telehealth continues to advance, special attention should be paid to bridging the digital divide; this will lead to optimizing access and knowledge regarding telehealth services, and ultimately bolster health equity.

- Medical management may fail to achieve weight loss in some patients with severe obesity and comorbid conditions despite a multidisciplinary team approach. Physicians should provide personalized counseling regarding risks and benefits of metabolic bariatric surgery and address potential barriers related to health disparities.

- Reviewing and addressing various social determinants of health (ie, transportation, insurance, health literacy) with patients during visits may help decrease future no-show rates.

DISCLOSURE

The authors have nothing to disclose.

REFERENCES

1. Sokol R, Austin A, Chandler C, et al. Screening children for social determinants of health: a systematic review. Pediatrics 2019;144(4):e20191622.
2. Tai DBG, Shah A, Doubeni CA, et al. The disproportionate impact of COVID-19 on racial and ethnic minorities in the United States. Clin Infect Dis 2020;72(4):703–6.
3. Fraiman YS, Litt JS, Davis JM, et al. Racial and ethnic disparities in adult COVID-19 and the future impact on child health. Pediatr Res 2021;89(5):1052–4.
4. Shonkoff JP, Garner AS. The lifelong effects of early childhood adversity and toxic stress. Pediatrics 2012;129(1):e232–46.
5. Martin P, DiMartini A, Feng S, et al. Evaluation for liver transplantation in adults: 2013 practice guideline by the American Association for the Study of Liver Diseases and the American Society of Transplantation. Hepatology 2014;59(3): 1144–65.
6. Ladin K, Emerson J, Butt Z, et al. How important is social support in determining patients' suitability for transplantation? Results from a National Survey of Transplant Clinicians. J Med Ethics 2018;44(10):666.
7. Berry KN, Daniels N, Ladin K. Should lack of social support prevent access to organ transplantation? Am J Bioeth 2019;19(11):13–24.
8. Ross K, Patzer RE, Goldberg DS, et al. Sociodemographic determinants of waitlist and posttransplant survival among end-stage liver disease patients. Am J Transpl 2017;17(11):2879–89.
9. Eberhardt MS, Pamuk ER. The importance of place of residence: examining health in rural and nonrural areas. Am J Public Health 2004;94(10):1682–6.
10. Singh GK, Siahpush M. Widening rural–urban disparities in life expectancy, U.S., 1969–2009. Am J Prev Med 2014;46(2):e19–29.
11. Loccoh E, Joynt Maddox KE, Xu J, et al. Rural-urban disparities in all-cause mortality among low-income medicare beneficiaries, 2004–17. Health Aff 2021;40(2): 289–96.
12. John BV, Love E, Dahman B, et al. Use of telehealth expedites evaluation and listing of patients referred for liver transplantation. Clin Gastroenterol Hepatol 2020;18(8):1822–30.e1824.
13. Norris P. Digital divide: civic engagement, information poverty, and the internet worldwide. Cambridge: Cambridge University Press; 2001.
14. Falling through the net [microform]: a survey of the "have nots" in rural and urban America. Washington, DC: U.S. Dept. of Commerce, National Telecommunications and Information Administration; 1995.
15. Ramsetty A, Adams C. Impact of the digital divide in the age of COVID-19. J Am Med Inform Assoc 2020;27(7):1147–8.
16. Wegermann K, Wilder JM, Parish A, et al. Racial and socioeconomic disparities in utilization of telehealth in patients with liver disease during COVID-19. Dig Dis Sci 2021. [Epub ahead of print].
17. Hirko KA, Kerver JM, Ford S, et al. Telehealth in response to the COVID-19 pandemic: implications for rural health disparities. J Am Med Inform Assoc 2020;27(11):1816–8.
18. Sewell JL, Velayos FS. Systematic review: the role of race and socioeconomic factors on IBD healthcare delivery and effectiveness. Inflamm Bowel Dis 2013; 19(3):627–43.

19. Nguyen GC, Chong CA, Chong RY. National estimates of the burden of inflammatory bowel disease among racial and ethnic groups in the United States. J Crohns Colitis 2014;8(4):288–95.

20. Dotson JL, Kappelman MD, Chisolm DJ, et al. Racial disparities in readmission, complications, and procedures in children with Crohn's disease. Inflamm Bowel Dis 2015;21(4):801–8.

21. Brant SR, Okou DT, Simpson CL, et al. Genome-wide association study identifies African-specific susceptibility loci in African Americans with inflammatory bowel disease. Gastroenterology 2017;152(1):206–17.e2.

22. Barnes EL, Kochar B, Long MD, et al. Minority pediatric patients with inflammatory bowel disease demonstrate an increased length of stay. Inflamm Bowel Dis 2017;23(12):2189–96.

23. Barnes EL, Loftus EV Jr, Kappelman MD. Effects of race and ethnicity on diagnosis and management of inflammatory bowel diseases. Gastroenterology 2021;160(3):677–89.

24. Dotson JL, Kappelman MD, Bricker J, et al. Multicenter evaluation of emergency department treatment for children and adolescents with crohn's disease according to race/ethnicity and insurance payor status. Inflamm Bowel Dis 2019;25(1): 194–203.

25. Benchimol EI, To TP, Griffiths AM, et al. Outcomes of pediatric inflammatory bowel disease: socioeconomic status disparity in a universal-access healthcare system. J Pediatr 2011;158(6):960–7.e964.

26. Skinner AC, Ravanbakht SN, Skelton JA, et al. Prevalence of obesity and severe obesity in US children, 1999-2016. Pediatrics 2018;141(3):e20173459. Pediatrics (Evanston). 2018;142(3):e20181916.

27. Mayer-Davis EJ, Lawrence JM, Dabelea D, et al. Incidence trends of type 1 and type 2 diabetes among youths, 2002–2012. N Engl J Med 2017;376(15):1419–29.

28. Messiah SE, Xie L, Atem F, et al. Disparity between United States adolescent class ii and iii obesity trends and bariatric surgery utilization, 2015-2018. Ann Surg 2020. [Epub ahead of print].

29. Inge TH, Laffel LM, Jenkins TM, et al. Comparison of surgical and medical therapy for type 2 diabetes in severely obese adolescents. JAMA Pediatr 2018; 172(5):452–60.

30. Inge TH, Courcoulas AP, Jenkins TM, et al. Five-year outcomes of gastric bypass in adolescents as compared with adults. N Engl J Med 2019;380(22):2136–45.

31. Perez NP, Westfal ML, Stapleton SM, et al. Beyond insurance: race-based disparities in the use of metabolic and bariatric surgery for the management of severe pediatric obesity. Surg Obes Relat Dis 2020;16(3):414–9.

32. Smith ED, Layden BI, Hassan C, et al. Surgical treatment of obesity in latinos and African Americans: future directions and recommendations to reduce disparities in bariatric surgery. Bariatric Surg Pract Patient Care 2018;13(1):2–11.

33. Mani J, Franklin L, Pall H. Impact of pre-procedure interventions on no-show rate in pediatric endoscopy. Children (Basel) 2015;2(1):89–97.

34. Andrews A, Franklin L, Rush N, et al. Age, gender, health insurance, and race associated with increased rate of emergent pediatric gastrointestinal procedures. J Pediatr Gastroenterol Nutr 2016;64(6):907–10.

35. May E, Brown O, Gracely E, et al. The role of health disparities and socioeconomic status in emergent gastrointestinal procedures. Health equity 2021;5(1): 27–276.

36. Faelker T, Pickett W, Brison RJ. Socioeconomic differences in childhood injury: a population based epidemiologic study in Ontario, Canada. Inj Prev 2000;6(3): 203–8.
37. Chung EK, Siegel BS, Garg A, et al. Screening for social determinants of health among children and families living in poverty: a guide for clinicians. Curr Probl Pediatr Adolesc Health Care 2016;46(5):135–53.
38. Philadelphia county census. 2019. Available at: https://www.census.gov/. Accessed May 15, 2019.
39. Philadelphia health tracts census. 2019. Available at: https://societyhealth.vcu.edu/work/the-projects/mapsphiladelphia.html2019. Accessed May 15, 2019.

COVID-19 and Pediatric Gastroenterology

Richard Taylor III, MD[a], Daniel Mallon, MD, MSHPEd[b],*

KEYWORDS

- COVID-19 • Pediatric gastroenterology • Telehealth • Endoscopy

KEY POINTS

- Coronavirus disease 2019 and multisystem inflammatory syndrome in children and adolescents can present with gastrointestinal symptoms and liver injury.
- Special populations of children and adolescents with chronic liver disease or immune suppression may be at greater risk of coronavirus disease 2019 or have attenuated responses to vaccination.
- Pediatric gastroenterologists have faced challenges of fewer patient care visits, delays in presentation of gastrointestinal illnesses, curtailed endoscopy, the adoption of telehealth, and fewer opportunities for clinical and research training.

INTRODUCTION

The novel coronavirus, severe acute respiratory syndrome coronavirus 2 (SARS-CoV-2), which is responsible for the coronavirus disease 2019 (COVID-19), was first recognized in Wuhan, China, in December 2019 and rapidly spread. Globally, there have been more than 127 million cases with 2.8 million deaths; the United States has contributed more than 30 million cases and 500,000 deaths as of April 2021. The impact of this disease cannot be understated, with far-reaching changes in the world and medicine. Our goal is to provide a review tailored to the pediatric gastroenterologist that focuses on caring for patients with COVID-19, preventing the disease in patients with chronic gastrointestinal (GI) and liver disorders, and adapting to the associated widespread changes to clinical practice and training.

[a] Pediatric Residency Program, Department of Pediatrics, Cincinnati Children's Hospital Medical Center, University of Cincinnati College of Medicine, 3333 Burnet Avenue, MLC 5018, Cincinnati, OH 45229, USA; [b] Department of Pediatrics, Division of Gastroenterology, Hepatology and Nutrition, Cincinnati Children's Hospital Medical Center, University of Cincinnati College of Medicine, 3333 Burnet Avenue, MLC 2010, Cincinnati, OH 45229, USA
* Corresponding author.
E-mail address: Daniel.Mallon@cchmc.org
Twitter: @dannymallon24 (D.M.)

Pediatr Clin N Am 68 (2021) 1157–1169
https://doi.org/10.1016/j.pcl.2021.07.003
pediatric.theclinics.com

EPIDEMIOLOGY

In children and adolescents, COVID-19 generally presents similar to a viral upper respiratory infection with the most common presenting symptoms being cough (48.5%), pharyngeal erythema (46.2%), fever (41.5%), diarrhea (8.8%), fatigue (7.6%), rhinorrhea (7.6%), and vomiting (6.4%).[1] When symptomatic, pediatric patients are more likely to have mild disease (53%) that can be managed in the outpatient setting.[2] A meta-analysis by Viner and colleagues[3] showed that children have a significantly lower susceptibility to COVID-19 infection with an odds ratio of 0.56 compared with adults. Saleh and colleagues[4] specifically investigated hospitalized children with COVID-19 and found that the most common presentations were fever (95%), headache (60.3%), fatigue (57.8%), and shock (21.8%). Acute pancreatitis (1.5%) was the most common atypical presentation of COVID-19 in this study.[4] Common laboratory abnormalities in hospitalized patients with COVID-19 include leukopenia, lymphopenia, elevated inflammatory markers, and abnormal liver tests.[4–6] Mortality rates remain low in children with 0.17 per 100,000 or 0.48% of the estimated total mortality from all causes in a normal year.[7] Older children have a higher mortality rate than young children; however, the rate is still low compared with adults.[7]

PATHOPHYSIOLOGY

SARS-CoV-2 is a positive-sense single-stranded RNA virus.[8] It enters target cells via interaction between the viral spike protein and angiotensin-converting enzyme 2 (ACE-2) receptors. Injury is likely due to direct cytotoxic effect of the virus, dysregulation of the renin–angiotensin–aldosterone system, cell endothelial damage, thromboinflammation, and a dysregulated immune response (**Fig. 1**).[9]

GI injury is multifactorial. There is a high prevalence of ACE-2 receptors in enterocytes with known viral replication in the GI tract given the presence of live virus in patient

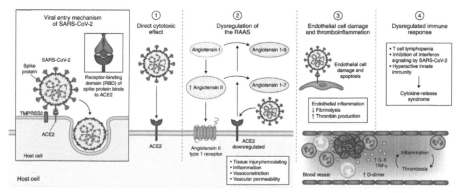

Fig. 1. SARS-CoV-2 enters host cells through interaction of its spike protein with the entry receptor ACE2 in the presence of TMPRSS2 (*far left*). Proposed mechanisms for COVID-19 caused by infection with SARS-CoV-2 include (1) direct virus-mediated cell damage; (2) dysregulation of the renin–angiotensin–aldosterone system (RAAS) as a consequence of downregulation of ACE2 related to viral entry, which leads to decreased cleavage of angiotensin I and angiotensin II; (3) endothelial cell damage and thromboinflammation; and (4) dysregulation of the immune response and hyperinflammation caused by inhibition of interferon signaling by the virus, T-cell lymphodepletion, and the production of proinflammatory cytokines, particularly IL-6 and tumor necrosis factor (TNF)-α. (*From* Gupta A, Madhavan MV, et al. Extrapulmonary Manifestations of COVID-19. Nat Med. 2020; 26: 1017-2032, with permission.)

stool.[9,10] There is also diffuse microvascular small bowel injury and inflammation-mediated tissue damage of the stomach, duodenum, and rectum.[9] Hepatobiliary injury is also multifactorial and may be due to ACE-2–mediated entry of SARS-CoV-2 directly into cholangiocytes damaging the biliary ducts.[9,11] Although some series reported that up to 37% of patients had abnormal liver tests,[12] a pooled data meta-analysis indicated no greater risk of abnormal transaminases or total bilirubin.[13] Drug-induced hepatic injury related to COVID-19 treatment is also possible. Some early reports of remdesivir treatment for COVID-19 included increased transaminases and bilirubin,[14] but a meta-analysis of multiple reports[15] and studies in the pediatric[16] and transplant populations[17,18] found no increased risk of liver injury. Pancreatic injury is also multifactorial and hypothetically due to cytotoxicity of the virus via ACE-2 receptors in the pancreas, drug-induced injury, and damage secondary to the cytokine storm caused by immune dysregulation in severe infections.[19] Of note, pancreas injury secondary to SARS-CoV-2 is controversial, although the pathophysiology is plausible.[19–21]

COMPLICATIONS

Although the risk of serious illness is highest in the elderly, children are not exempt from serious illness. A later consequence of COVID-19 infection is multisystem inflammatory syndrome in children (MIS-C). The Centers for Disease Control and Prevention diagnostic criteria for MIS-C are fever greater than 38 °C for at least 24 hours or subjective fever of at least 24 hours, laboratory evidence of inflammation (elevated C-reactive protein, erythrocyte sedimentation rate, ferritin, etc), a minimum of 2 organ systems involved, and recent or current SARS-CoV-2 infection or exposure.[22] This syndrome typically occurs 2 to 4 weeks after COVID-19 infection and rapid deterioration is common.[23] Treatment is currently focused on decreasing this dysregulated inflammatory response and cytokine storm with intravenous immune globulin, and steroids, as well as other biologic agents if needed.[24]

Of particular interest to the pediatric gastroenterologist is the high prevalence of GI manifestations, which is the most common organ system involved.[23] The most common GI manifestations are abdominal pain, diarrhea, and nausea and vomiting.[25] These symptoms are secondary to inflammation along the GI tract, with the ileum and colon most commonly effected.[25] In severe cases there can be bowel wall thickening, causing luminal narrowing and obstruction. Fortunately, most children will have resolution of their manifestations with appropriate medical management; however, rarely patients have required surgical resection.[25] Interestingly, when patients with severe abdominal pain underwent computed tomography imaging, approximately 85% showed inflammatory bowel changes including marked terminal ileitis, inflammation of the cecum, and mesenteric fat stranding.[25] Mucosal hyperenhancement, fibrostenosis, and penetrating lesions were not seen. On histopathologic assessment of the surgically removed tissue, there was noted to be marked transmural lymphocytic inflammation, venous microthrombi, arteritis, and necrotizing lymphadenitis, which was distinct from chronic inflammatory bowel disease (IBD).[25]

Acute hepatitis and pancreatitis have also been linked to MIS-C. Previous studies in adults have shown that as many as 43% of patients with MIS-C have hepatitis during the course of their illness.[26] Patients with hepatitis were noted to have more severe disease with higher inflammatory cytokine levels, longer hospitalizations, and increased respiratory support.[26] Although long-term data are not available currently, more than 50% of patients had persistent aspartate aminotransferase and alanine aminotransferase elevation at 1-month follow-up visits.[26] There is less literature on pancreatitis during MIS-C; however, adult studies have reported a 3% prevalence.[23]

DISCUSSION
Special Populations

Inflammatory bowel disease

Patients with IBD who are on immunosuppressive medication are at greater risk for infections. Comorbidities are a risk factor for severe COVID-19 infection, so there is particular concern for worse outcomes in pediatric patients with IBD. Fortunately, current pediatric data are encouraging, showing that COVID-19 is well-tolerated in this population.[27] Large tertiary care centers in the United States, China and, Italy have reported low rates of COVID-19 infection in pediatric patients with IBD and when symptomatic the vast majority of cases have been mild.[27,28] There is also no difference in severity of COVID-19 infection between patients with Crohn's disease, ulcerative colitis, or unspecified IBD.[27,28]

Mesalamine and chronic steroids confer an increased risk of COVID-19 infection, with steroids conferring the highest risk.[29–31] Other risk factors associated with COVID-19 incidence and severity in a mixed population of adults and children were older age, male sex, and comorbidities such as cardiovascular disease and diabetes.[31] Immunomodulators and biologic medications including infliximab and vedolizumab for IBD do not confer an increased risk of COVID-19 infection or increased severity when contracted.[31,32] The most common complication recognized in patients with IBD was not related to COVID-19 specifically, but rather delays in therapy or follow-up owing to changes in hospital policies or parental concerns.[28] Patients should receive their regularly scheduled infusions during the pandemic, because a delay increases the risk for exacerbation of the underlying disease.[28] Interestingly, biologics may be protective against severe COVID-19 infection and many immunomodulators are currently under investigation as possible treatments for the aberrant inflammatory response caused by COVID-19.[27]

One of the most pressing issues for pediatric gastroenterologist is whether they should be recommending the COVID-19 vaccine to their patients with IBD. Multiple vaccines have been approved and have shown excellent efficacy and safety in the general population.[33,34] A recent study by Kennedy and colleagues[35] investigated the COVID-19 vaccine in patients with IBD treated with infliximab and found that, similar to other vaccines, infliximab is associated with an attenuated immune response; however, most patients will still have seroconversion after a second dose of the vaccine. The International Organization for the Study of Inflammatory Bowel Disease has recommended providers give the COVID-19 vaccination to patients with IBD because the benefits of COVID-19 prevention outweigh the risks of the vaccine.[36]

Chronic liver disease

Overall, chronic liver disease from any cause is likely a risk factor for severe COVID-19 infection, although the literature in pediatrics is mixed. The adult data support chronic liver disease as a risk factor; Singh and colleagues[37] report an increased relative risk of mortality as compared with propensity-matched patients. Kehar and colleagues[38] examined pediatric chronic liver disease in comparison with liver transplant recipients. Their reported data are similar to adults, with higher admission rates, pediatric intensive care management, mechanical ventilation, and death in patients with chronic liver disease as compared with liver transplant recipients. An observational cohort study by Di Giorgio and colleagues[39] contradicted this result. Their data showed no difference in the severity of COVID-19 in patients with liver disease; however, they did show a higher observed incidence of infection than the estimated incidence in the population. Of note, their study reported 12% of their population as symptomatic for COVID-19 based on exposures; however, only 0.5% of patients had a confirmed case via testing, causing these data to be difficult to interpret. Regardless of the potential increased risk, treating patients with preexisting liver disease is further complicated by the hepatotoxicity of many of the medications used to treat COVID-19.[9,11] The adult data support cirrhosis as a risk factor for severe disease; however, again, the data in pediatrics are unclear.[38,39] When investigating autoimmune hepatitis as compared with other etiologies of liver disease, there was no difference in rate of severe disease.[40] Similar to IBD, immunosuppression with biologic agents was not a risk factor for severe disease secondary to COVID-19 for patients with autoimmune hepatitis.[40]

Metabolic-associated fatty liver disease

Similar to other chronic liver diseases, metabolic-associated fatty liver disease (MAFLD), formerly known as nonalcoholic fatty liver disease, has been shown to have higher risk of disease progression and longer viral shedding as compared with patients without MAFLD, although specific pediatric data are lacking.[41] Obesity, diabetes, and hypertension are all prominent risk factors for severe COVID-19 infection and are common comorbidities in patients with MAFLD.[11] Patients with MAFLD may have more severe COVID-19 infections owing to inflammation-suppressing M2 macrophages activation rather than M1 macrophages; however, this correlation is hypothetical.[11] Pediatric gastroenterologists should be prepared to see a to higher prevalence and worsening severity of MAFLD because the COVID-19 pandemic has caused a significant decrease in activity for many children that could worsen patients' obesity.[42] It is vital for pediatric gastroenterologist to help families identify safe effective ways to increase physical activity to help delay and potentially reverse the progression of MAFLD.

Liver transplantation

The risk of infection with SARS-CoV-2 in liver transplant recipients is unclear.[11,38] The literature is limited, and results are mixed. Large adult registry data around the world have shown no increased incidence of infection, but higher mortality rates.[11] Colmenero and colleagues[43] reported the opposite of this finding in their prospective cohort study with a higher incidence of COVID-19 infections, but a lower mortality rate as compared with matched members of the general population. Two case reports of COVID-19 and MIS-C in pediatric liver transplant recipients had poor outcomes[44,45]; however, the observational cohort study by Kehar and colleagues[38] specifically assessing pediatric liver transplant recipients showed improved outcomes as compared with patients with chronic liver disease. Consistent with data in other diseases, immunosuppression has not been shown to be a risk factor for increased severity of COVID-19 infection.[11,43] There has been a decrease in all solid organ transplants since the start of the COVID-19 pandemic.[46]

Early research into the COVID-19 vaccine for solid organ transplant recipients is encouraging. Multiple studies have shown that the vaccine is safe and effective, although the immune response is attenuated as compared with the general population.[47–49] The COVID-19 vaccine is recommended for solid organ transplant recipients, pretransplant patients, and all close contacts of solid organ transplant recipients by numerous societies, including the International Liver Transplantation society.[50–52]

IMPACT ON CLINICAL PRACTICE
Fewer Patient Visits

When the pandemic was identified and advice to decrease in-person visits to health care facilities and postpone elective surgical procedures, it had a large impact on pediatric gastroenterology practices. Outpatient visits decreased,[8,53] and most endoscopic procedures came to a halt.[54] Pediatric gastroenterologists considered the risk of transmission of SARS-CoV-2 to patients, staff, and themselves; the risk of delayed diagnosis for new patients; the jeopardized health of children with chronic disease owing to delays in follow-up care; medication or dietary adherence; fewer clinical opportunities for trainees; and the financial impact of fewer visits and endoscopies. Concerns about delays in diagnosis were realized in reports of severe illness and deaths owing to diabetic ketoacidosis, pyloric stenosis, sepsis, and cancer in children presenting to the hospital after delays attributed to fear of COVID-19 and decreased access to care.[55,56] Delays in presentation were suspected to contribute to an increase the rate of complicated appendicitis in more than 1 series.[56–59] A study of a large sample of emergency departments in the United States revealed a decrease in pediatric visits by up to 72%, compared with the same week 1 year prior.[60] Comparing the same 3-month period, March to June, there was a 22% decrease in visits for serious conditions, including appendicitis and intussusception, and a 62% decrease in visits for abdominal pain.[60] Patients were not visiting the gastroenterology clinic either; the largest pediatric GI practice in Iowa saw 20% and 90% decreases in face-to-face encounters in March and April 2020, respectively, compared with 2019.[53] That report and others highlighted the pivot to telehealth to see patients.[53,61,62]

Telehealth

Telehealth use increased in response to the pandemic,[63] facilitated by the relaxation of some regulatory requirements and affirmations of reimbursement by public and private payers.[64] Pediatric gastroenterology practices used existing and new technology via electronic health records and mobile and computer teleconferencing applications. A timely publication offered guidance specifically to pediatric gastroenterologists adopting telehealth.[62] A few centers have reported successful experiences using telehealth, including adapting multidisciplinary subspecialized disease based clinics,[65] and an approach to triaging referrals as e-consults, telehealth, or in-person visits.[66] Several studies have demonstrated the usefulness of telehealth for pediatric primary and subspecialty care,[67,68] but inequities in use and technology have been seen and merit addressing.[69,70]

The future of telehealth beyond the pandemic is bright, but some uncertainty remains. According to a survey of large employers, 53% of employers plan to implement more virtual care solutions for their health plans.[71] The increased access to coverage for telehealth for Medicare beneficiaries has depended on a temporary waiver during the public health emergency and will continue through the end of the calendar year of the end of the public health emergency. Medicaid rules can vary by state, but some have continued coverage beyond the initial emergency period.[72] Some expanded telehealth services for rural communities were made permanent in the Centers for Medicare and Medicaid Services Physician Fee Schedule final rule released in December 2020.[73] Although the pandemic helped to demonstrate the usefulness and feasibility of telehealth, the permanent and widespread adoption of expanded coverage for telehealth services is complex and faces several hurdles.[74]

Endoscopy

Several considerations related to the risk of transmission or patient complications owing to SARS-CoV-2 infection led to massive disruption of pediatric GI endoscopy. With the stay-at-home orders that were enacted in the spring of 2020, all but urgent and emergent endoscopies came to a halt. Recognizing that endoscopy can aerosolize patients' mucosal secretions, and because SARS-CoV-2 is frequently present in the stool of infected patients, upper endoscopies and colonoscopies carried a possibly higher risk of transmission of virus. Early guidance for weighing risks and benefits of performing a procedure, the implementation of screening and testing patients for SARS-CoV-2 infection, and the effective use of personal protective equipment came from the North American Society for Pediatric Gastroenterology, Hepatology and Nutrition.[54] This initial guidance aligned with American Gastroenterological Association recommendations in recommending N95 masks rather than standard surgical masks and using negative pressure rooms, in part based on concerns that children with SARS-CoV-2 infection may not have symptoms, testing may not be available or perfectly sensitive to detect infection, and the virus can be shed in stool beyond the period it is found in the nasopharynx. Subsequently, Hsu and colleagues,[75] proposed an alternative perspective reporting institutional practice of universal preprocedure polymerase chain reaction–based testing, to allow standard personal protective equipment, including surgical masks, for patients who test negative. A report from an endoscopy unit in Wuhan, China, described experience performing 159 endoscopies, including 17 in patients previously infected or thought to be carriers of the virus, and no cases of transmission were identified.[76] A more recent set of recommendations from the American Gastroenterological Association suggests using a preprocedure testing based on estimated local prevalence of asymptomatic infection.[77] To date, we found no reports of transmission of virus to health care workers attributed to an endoscopic procedure.

With the decrease in endoscopic procedures, outpatient visits, and hospital admissions, the opportunities for the typical clinical training of fellows were diminished during the first several months of the pandemic.[61,78] A survey of program directors revealed that endoscopy and typical outpatient clinical experiences were drastically decreased, but fellows were included with the rapid adoption of telehealth for outpatient visits.[61] Fellows' research activities were curtailed owing to a lack of access to

Table 1
Special population considerations and recommendations

IBD	There is no apparent increased risk of COVID-19 infection owing to IBD, but oral corticosteroids do increase the risk of severe COVID-19. There is no difference in disease severity between ulcerative colitis, Crohn's disease, or unspecified IBD. Immunosuppression is safe and regimens should not be changed prophylactically, except to minimize steroid use. COVID-19 vaccine is strongly recommended for patients with IBD.
Chronic liver disease	There is significantly increased risk of COVID-19 infection, particularly in patients with MAFLD. The treatment of COVID-19 infection is complicated by the hepatotoxic effects of medications. The incidence of MAFLD likely increased during the pandemic owing to decreased exercise.
Liver transplant	There is an increased risk of COVID-19 infection, however it is less than patients with chronic liver disease. Immunosuppression is safe and regimens should not be changed prophylactically, except to minimize steroid use. Vaccination is recommended for recipients, candidates, and close contacts.

research subjects and to the laboratory. Indeed, many fellows altered their research methodology or refocused on an alternative project. When fellows were surveyed, large proportions reported subjective negative impact on clinical (52%), research (46%), and procedural confidence (41%).[78] A small but important proportion of fellows graduating in the summer of 2020 reported that their postfellowship employment contracts were altered or rescinded owing to hiring freezes attributed to the pandemic. Fellows in their first and second years of 3-year fellowships reported high levels of concern in finding a job after graduation.

SUMMARY

Pediatric gastroenterologists took on a variety of challenges during the COVID-19 pandemic, including learning about a new disease and how to recognize and manage it, prevent its spread among their patients and health professions colleagues, and make decisions about managing patients with chronic GI and liver problems considering the threat (**Table 1**). They adapted their practice to accommodate drastically reduced in-person visits, adopting telehealth, and instituting new protocols to perform endoscopies safely. The workforce pipeline was also affected by the pandemic because of its impact on trainee education, clinical experience, research, and job searches.

FUTURE DIRECTIONS

Driven by vaccinations against COVID-19, the rate of infections in the United States is decreasing,[79] and public health measures such as mask mandates and restrictions on public gatherings are being lifted. As patients have returned to clinics, hospitals have filled again and procedures have resumed, pediatric gastroenterologists will consider ways to integrate telehealth into future practice, address questions about vaccinating and possibly revaccinating patients and continue to consider COVID-19 as a potential cause of GI illness.

CLINICS CARE POINTS

- COVID-19 infection and MIS-C often have GI manifestations that can be severe and the initial presenting symptoms.
- Patients requiring immunosuppression should not have their regimens altered prophylactically, except to minimize chronic steroid use, because the risk of underlying disease exacerbation greatly outweighs COVID-19 infection risk.
- The COVID-19 vaccination should be given to all patients; however, those with chronic disease and immunosuppression are likely to have an attenuated immune response.
- Office visits and procedures significantly decreased during the pandemic and are slowly returning to normal volumes.
- Telehealth greatly expanded over the last year and is likely to continue to be a popular visit option for patients.
- Typical training experiences were decreased for fellows with lower patient volumes, procedures, and research opportunities during the start of the pandemic.

DISCLOSURE

The authors have nothing to disclose.

REFERENCES

1. Lu X, Zhang L, Du H, et al. SARS-CoV-2 infection in children. N Engl J Med 2020; 382(17):1663–5.
2. Dong Y, Mo X, Hu Y, et al. Epidemiology of COVID-19 among children in China. Pediatrics 2020;145(6):e20200702.
3. Viner RM, Mytton OT, Bonell C, et al. Susceptibility to SARS-CoV-2 infection among children and adolescents compared with adults: a systematic review and meta-analysis. JAMA Pediatr 2021;175(2):143–56.
4. Saleh NY, Aboelghar HM, Salem SS, et al. The severity and atypical presentations of COVID-19 infection in pediatrics. BMC Pediatr 2021;21(1):144.
5. Cai Q, Huang D, Yu H, et al. COVID-19: abnormal liver function tests. J Hepatol 2020;73(3):566–74.
6. Qi X, Liu C, Jiang Z, et al. Multicenter analysis of clinical characteristics and outcomes in patients with COVID-19 who develop liver injury. J Hepatol 2020;73(2): 455–8.
7. Bhopal SS, Bagaria J, Olabi B, et al. Children and young people remain at low risk of COVID-19 mortality. Lancet Child Adolesc Health 2021;5(5):e12–3.
8. Murray KF, Gold BD, Shamir R, et al. Coronavirus disease 2019 and the pediatric gastroenterologist. J Pediatr Gastroenterol Nutr 2020;70(6):720–6.
9. Gupta A, Madhavan MV, Sehgal K, et al. Extrapulmonary manifestations of COVID-19. Nat Med 2020;26(7):1017–32.
10. Santos VS, Gurgel RQ, Cuevas LE, et al. Prolonged fecal shedding of SARS-CoV-2 in pediatric patients: a quantitative evidence synthesis. J Pediatr Gastroenterol Nutr 2020;71(2):150–2.
11. Mohammed A, Paranji N, Chen PH, et al. COVID-19 in chronic liver disease and liver transplantation: a clinical review. J Clin Gastroenterol 2021;55(3):187–94.
12. Fan Z, Chen L, Li J, et al. Clinical features of COVID-19-related liver functional abnormality. Clin Gastroenterol Hepatol 2020;18(7):1561–6.
13. Bzeizi K, Abdulla M, Mohammed N, et al. Effect of COVID-19 on liver abnormalities: a systematic review and meta-analysis. Sci Rep 2021;11(1):10599.
14. Spinner CD, Gottlieb RL, Criner GJ, et al. Effect of remdesivir vs standard care on clinical status at 11 days in patients with moderate COVID-19: a randomized clinical trial. JAMA 2020;324(11):1048–57.
15. Tasavon Gholamhoseini M, Yazdi-Feyzabadi V, Goudarzi R, et al. Safety and efficacy of remdesivir for the treatment of COVID-19: a systematic review and meta-analysis. J Pharm Pharm Sci 2021;24:237–45.
16. Méndez-Echevarría A, Pérez-Martínez A, Gonzalez Del Valle L, et al. Compassionate use of remdesivir in children with COVID-19. Eur J Pediatr 2021;180(4): 1317–22.
17. Dale M, Sogawa H, Seyedsaadat SM, et al. Successful management of COVID-19 infection in 2 early post-liver transplant recipients. Transplant Proc 2021;53(4): 1175–9.
18. Meshram HS, Kute VB, Patel H, et al. Feasibility and safety of remdesivir in SARS-CoV2 infected renal transplant recipients: a retrospective cohort from a developing nation. Transpl Infect Dis 2021;e13629. https://doi.org/10.1111/tid.13629.
19. Samanta J, Gupta R, Singh MP, et al. Coronavirus disease 2019 and the pancreas. Pancreatology 2020;20(8):1567–75.
20. Inamdar S, Benias PC, Liu Y, et al. Prevalence, risk factors, and outcomes of hospitalized patients with coronavirus disease 2019 presenting as acute pancreatitis. Gastroenterology 2020;159(6):2226–8.e2.

21. de-Madaria E, Capurso G. COVID-19 and acute pancreatitis: examining the causality. Nat Rev Gastroenterol Hepatol 2021;18(1):3–4.
22. Centers for Disease Control and Prevention (CDC). Multisystem inflammatory syndrome in children (MIS-C) associated with coronavirus disease 2019 (COVID-19). Available at: https://emergency.cdc.gov/han/2020/han00432.asp. Accessed May 8, 2021.
23. Feldstein LR, Rose EB, Horwitz SM, et al. Multisystem inflammatory syndrome in U.S. children and adolescents. N Engl J Med 2020;383(4):334–46.
24. American Academy of Pediatrics. Multisystem inflammatory syndrome in children (MIS-C) interim guidance. Available at: https://services.aap.org/en/pages/2019-novel-coronavirus-covid-19-infections/clinical-guidance/multisystem-inflammatory-syndrome-in-children-mis-c-interim-guidance/#:~:text=Patients%20with%20MIS%2DC%20are,the%20infusion%20of%20IVIG%20therapy. Accessed May 8, 2021.
25. Sahn B, Eze OP, Edelman MC, et al. Features of intestinal disease associated with COVID-related multisystem inflammatory syndrome in children. J Pediatr Gastroenterol Nutr 2021;72(3):384–7.
26. Cantor A, Miller J, Zachariah P, et al. Acute hepatitis is a prominent presentation of the multisystem inflammatory syndrome in children: a single-center report. Hepatology 2020;72(5):1522–7.
27. Sultan K, Mone A, Durbin L, et al. Review of inflammatory bowel disease and COVID-19. World J Gastroenterol 2020;26(37):5534–42.
28. Turner D, Huang Y, Martín-de-Carpi J, et al. Corona virus disease 2019 and paediatric inflammatory bowel diseases: global experience and provisional guidance (March 2020) from the Paediatric IBD Porto Group of European Society of Paediatric Gastroenterology, Hepatology, and Nutrition. J Pediatr Gastroenterol Nutr 2020;70(6):727–33.
29. Brenner EJ, Pigneur B, Focht G, et al. Benign evolution of SARS-Cov2 infections in children with inflammatory bowel disease: results from two international databases. Clin Gastroenterol Hepatol 2021;19(2):394–6.e5.
30. Khan N, Mahmud N, Trivedi C, et al. Risk factors for SARS-CoV-2 infection and course of COVID-19 disease in patients with IBD in the Veterans Affair Healthcare System. Gut 2021. https://doi.org/10.1136/gutjnl-2021-324356.
31. Sperger J, Shah KS, Lu M, et al. Development and validation of multivariable prediction models for adverse COVID-19 outcomes in IBD patients. medRxiv 2021. https://doi.org/10.1101/2021.01.15.21249889.
32. D'Arcangelo G, Distante M, Raso T, et al. Safety of biological therapy in children with inflammatory bowel disease. J Pediatr Gastroenterol Nutr 2021;72(5):736–41.
33. D'Amico F, Rabaud C, Peyrin-Biroulet L, et al. SARS-CoV-2 vaccination in IBD: more pros than cons. Nat Rev Gastroenterol Hepatol 2021;18(4):211–3.
34. Olliaro P, Torreele E, Vaillant M. COVID-19 vaccine efficacy and effectiveness—the elephant (not) in the room. Lancet Microbe 2021;2(7):e279–80.
35. Kennedy NA, Lin S, Goodhand JR, et al. Infliximab is associated with attenuated immunogenicity to BNT162b2 and ChAdOx1 nCoV-19 SARS-CoV-2 vaccines in patients with IBD. Gut 2021. https://doi.org/10.1136/gutjnl-2021-324789.
36. Siegel CA, Melmed GY, McGovern DP, et al. SARS-CoV-2 vaccination for patients with inflammatory bowel diseases: recommendations from an international consensus meeting. Gut 2021;70(4):635–40.
37. Singh S, Khan A. Clinical characteristics and outcomes of coronavirus disease 2019 among patients with preexisting liver disease in the United States: a multicenter research network study. Gastroenterology 2020;159(2):768–71.e3.

38. Kehar M, Ebel NH, Ng VL, et al. SARS-CoV2 infection in children with liver transplant and native liver disease: an international observational registry study. J Pediatr Gastroenterol Nutr 2021;72(6):807–14.

39. Di Giorgio A, Nicastro E, Arnaboldi S, et al. Health status of children with chronic liver disease during the SARS-CoV-2 outbreak: results from a multicentre study. Clin Res Hepatol Gastroenterol 2021;45(2):101610.

40. Marjot T, Buescher G, Sebode M, et al. SARS-CoV-2 infection in patients with autoimmune hepatitis. J Hepatol 2021;74(6):1335–43.

41. Ji D, Qin E, Xu J, et al. Non-alcoholic fatty liver diseases in patients with COVID-19: a retrospective study. J Hepatol 2020;73(2):451–3.

42. Zhou YH, Rios RS, Zheng KI, et al. Recommendations and clinical guidance for children with metabolic-associated fatty liver disease during the COVID-19 pandemic. J Clin Transl Hepatol 2021;9(1):1–2.

43. Colmenero J, Rodríguez-Perálvarez M, Salcedo M, et al. Epidemiological pattern, incidence, and outcomes of COVID-19 in liver transplant patients. J Hepatol 2021;74(1):148–55.

44. Nikoupour H, Kazemi K, Arasteh P, et al. Pediatric liver transplantation and COVID-19: a case report. BMC Surg 2020;20(1):224.

45. Petters LM, Vogel TP, Munoz FM, et al. Multisystem inflammatory syndrome in children associated with SARS-CoV-2 in a solid organ transplant recipient. Am J Transplant 2021;21(7):2596–9.

46. Doná D, Torres Canizales J, Benetti E, et al. Pediatric transplantation in Europe during the COVID-19 pandemic: early impact on activity and healthcare. Clin Transpl 2020;34(10):e14063.

47. Rabinowich L, Grupper A, Baruch R, et al. Low immunogenicity to SARS-CoV-2 vaccination among liver transplant recipients. J Hepatol 2021;75(2):435–8.

48. Boyarsky BJ, Werbel WA, Avery RK, et al. Antibody response to 2-dose SARS-CoV-2 mRNA vaccine series in solid organ transplant recipients. JAMA 2021; 325(21):2204–6.

49. Peled Y, Ram E, Lavee J, et al. BNT162b2 vaccination in heart transplant recipients: clinical experience and antibody response. J Heart Lung Transplant 2021; 40(8):759–62.

50. American Society of Transplantation. Statement on COVID-19 vaccination in solid organ transplant recipients. 2021. Available at: https://www.myast.org/statement-covid-19-vaccination-solid-organ-transplant-recipients#. Accessed May 29, 2021.

51. Cornberg M, Buti M, Eberhardt CS, et al. EASL position paper on the use of COVID-19 vaccines in patients with chronic liver diseases, hepatobiliary cancer and liver transplant recipients. J Hepatol 2021;74(4):944–51.

52. Fix OK, Blumberg EA, Chang KM, et al. AASLD Expert Panel Consensus Statement: vaccines to prevent COVID-19 infection in patients with liver disease. Hepatology 2021. https://doi.org/10.1002/hep.31751.

53. Kriem J, Rahhal R. COVID-19 pandemic and challenges in pediatric gastroenterology practice. World J Gastroenterol 2020;26(36):5387–94.

54. Walsh CM, Fishman DS, Lerner DG. Pediatric endoscopy in the era of coronavirus disease 2019: a North American Society for Pediatric Gastroenterology, Hepatology, and Nutrition position paper. J Pediatr Gastroenterol Nutr 2020;70(6): 741–50.

55. Lazzerini M, Barbi E, Apicella A, et al. Delayed access or provision of care in Italy resulting from fear of COVID-19. Lancet Child Adolescent Health 2020;4(5): e10–1.

56. Ding YY, Ramakrishna S, Long AH, et al. Delayed cancer diagnoses and high mortality in children during the COVID-19 pandemic. Pediatr Blood Cancer 2020;67(9):e28427.
57. Bonilla L, Gálvez C, Medrano L, et al. [Impact of COVID-19 on the presentation and course of acute appendicitis in paediatrics]. An Pediatr (Engl Ed) 2021; 94(4):245–51.
58. Delgado-Miguel C, Muñoz-Serrano AJ, Miguel-Ferrero M, et al. Complicated acute appendicitis during COVID-19 pandemic: the hidden epidomic in children. Eur J Pediatr Surg 2021. https://doi.org/10.1055/s-0041-1723992.
59. Snapiri O, Rosenberg Danziger C, Krause I, et al. Delayed diagnosis of paediatric appendicitis during the COVID-19 pandemic. Acta Paediatr 2020;109(8): 1672–6.
60. Pines JM, Zocchi MS, Black BS, et al. Characterizing pediatric emergency department visits during the COVID-19 pandemic. Am J Emerg Med 2021;41: 201–4.
61. Mallon D, Pohl JF, Phatak UP, et al. Impact of COVID-19 on pediatric gastroenterology fellow training in North America. J Pediatr Gastroenterol Nutr 2020; 71(1):6–11.
62. Berg EA, Picoraro JA, Miller SD, et al. COVID-19 - a guide to rapid implementation of telehealth services: a playbook for the pediatric gastroenterologist. J Pediatr Gastroenterol Nutr 2020;70(6):734–40.
63. Wosik J, Fudim M, Cameron B, et al. Telehealth transformation: COVID-19 and the rise of virtual care. J Am Med Inform Assoc 2020;27(6):957–62.
64. Centers for Medicare and Medicaid Services. Medicare and Medicaid programs; policy and regulatory revisions in response to the COVID-19 public health emergency. Available at: https://www.cms.gov/files/document/covid-final-ifc.pdf. Accessed April 19, 2020.
65. Verstraete SG, Sola AM, Ali SA. Telemedicine for pediatric inflammatory bowel disease in the era of COVID-19. J Pediatr Gastroenterol Nutr 2020;70(6):e140.
66. Leinwand K, Blodgett N, Ramraj R. Telehealth in pediatric gastroenterology can be a sustainable long-term option: a single-center experience. Permanente J 2021;25:1.
67. Shah AC, Badawy SM. Telemedicine in pediatrics: systematic review of randomized controlled trials. JMIR Pediatr parenting 2021;4(1):e22696.
68. Haynes SC, Marcin JP, Dayal P, et al. Impact of telemedicine on visit attendance for paediatric patients receiving endocrinology specialty care. J Telemed Telecare 2020. https://doi.org/10.1177/1357633X20972911. 1357633x20972911.
69. Eberly LA, Kallan MJ, Julien HM, et al. Patient characteristics associated with telemedicine access for primary and specialty ambulatory care during the COVID-19 pandemic. JAMA Netw Open 2020;3(12):e2031640.
70. Ray KN, Mehrotra A, Yabes JG, et al. Telemedicine and outpatient subspecialty visits among pediatric Medicaid beneficiaries. Acad Pediatr 2020;20(5):642–51.
71. Business Group on Health. 2021 large employers' health care strategy and plan design survey. August 2020. Available at: https://www.businessgrouphealth.org/resources/2021-large-employers-health-care-strategy-and-plan-design-survey. Accessed May 8, 2021.
72. Ohio Department of Medicaid. Telehealth billing guidelines 2020. Available at: https://medicaid.ohio.gov/Portals/0/Providers/COVID19/Telehealth-Billing-Guidelines-on-or-after-11-15-2020.pdf.
73. Centers for Medicare and Medicaid Services (CMS): Trump Administration Finalizes Permanent Expansion of Medicare Telehealth Services and Improved

Payment for Time Doctors Spend with Patients [press release]. December 2020. Available at: https://www.cms.gov/newsroom/press-releases/trump-administration-finalizes-permanent-expansion-medicare-telehealth-services-and-improved-payment. Accessed May 8, 2021.

74. Turner Lee N, Karsten J, Roberts J. Removing regulatory barriers to telehealth before and after COVID-19. May 2020. Available at: https://www.brookings.edu/research/removing-regulatory-barriers-to-telehealth-before-and-after-covid-19. Accessed May 8, 2020.

75. Hsu EK, Ambartsumyan L, Wahbeh GT, et al. Pediatric endoscopy during the COVID-19 pandemic: addressing the implications of universal preprocedural testing for PPE utilization. J Pediatr Gastroenterol Nutr 2021;72(1):e25–6.

76. Yu Q, Xu P, Gan H, et al. Comprehensive gastroenterology endoscopy unit workflow and infection prevention during the COVID-19 pandemic: experience with 159 cases in Wuhan, China. Dig Endosc 2021;33(1):195–202.

77. Sultan S, Siddique SM, Altayar O, et al. AGA Institute Rapid Review and Recommendations on the role of pre-procedure SARS-CoV-2 testing and endoscopy. Gastroenterology 2020;159(5):1935–48.e5.

78. Irastorza LE, Hopson P, Ta A, et al. The impact of COVID-19 on job prospects and educational training for pediatric gastroenterology fellows. J Pediatr Gastroenterol Nutr 2021;72(4):514–9.

79. CDC. COVID data tracker. 2021. 2021. Available at: https://covid.cdc.gov/covid-data-tracker/#trends_dailytrendscases. Accessed May 26, 2021.

Precision Medicine in Pediatric Inflammatory Bowel Disease

Elizabeth A. Spencer, MD, Marla C. Dubinsky, MD*

KEYWORDS

- Precision medicine • Inflammatory bowel disease • Crohn's disease
- Ulcerative colitis • Pediatrics • Therapeutic drug monitoring • Prevention

KEY POINTS

- Precision medicine in pediatric IBD is the use of individual patient data to determine the **right** patient, **right** therapy, **right** dose, **right** time, and **right** strategy.
- There is a growing body of evidence to incorporate multi'omic data into precision medicine strategies in the clinic to improve the care of patients with pediatric IBD.
- This multi'omic data may be difficult to interpret for individual clinicians, making the co-development and implementation of machine learning approaches and electronic medical record-integrated clinical decision support tools vital.
- Precision medicine holds promise to be not only the tool that breaks our current therapeutic ceiling but the key that unlocks currently unattainable goals like prevention.

INTRODUCTION

Inflammatory bowel disease (IBD) has been rising in prevalence across the world since the start of the industrial revolution,[1] and IBD is diagnosed before the age of 20 in about a quarter of patients, making it commonly a disease of childhood.[2] While the incidence has stabilized in North America and Western Europe, the prevalence is compounding from the pre-existing, aging IBD population,[3,4] and, in newly industrialized countries, the incidence is accelerating.[5,6] With these combined effects, the global

Funding: Dr E.A. Spencer is supported on an NIH T32 training grant; there has been no other funding from any agency in the public, commercial, or not-for-profit sector for this research.
Conflicts of Interest: M.C. Dubinsky; Consultant for Janssen, Abbvie, UCB, Takeda, Pfizer, Prometheus labs, Genentech, Salix, Celgene Research support; Takeda, Pfizer, Janssen. Co-Founder and shareholder Trellus Health. Co-inventor Patent pending PROSPECT Tool licensed to Takeda.
Department of Pediatrics, Mount Sinai Kravis Children's Hospital, Susan and Leonard Feinstein Inflammatory Bowel Disease Clinical Center, Mount Sinai Hospital, Icahn School of Medicine, 1 Gustave L. Levy Place, Box 1656, New York, NY 10029, USA
* Corresponding author.
E-mail address: Marla.Dubinsky@mssm.edu

burden of IBD is increasing, and, because it is a disease with significant morbidity and high health care costs, it is putting a strain both on the affected patients and the health care systems that take care of them. Precision medicine (PM) is vital to improve and create efficiencies within care for this burgeoning disease, as well as to identify tactics to achieve prevention to drive down incidence.

PM is, further, one of the five focus areas proposed by the Crohn's and Colitis Foundation as a "Challenge in IBD" that deserves dedicated research.[7] There is widely considered to be a therapeutic ceiling in IBD, where all therapies, old and new, result in remission in 20% to 50% of patients with further loss of response over time in those who initially respond.[8-11] To break this ceiling, optimization of therapies using therapeutic drug monitoring (TDM), the rational selection of initial therapy to avoid reduction in effectiveness due to the sequence of the therapy,[12] and the use of combinations of biologics or small molecules have all been proposed.[13] With each successive trial and failure of medical therapy, there is on-going inflammation and accrual of bowel wall damage, which can occur in all types of IBD; intervening as early as possible with an effective therapy tailored to a patient profile and achieving endoscopic remission rapidly could lead to a reduction in negative outcomes, such as hospitalization, surgery, complication, fibrosis, disability, including psychological disability, and colorectal cancer.[14-17]

While there is a clear need for PM, it is an incredibly complex undertaking due to the multifactorial pathogenesis of IBD, where summative effects from variable combinations of genetic, microbial, immunologic, and environmental factors lead to the development of overt disease.[18] There is also interplay between these factors further complicating matters. The increasingly diverse worldwide IBD population poses additional hurdles for a PM-approach because multi'omic coverage of this diversity is still lacking.[19] All of this makes characterization of a specific patient's precision profile a labyrinthian task, requiring large existing data sets describing these contributing factors across diverse populations.[19]

Despite this complexity, the long-established core tenets of PM of **right patient, right therapy, right dose, and right time** are fitting for IBD and a good starting point for the real-world application of PM principles. One additional goal of the **right strategy** is also needed because pediatric IBD is a chronic, lifelong condition without a cure, making attainment of disease-modifying goals (treat-to-target) and maintaining them through close monitoring (tight control) foundational to precision IBD care (**Fig. 1**). Finally, an aspirational goal of PM in IBD is to unlock **prevention** as an achievable target through identification of those at high risk for IBD.[20] While PM is a rapidly changing art, this review will strive to detail the current state and future directions of PM in pediatric IBD.

RIGHT PATIENT

Pediatric IBD is extremely heterogenous with a variety of subtypes and complicating extraintestinal manifestations (EIMs), and the clinical features of pediatric IBD, particularly phenotypic differences of subtypes, are detailed by both the North American and European societies for Pediatric Gastroenterology, Hepatology, and Nutrition (NASPGHAN and ESPGHAN).[21-24] The initiation of effective therapy early is ideal,[25] making distinguishing who among this extremely heterogenous set of patients are at low and high risk for progression and complication very important to guide initial selection of therapy.

Currently, clinical and laboratory features, including serologic response to enteric pathogens, are assessed crudely by clinicians to determine risk of progression. In

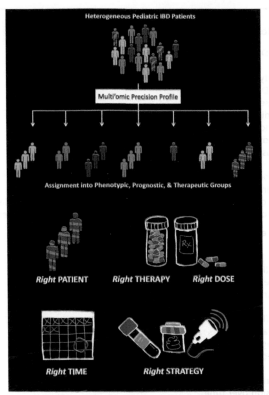

Fig. 1. Precision medicine in pediatric IBD. With heterogenous IBD population, precision medicine may be used to assign patients into phenotypic, prognostic, and therapeutic groups to then apply the RIGHT principles of precision medicine: Right Patient, Right Therapy, Right Dose, Right Time, and Right Strategy.

future, the large-scale databases of genomic, proteomic, microbial, and metabolomic signatures will continue to be expanded and refined and become incorporated into models of risk prognostication, and clinicians, aided by artificial intelligence and machine learning, may use these more precise risk models to better identify patients at high risk of progression to intervene early with more aggressive therapy and alternatively to identify patients at low risk of progression, where aggressive intervention is not needed.

Clinical and Laboratory Features

Clinical features and routine laboratory findings have been associated with complicated disease and/or surgery in both Crohn's disease (CD) and ulcerative colitis (UC) (**Box 1**).[26] Growth, Relapse and Outcomes With Therapy CD, a large pediatric CD inception cohort, has shown that stricturing disease at baseline and Pediatric CD Activity Index (PCDAI) > 10 at week 12 after therapy were predictors for early surgery.[23] In a recent retrospective pediatric cohort, longer disease duration and younger age of diagnosis were associated with endoscopic recurrence after ileocecal resection, which occurred commonly (46% at 2 years) despite the frequent use of biologics.[27] Furthermore, a recent meta-analysis demonstrated that ileal disease location and older age at diagnosis were both associated with increased risk of

---

Box 1
Clinical & Laboratory Predictors of Prognosis

Pediatric Crohn's Disease
Severe Disease
  ASCA positivity
  Complicated Disease
Complicated Disease
  Small bowel disease
  African American Race (*penetrating disease*)
  ASCA/CBir1 positivity
  Perianal disease
Surgery
  Ileal disease location
  Growth impairment at diagnosis
  Diagnosis in adolescence (>13 years) associated with surgery early in disease course
  Diagnosis in younger children (<12–14) associated with recurrence after surgery

Pediatric Ulcerative Colitis
Severe Disease
  Pancolitis
  Severe colitis (PUCAI >65) at diagnosis
  Hypoalbuminemia at diagnosis
  PUCAI score greater than 10 3 months following therapy
Colectomy
  Severe colitis (PUCAI >65) at diagnosis
  Extensive disease
  Anemia at diagnosis
  C difficile infection
  Poor response to corticosteroids
  Neutrophilic infiltration of stomach and duodenum
  Disease extension over time

---

complication and/or surgery.[26] Higher ($\geq$5 mg/dL) C-reactive protein (CRP), an IL-6 dependent acute-phase reactant, has also been associated with moderate-severe disease.[26,28,29] Furthermore, in a multicenter, pediatric UC inception cohort (PROTECT), higher baseline albumin levels and Pediatric UC Activity Index (PUCAI) < 10 4 weeks into therapy were both associated with response to therapy.[30]

Serologic Markers

Serologic response to enteric pathogens, notably anti-*Saccharomyces cerevisiae* antibody (ASCA), antibody to *Escherichia coli* outer-membrane porin C (OmpC), and antibody to flagellin (CBir1), as well as perinuclear antineutrophil antibody (pANCA) have been used to prognosticate risk. It was initially demonstrated in a large pediatric cohort that the rate of complicated and progressive CD increases as immune reactivity increases,[31] and there is a large body of literature validating and supporting this concept of more complicated disease with increasing immune reactivity.[32,33] In a pediatric CD inception cohort, the Risk Stratification and Identification of Immunogenetic and Microbial Markers of Rapid Disease Progression in Children with CD (RISK) study, patients positive for two or more serologic markers (ASCA, OmpC, and/or CBir1) progressed to complicated disease more quickly than those with only one serologic marker.[34] In UC, high-titer (>100 EU/mL) pANCA has been found to be associated with pancolitis,[35] as well as chronic pouchitis after IPAA.[36]

Genetic Risk Loci and Risk Scores

Large GWAS studies in IBD have identified risk loci that are associated with a complicated course. The first, and to this day the strongest, identified risk allele is nucleotide binding oligomerization domain containing 2 (NOD2), and it was initially shown to be associated with complicated CD, defined as development of stricture and need for surgery.[37] However, RISK did not find an association of NOD2 or a polygenic risk score with stricturing or fistulizing CD,[34] and a large genotype-phenotype study showed that NOD2's association with complicated disease was more likely due to its association with younger age of diagnosis and stricturing disease.[38] There have since been other risk loci (FOXO3, XACT, IGFBP1, and the MHC region between HLA-B and HLA-DR) identified as associated with poor prognosis; however, they currently require further validation.[39] In UC, the HLA DRB1*0103 allele is associated with pancolitis and the need for colectomy.[40,41]

A genome-wide polygenic risk score (GRS) incorporates the additive effects of genetic variants weighted by effect size to estimate the risk of a certain phenotype based on genotype. IBD was one of five diseases used to demonstrate this technique, with area under the curve (AUC) of 0.63 in both the testing (95% confidence interval [CI]: 0.62–0.65) and validation (95% CI: 0.62–0.64) data sets. The predictive value of this risk score is improved with the increased incorporation of diverse racial population data.[19] These risk scores are promising and may allow for improved predictive power compared with high-risk variants alone.

Proteomics

An important goal for PM in IBD is the identification of a biomarker or biomarkers that can surpass fecal calprotectin (FC) in ability to discern endoscopic findings without the attendant issue of patient dissatisfaction and/or nonadherence. Proteomics holds significant promise in allowing for more precise characterization of the individual patient, and the use of proteomics has already been established with more sophisticated panels already in clinical use. In the RISK cohort, using a panel of blood proteomic markers, five proteins were associated with B3 complications (AUC 0.79, 95% CI: 0.76–0.82), and four proteins were associated with B2 complications (AUC 0.68, 95% CI: 0.65–0.71).[42] Additionally, collagen Type III alpha 1 chain (COL3A1) levels at diagnosis were higher in patients who went on to develop stricture in RISK.[43] A panel of 13 protein markers, called a serum endoscopic healing index (Monitr, Prometheus Biosciences, San Diego, CA) has been validated in CD to distinguish endoscopic activity comparable to FC and superior to CRP,[44] and this same panel has preliminary data in UC demonstrating success in distinguishing moderate-to-severe disease activity.[45]

Gene Expression

Specific gene expression profiles have been implicated in IBD prognosis and phenotype. For example, in CD, in the RISK cohort, RNA sequencing was used to characterize gene expression of biopsy specimens, and they found that high ileal expression of extracellular matrix genes was associated with later development of stricture, which corresponds with the finding of elevation of COL3A1 at diagnosis.[34] A transcriptional risk score, which was a summative score of gene expression associated with known IBD-risk alleles, was also derived from the RISK cohort data and shown to have promise in identification of CD patients and distinguishing which patients may complicate over time.[46] A commercially available transcriptional signature in peripheral CD8 T cells associated with T cell exhaustion (PredictSURE,

PredictImmune, Cambridge) has further had promising initial results as a potential predictor of more aggressive disease, and it is currently undergoing validation.[47,48]

In UC, a type 2 gene expression pattern was associated with a higher likelihood of achieving clinical remission[49]; similarly, a higher eosinophil count in PROTECT was associated with lesser likelihood of escalation from 5-ASA to antitumor necrosis factor α (anti-TNF) therapy.[30] Pre-treatment rectal UC gene expression signatures from PROTECT were associated with disease severity and corticosteroid response, and, interestingly, gene sets dysregulated in severe disease had been previously seen in adenocarcinoma. Further, the pathways enriched in disease severity and treatment response were also linked with disease-associated microbial taxa.[50]

Microbial Dysbiosis

An imbalance in microbial composition compared with healthy controls, called dysbiosis, is commonly found in IBD; this dysbiosis is characterized by decreased bacterial diversity and abundance in those with IBD, as well as increasing evidence for a role for fungi and viruses.[51] Adding further complexity, metagenomics and metabolomics have revealed changes in the composition and microbial metabolites in patients with IBD.[52] In a pediatric IBD cohort, severe microbial dysbiosis, or imbalanced intestinal microbiota, was associated with extensive and/or complicated phenotypes, use of biologic therapy, and failure to achieve mucosal healing.[53] Additionally, classifiers describing the microbiome structure and metabolic activity are associated with IBD status.[52] Further refinement and incorporation of these microbial profiles are likely to be an important part of PM in IBD and offer new targeted treatment strategies aimed at the microbiome and stool metabolome.[54]

Putting It All Together: Clinical Decision Support Tools

Increasingly, all of these features are being incorporated into comprehensive clinical decision support tools (CDSTs). CDST can be incorporated directly into the electronic medical record (EMR), making interpretation of these predictors easier for the clinician directing the initial choice of therapy. Currently, there is a commercially available tool for CD, CD-PATH, which places patients into low-, medium-, and high-risk groups based on a combination of clinical, serologic, and genetic markers with predictive accuracy of 75% in children.[55] For vedolizumab, a CDST made of clinical and laboratory findings was able to identify patients likely to achieve corticosteroid-free remission in addition to differentiating those who would need interval shortening.[56]

RIGHT THERAPY

Selection of therapy is currently based on clinical factors such as risk of progression and disease location, severity, and activity.[57]

While the number of available IBD therapies has increased over time, the first biologic, regardless of choice, has the highest probability of success. The sequence of therapies can also determine the effectiveness of a therapy; for example, in UC, vedolizumab (VDZ, Entyvio) is less effective if it is given after anti-TNF therapy, and this negative effect of a prior anti-TNF is not as marked with ustekinumab (UST; Stelara).[12,58] Additionally, with each successive trial of a therapy, patients experience symptoms while awaiting response, which can lead to disability, exposure to corticosteroids, and health care utilization. For all of these reasons, it is important to be thoughtful in the selection of an initial therapy, and a PM approach to better select a therapy tied to patient characteristics, reflective of the biology underpinning their IBD, can minimize time to remission and reduce morbidity.

Anti-Tumor Necrosis Factor α Therapies

Several *baseline* gene expression profiles have been identified in patients with IBD treated with anti-TNF that are associated with *later* nonresponse to therapy. Higher expression of Oncostatin M (OSM), a member of the IL-6 proinflammatory cytokine family, was associated with anti-TNF nonresponse (relative risk [RR] = 5, 95% CI: 1.4–17.9) with an impressive AUC of 0.99[59]; however, it is unclear if this is simply reflective of a higher inflammatory burden being linked to nonresponse. Low level expression of triggering receptor expressed on myeloid cells 1 (TREM-1) has also been associated with nonresponse to anti-TNF in both CD and UC.[60] Upregulation of TREM-1 and CCR-CCL7, has also been shown to be associated with anti-TNF nonresponse, both lead to an increase in inflammatory macrophages.[61] These serum gene expression profiles may be incorporated in future into CDSTs aimed at therapeutic selection. Finally, a cellular module was identified, using single cell seq, in a cohort of patients with ileal CD, comprised IgG plasma cells, inflammatory mononuclear phagocytes, activated T cells, and stromal cells which was found to be associated with failure to achieve steroid-free clinical remission on anti-TNF therapy.[62]

Anti-Integrin Therapies

In a retrospective cohort of 251 patients with IBD, pretreatment colonic mucosal eosinophilia predicted nonresponse to VDZ at 6 months.[63] Circulating $\alpha_4\beta_7$ may also be a marker of VDZ response, with on-going studies developing this further.[64] VedoNet, a neural network algorithm to predict clinical remission at Week 14 on VDZ, had improved predictive power when microbial data were combined with clinical data (clinical data alone: AUC = 0.619; clinical and microbial data: AUC = 0.872). Importantly, increased microbial diversity at baseline was associated with response to VDZ.[65] EUCALYPTUS, a phase II trial for the anti-integrin, etrolizumab, αE gene expression (ITGAE) could stratify participants by likelihood of achieving Week 10 clinical remission.[66]

Anti-IL-12 and IL-23 Therapies

In a clinical trial of brazikumab (an anti-interleukin-23 (IL-23) therapy) for CD, concentrations of interleukin-22 (IL-22), an upstream regulator of IL-23 signaling, were measured at baseline, and levels higher than a cut-point of 15.6 pg/mL were associated with an increased likelihood of clinical remission at week 8.[67] In EMerging BiomARKers in IBD (EMBARK), a study correlating biomarkers with endoscopy and imaging, IL-22, along with FC and matrix metalloproteinase 9 (MMP9), was also associated, in CD, with a composite inflammation score derived from combining colonoscopy and computed tomography enterography scores into a single score; FC and MMP were most closely associated with this composite inflammation score in UC.[68]

There is an increased rate of psoriasis in IBD compared with the general population, and there is also a higher incidence of a family history of psoriasis in CD and UC.[69] Further reinforcing this connection, there are variants in the IL23 R gene that confer protection in both psoriasis and IBD,[70] and therapy targeting this pathway, such as ustekinumab, has proven efficacious in both psoriasis and IBD.[71–73] Assessing for a family history of psoriasis may allow for assessment for this shared genetic link and associated biologic pathway, which could inform therapeutic choice.

Clinical Decision Support Tools and Multi-Omic Analysis

As previously noted, CDSTs will play an important role in incorporating these novel markers of response to therapy.[74–76] As an example, the PROTECT investigators combined gene expression profiles and microbial composition to create a signature associated with early responders to therapy.[77] Multi-omic Factor Analysis (MOFA) has also been used to integrate "-omic" data; one such MOFA was developed for prediction of Week 24 endoscopic response to ustekinumab with 98% accuracy.[78]

Pharmacogenomics

Thiopurines, which include 6-mercaptopurine (6-MP) and AZA, are some of the first medications used for IBD. They are associated with potentially life-threatening side effects, which include leukopenia and pancreatitis. Thiopurines are metabolized by the enzyme thiopurine methyltransferase (TPMT). Perhaps, the longest-standing PM tactic in IBD is the use of TPMT genotyping or the associated enzyme level to determine dosing of thiopurines.[79]

Homozygosity for a mutation in TPMT resulting in decreased activity leads to increased accumulation of the active metabolites and resultant leukopenia, which can be severe and even require hospitalization.[80,81] In a large Dutch study, TPMT variant carriers with an a priori dose reduction had a 10-fold reduction in leukopenic events (RR: 0.11; 95% CI: 0.01–0.85).[82] Another genetic variant in Nudix hydrolase 15 (NUDT15) has also been identified as associated with increased risk of leukopenia with thiopurines, and it can be additive with variants in TPMT.[83] Currently, it is advised to check both TPMT (either genotype or activity level) and NUDT15 (genotype) before initiation of thiopurine therapy to guide dosing or potentially preclude usage of thiopurines in a small high-risk subset.

The Personalizing Anti-TNF Therapy in CD consortium have suggested that the allele group HLA-DQA1*05 is associated with time to development of antidrug antibody to anti-TNF therapies (hazard ratio: 1.90, 95% CI: 1.60–2.25).[84] This is now commercially available to use clinically (*RiskImmune*, Prometheus Biosciences, San Diego, CA); there is currently on-going work to understand the complexities of the various HLA-DQA1*05 alleles, which may have distinct impacts on immunogenicity and may be variably associated by anti-TNF type.[85]

There are other genetic variants associated with adverse outcomes that are not currently used clinically. For example, a polymorphism in the HLA class II region (rs2647087) was identified that is, associated with an increased risk of pancreatitis with thiopurines; patients homozygous for this gene have a 17% risk of developing pancreatitis.[86,87] Additionally, a small study identified a potential risk allele and protective allele associated with developing adverse dermatologic reactions with anti-TNF therapy.[88] Variants like this may, in future, be gathered together into a large IBD pharmacogenomic panel done at disease diagnosis and used to guide therapeutic choice. Furthermore, a universal IBD pharmacogenomic panel may incorporate pre-existing panels aimed at common comorbid conditions, such as anxiety and depression, as we move toward a 360° care model of IBD aimed at treating the whole patient.

RIGHT DOSE
Therapeutic Drug Monitoring

As previously noted, given that IBD therapies are finite, therapy must be rationally selected but also optimized to maximize the therapeutic effect and verify that pharmacokinetic parameters are not limiting effectiveness. This optimization entails dose and interval adjustments or the addition of a medication to use in combination and is often based on TDM.

TDM is used to optimize both thiopurines and biologics. With thiopurines, TDM has long been accepted; when used in monotherapy, one can check thiopurine metabolite levels and aim to adjust the dose to achieve a 6-TGN level of$\geq$235 while maintaining a 6-MMP level less than 5700.[81] For biologic therapies, TDM is recommended to achieve target drug concentrations.[89] In 2019, the Building Research in IBD Globally group presented an expert consensus statement on the appropriate use of TDM and target ranges for biologic therapies based on the currently available medical literature; they additionally developed a web-based tool to assist in choosing target drug concentrations based on patient characteristics.[90,91] If these targets are not achieved, the physician should weigh the relative feasibility and benefits of dose escalation, and/or interval shortening. In the case of anti-TNF therapy, the addition of an immunomodulator may also be considered. Drug concentration should continue to be reassessed with adjustments made until the target is reached. In the case of monotherapy with an anti-TNF careful attention should be paid to the drug concentrations during induction to assure appropriate levels and avoid the formation of antidrug antibodies; this practice, known as optimized monotherapy, has been shown to be effective in the prevention of antidrug antibodies.[92]

There is still much debate about the use of reactive versus proactive TDM; reactive TDM is the practice of obtaining a drug concentration in response to clinical or laboratory findings, and proactive TDM is when drug concentrations are checked at regular intervals without any clinical or biomarker impetus for the test. Analysis of clinical trial data has revealed improved outcomes with higher serum drug concentrations. However, two large RCTs, Trough Level Adapted infliximab (IFX, Remicade) Treatment (TAXIT) and Drug concentration versus Symptom-driven Dose Adaptation of IFX in patients with active CD (TAILORIX), were inconclusive about the benefit of proactive monitoring, but they both had methodological issues (eg optimization of *all* patients in TAXIT prior to randomization).[93,94] In TAXIT, several of the secondary outcomes favored proactive TDM,[93] and higher levels during induction in TAILORIX were associated with early endoscopic remission at week 12.[95] In pediatrics, Pediatric CD Adalimumab-Level-based Optimization Treatment, a study of TDM in a cohort of biologic-naïve pediatric patients with CD started on adalimumab, revealed that proactive TDM was more likely to lead to corticosteroid-free clinical remission through Week 72 when compared with reactive TDM.[96] Beyond clinical benefit, there is also growing evidence that TDM is more cost-effective than empirical adjustments of biologic therapy.[97,98]

Dashboard-guided adaptive dosing of biologics based on clinical and laboratory parameters, including drug concentration, from an individual patient are also on the horizon for use in clinical practice. This has been shown to be feasible with anti-TNF and led to lower rates of antidrug antibodies ($P < .002$) and increased rates of CRP normalization ($P = .002$).[99,100] In the PRECISION trial, which randomized patients to receive dashboard-guided dosing targeting a trough of 3 ug/ml or standard dosing without dose adjustments, the patients with the guided dosing were significantly more likely to be in clinical remission at 1 year (88% vs 64%, $P = .017$).[101] These dashboards are of particular importance in pediatrics as it has previously been observed that subtherapeutic infliximab levels are common in pediatric patients,[100,102] and, in a pediatric real-world study of dashboard dosing, age (<10) and weight (<30 kg) were predictors of subtherapeutic levels.[100]

RIGHT TIME
Early Effective Intervention

Within CD, early effective intervention is currently the model of choice for the administration of therapy. This means a medical intervention targeted at the patient's specific factors from disease outset to rapidly achieve targets of therapy rather than putting the patient through needless trials of ineffective therapies. Data from randomized clinical trials, as well as observational cohort studies have shown that early intervention with biologic therapies can slow progression in CD with improvement in long-term outcomes.[25] Within the RISK pediatric cohort, remission at 1 year was more likely with early treatment with anti-TNF therapy than early treatment with an immunomodulator (85.3% vs 60.3% in remission; RR: 1.41; 95% CI: 1.14–1.75; P = .0017).[103] A randomized clinical trial in pediatric CD similarly showed the early treatment with anti-TNF led to faster remission than conventional therapy (induction with exclusive enteral nutrition or prednisone and maintenance with thiopurine), and many in the conventional arm needed escalation to anti-TNF during the course of the study.[104] The data in pediatric UC are still somewhat limited; however, in PROTECT, nearly 20% of patients with UC with moderate-to-severe disease at baseline escalated to anti-TNF therapy within the first 4 weeks of therapy compared with 0% of those with mild disease; a further 20% of those with moderate-to-severe disease escalated to anti-TNF within the first year of therapy, signifying a potential role for the early use of biologic therapy in pediatric UC patients with moderate-to-severe disease.[30]

RIGHT STRATEGY
Treat-To-Target & Tight Control

Based on strategies within the fields of rheumatoid arthritis and diabetes, where specific treatment goals were created to improve outcomes and minimize end-organ damage, the field of IBD now uses a treat-to-target (T2T) approach. T2T defines discrete goals of therapy and a timeline in which to achieve them, and, if these goals are not met, the therapeutic strategy must be reconsidered. The process of using a close monitoring strategy to attain and sustain these goals is called tight control.

The landmark CALM trial, a randomized, controlled trial of patients with moderate-to-severe CD treated with anti-TNF early in their disease course, used a tight control strategy aimed at achieving and maintaining target goals. In the study, escalation of anti-TNF and thiopurine therapy based on clinical symptoms and/or lab markers of inflammation (FC≤250 ug/g and CRP≤5) resulted in more patients achieving mucosal healing at week 48 compared with clinical symptoms alone (46% vs 30%).[105] While the rates of remission were higher in the tight control group, they still did *not* result in most patients achieving the desired end point of remission; this may be due to the limitations of the tight control strategy utilized because it relied heavily on CRP and FC and did not incorporate TDM. The long-term extension of CALM then went on to show that realization of target goals of either endoscopic (CD Endoscopic Index of Severity (CDEIS) < 4 with no deep ulcerations) or deep (CD Activity Index < 150, CDEIS less than 4 with no deep ulcerations, and no steroids for≥8 weeks) remission by week 48 was associated with a reduction in the progression of disease (median 3 years follow-up).[106]

The Selecting Therapeutic Targets in IBD (STRIDE) program, initiated by the International Organization for the Study of IBD (IOIBD), published initial guidelines (STRIDE) targeting clinical (with specific patient-reported-outcome goals for CD and UC) and endoscopic remission, with biomarkers as only an adjunct.[107] However, after the findings of the CALM study revealed the importance of biomarkers as a stepping stone to endoscopic remission, this guideline was reconsidered, and an updated (STRIDE-II) consensus statement was recently published which incorporated biomarkers, CRP and FC, as intermediate, short-term goals (**Box 2**).[108] There is now a progression from clinical to biomarker to endoscopic remission/restoration of growth with reconsideration of therapy at each successive level of remission if the target is not attained.

Box 2
Summarization of STRIDE-II

- **Immediate Treatment Target:**
  - Clinical Response
    - CD: Decrease in PCDAI≥12.5 and in wPCDAI≥17.5 points
    - UC: Decrease in PUCAI≥20 points
      Mean weeks until target vary by medication, ranging from 2 to 11 weeks in both CD and UC.

- **Intermediate Treatment Targets:**
  - Clinical Remission
    - CD: PCDAI less than 10 or less than 7.5 if height excluded; wPCDAI less than 12.5 points
    - UC: PUCAI less than 10
      Mean weeks until target vary by medication, ranging from 2 to 17 weeks in CD and 2 to 15 weeks in UC.
  - Normalization of Biomarkers
    - Normalization of CRP
    - Fecal Calprotectin less than 100 to 250 ug/g
      Mean weeks until target vary by medication, ranging from 5 to 17 weeks in CD and 5 to 15 weeks in UC.

- **Long Term Targets:**
  - Endoscopic Healing
    - CD: SES-CD less than 3 or SES-CD ulceration subscore = 0
    - UC: Mayo = 0 or UCEIS≤1
  - Restoration of Normal Growth
    Mean weeks until target vary by medication, ranging from 13 to 24 weeks in CD and 11 to 20 weeks in UC.

- **Aspirational Targets:**
  Not current targets of therapy, but can be used to determine depth of remission, which may speak to durability of remission.
  - Histologic remission
  - Transmural healing

Abbreviations: PCDAI, Pediatric Crohn's Disease Activity Index; PUCAI, Pediatric Ulcerative Colitis Activity Index; wPCDAI, weighted PCDAI; SES-CD, Simple Endoscopic Score for Crohn Disease; UCEIS, Ulcerative Colitis Endoscopic Index of Severity.

There are moreover two emerging targets of therapy beyond endoscopic remission: histologic remission and transmural healing. There is evolving evidence that these targets may lead to improved long-term outcomes and, perhaps, in conjunction with the incorporation of novel biomarkers, allow for target achievement in a definitive majority of patients with IBD, unlike CALM. Presently, however, there remains debate if these two targets lead to sufficient gains to offset the burdens and risks of the therapeutics used to achieve them.[108]

Notably, ultrasound of the small and large bowel, which allows for noninvasive and inexpensive evaluation of a number of measures of transmural inflammation (eg bowel wall thickness, doppler signal, and wall layer stratification), was explored in the STRIDE-II consensus as an important developing modality for target assessment.[108] Intestinal ultrasound has already proven to be a successful tool for monitoring disease activity in both CD and UC with the unique benefit of being a real-time assessment in clinic.[109,110] In a serial, tight control strategy, a transmural assessment like ultrasound that is, both quick and inexpensive to perform is ideal.

On achieving target goals, it has been proposed that patients continue to be monitored serially every 3 to 6 months with clinical assessment and noninvasive biomarkers or point-of-care ultrasound as part of a tight control maintenance strategy. Importantly, FC has been shown to rise approximately 3 months before clinical relapse, making it a useful predictive biomarker even during remission.[111] Combining TDM and FC is particularly useful to assess for a possible pharmacokinetic cause of relapse, and this may be of special importance in pediatrics where periods of growth may affect drug pharmacokinetics.[95,112] Additionally, many of the precision techniques previously mentioned have potential to serve as superior targets compared with FC or CRP for purposes of serial monitoring.

Finally, to take a step beyond STRIDE goals, the IOIBD group noted that the ultimate goal of IBD care is not necessarily to achieve remission in the eyes of the clinician but rather to minimize the impact of IBD on a patient's life. While these two goals are often aligned, they are distinctly different concepts. Within rheumatology, Outcome Measures in Rheumatology (OMERACT) clearly defined outcome measures aimed at altering the disease course. IOIBD set out to create similar goals for IBD and recently published these recommendations from the groundbreaking SPIRIT initiative. These set disease modification goals, which should be incorporated into trials in IBD. These goals range from improving quality of life and minimizing disability to reducing complications such as bowel wall damage, surgery, hospitalization, disease extension in UC, EIM, dysplasia/cancer, and mortality. By placing an emphasis on achieving these end points that are truly meaningful to the patient, it may be possible to alter the current natural history of IBD.[113]

EMR-Embedded Dashboards and Machine Learning Approaches

TDM, T2T, and tight control strategies are not frictionless endeavors, they require quite a bit of buy-in and effort on the part of both patient and provider, which may hamper their universal implementation. For TDM, PK dashboards embedded in the EMR can take prepopulated clinical and laboratory characteristics and suggest changes to optimize dosing strategies.[99,100] Wearable devices are also being studied and may be incorporated into monitoring strategies, requiring no input from the patient and with associated artificial intelligence to minimize the noise for ease of physician or advanced practice provider interpretation.[114,115] Machine learning approaches could also work in real time to incorporate and refine monitoring by providing a method to interpret and clinically apply an increasing number of multi'omic and clinical inputs.

PREVENTION
Identification of Children at High-Risk to Develop IBD

The PREDICTS study, which examined prediagnosis sera from patients who developed CD in the US Department of Defense Serum Repository, found serologic antimicrobial antibodies in 65% of samples at the earliest prediagnosis time point (Median: 6 years; IQR: 5.6–8.2 years), indicating a possible role for serologies in the identification of high-risk individuals in whom to consider preventative strategies.[116] The Genetic, Environmental, Microbial (GEM) Study has been following family members of patients with IBD who carry a higher risk for IBD to identify the changes that occur prior to development of overt disease. They have identified increased intestinal permeability within family members who later go on to develop IBD; this permeability may explain the development of antimicrobial antibodies seen in PREDICTS.[117] Another cohort of very large families with multiple first-degree relatives with IBD has shown that serologic markers, GRS, degree of dysbiosis, and FC can be combined to predict IBD status.[118] Preventative measures could potentially be developed if identification of those at risk was improved through validation of these multi'omic scoring methods;

currently, the main, potentially modifiable preventative measures identified on a recent meta-analysis are breastfeeding and the avoidance of passive smoke exposure and unnecessary antibiotics.[119]

SUMMARY

Advances in technology and drug development have made PM possible and also necessary. The rise of PM heralds a new age for patients with IBD as we start to see cracks in the therapeutic ceiling that has constrained us from the initial introduction of IFX over 20 years ago. Continuing improvements in "-omic" technologies, generation of larger, diverse data sets, incorporation of big data methodologies, and ever-more-refined machine learning approaches will continue to push the field forward as we learn to incorporate these findings into clinical practice in a streamlined way using CDST and EMR integration.

CLINICS CARE POINTS

- Use of clinical characteristics and biomarkers associated with poor prognosis can help guide the choice of the most appropriate early effective intervention.
- A treat-to-target strategy is recommended to optimize management and outcomes of patients with pediatric IBD (see **Box 2**).
- Use of therapeutic drug monitoring is recommended with both thiopurine and biologic therapies.
- Genetic variants can help inform treatment selection and risk of adverse events (eg, variants in TMPT and NUDT15 can warn of an increased risk of severe leukopenia).

REFERENCES

1. Kaplan GG, Windsor JW. The four epidemiological stages in the global evolution of inflammatory bowel disease. Nat Rev Gastroenterol Hepatol 2021;18(1): 56–66.
2. Baldassano RN, Piccoli DA. Inflammatory bowel disease in pediatric and adolescent patients. Gastroenterol Clin North Am 1999;28(2):445–58.
3. Benchimol EI, Bernstein CN, Bitton A, et al. Trends in epidemiology of pediatric inflammatory bowel disease in Canada: distributed network analysis of multiple population-based provincial health administrative databases. Am J Gastroenterol 2017;112(7):1120–34.
4. Nguyen GC, Targownik LE, Singh H, et al. The impact of inflammatory bowel disease in Canada 2018: IBD in seniors. J Can Assoc Gastroenterol 2019;2(Suppl 1):S68–72.
5. Kotze PG, Underwood FE, Damião A, et al. Progression of inflammatory bowel diseases throughout Latin America and the Caribbean: a systematic review. Clin Gastroenterol Hepatol 2020;18(2):304–12.
6. Mokhtar NM, Nawawi KNM, Verasingam J, et al. A four-decade analysis of the incidence trends, sociodemographic and clinical characteristics of inflammatory bowel disease patients at single tertiary centre, Kuala Lumpur, Malaysia. BMC Public Health 2019;19(Suppl 4):550.
7. Denson LA, Curran M, McGovern DPB, et al. Challenges in IBD research: precision medicine. Inflamm Bowel Dis 2019;25(Suppl 2):S31–9.

8. Alsoud D, Verstockt B, Fiocchi C, et al. Breaking the therapeutic ceiling in drug development in ulcerative colitis. Lancet Gastroenterol Hepatol 2021;6(7): 589–95.

9. Hyams J, Crandall W, Kugathasan S, et al. Induction and maintenance infliximab therapy for the treatment of moderate-to-severe Crohn's disease in children. Gastroenterology 2007;132(3):863–73, quiz 1165–1166.

10. Ruemmele FM, Lachaux A, Cézard JP, et al. Efficacy of infliximab in pediatric Crohn's disease: a randomized multicenter open-label trial comparing scheduled to on demand maintenance therapy. Inflamm Bowel Dis 2009;15(3): 388–94.

11. Hyams JS, Griffiths A, Markowitz J, et al. Safety and efficacy of adalimumab for moderate to severe Crohn's disease in children. Gastroenterology 2012;143(2): 365–74.e362.

12. Jossen J, Kiernan BD, Pittman N, et al. Anti-tumor necrosis factor-alpha exposure impacts vedolizumab mucosal healing rates in pediatric inflammatory bowel disease. J Pediatr Gastroenterol Nutr 2020;70(3):304–9.

13. Colombel JF, Narula N, Peyrin-Biroulet L. Management strategies to improve outcomes of patients with inflammatory bowel diseases. Gastroenterology 2017;152(2):351–61.e355.

14. Oussalah A, Evesque L, Laharie D, et al. A multicenter experience with infliximab for ulcerative colitis: outcomes and predictors of response, optimization, colectomy, and hospitalization. Am J Gastroenterol 2010;105(12):2617–25.

15. Gordon IO, Agrawal N, Willis E, et al. Fibrosis in ulcerative colitis is directly linked to severity and chronicity of mucosal inflammation. Aliment Pharmacol Ther 2018;47(7):922–39.

16. Le Berre C, Ananthakrishnan AN, Danese S, et al. Ulcerative colitis and Crohn's disease have similar burden and goals for treatment. Clin Gastroenterol Hepatol 2020;18(1):14–23.

17. El-Matary W, Bernstein CN. Cancer risk in pediatric-onset inflammatory bowel disease. Front Pediatr 2020;8:400.

18. Sartor RB. Mechanisms of disease: pathogenesis of Crohn's disease and ulcerative colitis. Nat Clin Pract Gastroenterol Hepatol 2006;3(7):390–407.

19. Gettler K, Levantovsky R, Moscati A, et al. Common and rare variant prediction and penetrance of IBD in a large, multi-ethnic, health system-based biobank cohort. Gastroenterology 2021;160(5):1546–57.

20. Torres J. Prediction of inflammatory bowel disease: a step closer? Gastroenterology 2020;158(1):278–9.

21. Birimberg-Schwartz L, Zucker DM, Akriv A, et al. Development and validation of diagnostic criteria for IBD subtypes including IBD-unclassified in children: a multicentre study from the pediatric IBD porto group of ESPGHAN. J Crohns Colitis 2017;11(9):1078–84.

22. Bousvaros A, Antonioli DA, Colletti RB, et al. Differentiating ulcerative colitis from Crohn disease in children and young adults: report of a working group of the North American Society for Pediatric Gastroenterology, Hepatology, and Nutrition and the Crohn's and Colitis Foundation of America. J Pediatr Gastroenterol Nutr 2007;44(5):653–74.

23. Levine A, Koletzko S, Turner D, et al. ESPGHAN revised porto criteria for the diagnosis of inflammatory bowel disease in children and adolescents. J Pediatr Gastroenterol Nutr 2014;58(6):795–806.

24. Isene R, Bernklev T, Høie O, et al. Extraintestinal manifestations in Crohn's disease and ulcerative colitis: results from a prospective, population-based European inception cohort. Scand J Gastroenterol 2015;50(3):300–5.

25. Danese S, Fiorino G, Peyrin-Biroulet L. Early intervention in Crohn's disease: towards disease modification trials. Gut 2017;66(12):2179–87.

26. Ricciuto A, Aardoom M, Orlanski-Meyer E, et al. Predicting outcomes in pediatric Crohn's disease for management optimization: systematic review and consensus statements from the pediatric inflammatory bowel disease-ahead program. Gastroenterology 2021;160(1):403–36.e426.

27. Spencer EA, Jarchin L, Rolfes P, et al. Su499 Long-term outcomes after primary ileocolic resection in pediatric crohn's disease in the biologic era: a single-center experience. Gastroenterology 2021;160(6). S-717.

28. Siegel CA, Whitman CB, Spiegel BMR, et al. Development of an index to define overall disease severity in IBD. Gut 2018;67(2):244–54.

29. Pepys MB, Hirschfield GM. C-reactive protein: a critical update. J Clin Invest 2003;111(12):1805–12.

30. Hyams JS, Davis Thomas S, Gotman N, et al. Clinical and biological predictors of response to standardised paediatric colitis therapy (PROTECT): a multicentre inception cohort study. Lancet 2019;393(10182):1708–20.

31. Dubinsky MC, Kugathasan S, Mei L, et al. Increased immune reactivity predicts aggressive complicating Crohn's disease in children. Clin Gastroenterol Hepatol 2008;6(10):1105–11.

32. Dubinsky MC. Serologic and laboratory markers in prediction of the disease course in inflammatory bowel disease. World J Gastroenterol 2010;16(21):2604–8.

33. Olbjørn C, Cvancarova Småstuen M, Thiis-Evensen E, et al. Serological markers in diagnosis of pediatric inflammatory bowel disease and as predictors for early tumor necrosis factor blocker therapy. Scand J Gastroenterol 2017;52(4):414–9.

34. Kugathasan S, Denson LA, Walters TD, et al. Prediction of complicated disease course for children newly diagnosed with Crohn's disease: a multicentre inception cohort study. Lancet 2017;389(10080):1710–8.

35. Elizabeth A, Spencer M, Sonia M, et al. Serologic reactivity reflects clinical expression of ulcerative colitis in children. IBD 2018;24(6):1335–43.

36. Fleshner PR, Vasiliauskas EA, Kam LY, et al. High level perinuclear antineutrophil cytoplasmic antibody (pANCA) in ulcerative colitis patients before colectomy predicts the development of chronic pouchitis after ileal pouch-anal anastomosis. Gut 2001;49(5):671–7.

37. Adler J, Rangwalla SC, Dwamena BA, et al. The prognostic power of the NOD2 genotype for complicated Crohn's disease: a meta-analysis. Am J Gastroenterol 2011;106(4):699–712.

38. Cleynen I, Boucher G, Jostins L, et al. Inherited determinants of Crohn's disease and ulcerative colitis phenotypes: a genetic association study. Lancet 2016;387(10014):156–67.

39. Lee JC. Genome-wide association study identifies distinct genetic contributions to prognosis and susceptibility in Crohn's disease. Nat Genet 2017;49(2):262–8.

40. Ahmad T, Armuzzi A, Neville M, et al. The contribution of human leucocyte antigen complex genes to disease phenotype in ulcerative colitis. Tissue Antigens 2003;62(6):527–35.

41. Roussomoustakaki M, Satsangi J, Welsh K, et al. Genetic markers may predict disease behavior in patients with ulcerative colitis. Gastroenterology 1997;112(6):1845–53.

42. Ungaro RC, Hu L, Ji J, et al. Machine learning identifies novel blood protein predictors of penetrating and stricturing complications in newly diagnosed paediatric Crohn's disease. Aliment Pharmacol Ther 2021;53(2):281–90.

43. Ballengee CR, Stidham RW, Liu C, et al. Association between plasma level of collagen type III alpha 1 chain and development of strictures in pediatric patients with Crohn's disease. Clin Gastroenterol Hepatol 2019;17(9):1799–806.

44. D'Haens G, Kelly O, Battat R, et al. Development and validation of a test to monitor endoscopic activity in patients with Crohn's disease based on serum levels of proteins. Gastroenterology 2020;158(3):515–26.e510.

45. Holmer A, Boland B, Singh S, et al. P302 Diagnostic accuracy of a serum-based biomarker panel for endoscopic activity in ulcerative colitis. J Crohns Colitis 2020;14(Supplement_1):S304.

46. Marigorta UM, Denson LA, Hyams JS, et al. Transcriptional risk scores link GWAS to eQTLs and predict complications in Crohn's disease. Nat Genet 2017;49(10):1517–21.

47. Biasci D, Lee JC, Noor NM, et al. A blood-based prognostic biomarker in IBD. Gut 2019;68(8):1386–95.

48. Parkes M, Noor NM, Dowling F, et al. PRedicting Outcomes For Crohn's dIsease using a moLecular biomarkEr (PROFILE): protocol for a multicentre, randomised, biomarker-stratified trial. BMJ open 2018;8(12):e026767.

49. Rosen MJ, Karns R, Vallance JE, et al. Mucosal expression of type 2 and type 17 immune response genes distinguishes ulcerative Colitis from colon-only Crohn's disease in treatment-naive pediatric patients. Gastroenterology 2017;152(6): 1345–57.e1347.

50. Haberman Y, Tickle TL, Dexheimer PJ, et al. Pediatric Crohn disease patients exhibit specific ileal transcriptome and microbiome signature. J Clin Invest 2014;124(8):3617–33.

51. Sartor RB, Wu GD. Roles for intestinal bacteria, viruses, and fungi in pathogenesis of inflammatory bowel diseases and therapeutic approaches. Gastroenterology 2017;152(2):327–39.e324.

52. Franzosa EA, Sirota-Madi A, Avila-Pacheco J, et al. Gut microbiome structure and metabolic activity in inflammatory bowel disease. Nat Microbiol 2019;4(2): 293–305.

53. Olbjørn C, Cvancarova Småstuen M, Thiis-Evensen E, et al. Fecal microbiota profiles in treatment-naïve pediatric inflammatory bowel disease - associations with disease phenotype, treatment, and outcome. Clin Exp Gastroenterol 2019;12:37–49.

54. Zhu W, Winter MG, Byndloss MX, et al. Precision editing of the gut microbiota ameliorates colitis. Nature 2018;553(7687):208–11.

55. Siegel CA, Horton H, Siegel LS, et al. A validated web-based tool to display individualised Crohn's disease predicted outcomes based on clinical, serologic and genetic variables. Aliment Pharmacol Ther 2016;43(2):262–71.

56. Dulai PS, Singh S, Casteele NV, et al. Development and validation of clinical scoring tool to predict outcomes of treatment with vedolizumab in patients with ulcerative colitis. Clin Gastroenterol Hepatol 2020;18(13):2952–61, e2958.

57. Agrawal M, Spencer EA, Colombel JF, et al. Approach to the management of recently diagnosed inflammatory bowel disease patients: a user's guide for adult and pediatric gastroenterologists. Gastroenterology 2021;161(1):47–65.

58. Biemans VBC, van der Woude CJ, Dijkstra G, et al. Ustekinumab is associated with superior effectiveness outcomes compared to vedolizumab in Crohn's

disease patients with prior failure to anti-TNF treatment. Aliment Pharmacol Ther 2020;52(1):123–34.

59. West NR, Hegazy AN, Owens BMJ, et al. Oncostatin M drives intestinal inflammation and predicts response to tumor necrosis factor-neutralizing therapy in patients with inflammatory bowel disease. Nat Med 2017;23(5):579–89.

60. Verstockt B, Verstockt S, Dehairs J, et al. Low TREM1 expression in whole blood predicts anti-TNF response in inflammatory bowel disease. EBioMedicine 2019; 40:733–42.

61. Gaujoux R, Starosvetsky E, Maimon N, et al. Cell-centred meta-analysis reveals baseline predictors of anti-TNFα non-response in biopsy and blood of patients with IBD. Gut 2019;68(4):604–14.

62. Martin JC, Chang C, Boschetti G, et al. Single-cell analysis of crohn's disease lesions identifies a pathogenic cellular module associated with resistance to anti-TNF therapy. Cell 2019;178(6):1493–508.e1420.

63. Kim EM, Randall C, Betancourt R, et al. Mucosal eosinophilia is an independent predictor of vedolizumab efficacy in inflammatory bowel diseases. Inflamm Bowel Dis 2020;26(8):1232–8.

64. Uzzan M, Tokuyama M, Rosenstein AK, et al. Anti-alpha4beta7 therapy targets lymphoid aggregates in the gastrointestinal tract of HIV-1-infected individuals. Sci Transl Med 2018;10(461):eaau4711.

65. Ananthakrishnan AN, Luo C, Yajnik V, et al. Gut Microbiome Function Predicts Response to Anti-integrin Biologic Therapy in Inflammatory Bowel Diseases. Cell host & microbe 2017;21(5):603–10, e603.

66. Vermeire S, O'Byrne S, Keir M, et al. Etrolizumab as induction therapy for ulcerative colitis: a randomised, controlled, phase 2 trial. Lancet 2014;384(9940): 309–18.

67. Sands BE, Chen J, Feagan BG, et al. Efficacy and safety of MEDI2070, an antibody against interleukin 23, in patients with moderate to severe Crohn's disease: A Phase 2a study. Gastroenterology 2017;153(1):77–86, e76.

68. Faubion WA Jr, Fletcher JG, O'Byrne S, et al. EMerging BiomARKers in Inflammatory Bowel Disease (EMBARK) study identifies fecal calprotectin, serum MMP9, and serum IL-22 as a novel combination of biomarkers for Crohn's disease activity: role of cross-sectional imaging. Am J Gastroenterol 2013; 108(12):1891–900.

69. Hemminki K, Li X, Sundquist K, et al. Familial association of inflammatory bowel diseases with other autoimmune and related diseases. Am J Gastroenterol 2010;105(1):139–47.

70. Fu Y, Lee CH, Chi CC. Association of psoriasis with inflammatory bowel disease: a systematic review and meta-analysis. JAMA Dermatol 2018;154(12):1417–23.

71. Sandborn WJ, Gasink C, Gao LL, et al. Ustekinumab induction and maintenance therapy in refractory Crohn's disease. N Engl J Med 2012;367(16):1519–28.

72. Sands BE, Sandborn WJ, Panaccione R, et al. Ustekinumab as induction and maintenance therapy for ulcerative colitis. New Eng J Med 2019;381(13): 1201–14.

73. Farhi D. Ustekinumab for the treatment of psoriasis: review of three multicenter clinical trials. Drugs Today (Barc) 2010;46(4):259–64.

74. Vande Casteele N, Jairath V, Jeyarajah J, et al. Development and validation of a clinical decision support tool that incorporates pharmacokinetic data to predict endoscopic healing in patients treated with infliximab. Clin Gastroenterol Hepatol 2020;19(6). 1209–1217.e2.

75. Dulai PS, Boland BS, Singh S, et al. Development and validation of a scoring system to predict outcomes of vedolizumab treatment in patients with Crohn's disease. Gastroenterology 2018;155(3):687–95.e610.

76. Dulai PS, Singh S, Casteele NV, et al. Development and validation of clinical scoring tool to predict outcomes of treatment with vedolizumab in patients with ulcerative colitis. Clin Gastroenterol Hepatol 2020;18(13). 2952–2961.e8.

77. Hyams JS, Davis S, Mack DR, et al. Factors associated with early outcomes following standardised therapy in children with ulcerative colitis (PROTECT): a multicentre inception cohort study. Lancet Gastroenterol Hepatol 2017;2(12): 855–68.

78. Verstockt B, Sudahakar P, Creyns B, et al. DOP70 An integrated multi-omics biomarker predicting endoscopic response in ustekinumab treated patients with Crohn's disease. J Crohns Colitis 2019;13(Supplement_1):S072–3.

79. Administration UFaD. Approved drug products with therapeutic equivalence evaluations (Orange Book). Available at: https://www.fda.gov/Drugs/ InformationOnDrugs/ucm129662.htm. Accessed May 19, 2019.

80. Weinshilboum RM, Sladek SL. Mercaptopurine pharmacogenetics: monogenic inheritance of erythrocyte thiopurine methyltransferase activity. Am J Hum Genet 1980;32(5):651–62.

81. Dubinsky MC, Lamothe S, Yang HY, et al. Pharmacogenomics and metabolite measurement for 6-mercaptopurine therapy in inflammatory bowel disease. Gastroenterology 2000;118(4):705–13.

82. Coenen MJ, de Jong DJ, van Marrewijk CJ, et al. Identification of patients with variants in TPMT and dose reduction reduces hematologic events during thiopurine treatment of inflammatory bowel disease. Gastroenterology 2015; 149(4):907–17.e907.

83. Walker GJ, Harrison JW, Heap GA, et al. Association of genetic variants in NUDT15 with thiopurine-induced myelosuppression in patients with inflammatory Bowel disease. JAMA 2019;321(8):773–85.

84. Sazonovs A, Kennedy NA, Moutsianas L, et al. HLA-DQA1*05 carriage associated with development of anti-drug antibodies to infliximab and adalimumab in patients with Crohn's disease. Gastroenterology 2020;158(1):189–99.

85. Powell Doherty RD, Liao H, Satsangi JJ, et al. Extended analysis identifies drug-specific association of 2 distinct HLA class ii haplotypes for development of immunogenicity to adalimumab and infliximab. Gastroenterology 2020;159(2): 784–7.

86. Heap GA, Weedon MN, Bewshea CM, et al. HLA-DQA1-HLA-DRB1 variants confer susceptibility to pancreatitis induced by thiopurine immunosuppressants. Nat Genet 2014;46(10):1131–4.

87. Wilson A, Jansen LE, Rose RV, et al. HLA-DQA1-HLA-DRB1 polymorphism is a major predictor of azathioprine-induced pancreatitis in patients with inflammatory bowel disease. Aliment Pharmacol Ther 2018;47(5):615–20.

88. Bucalo A, Rega F, Zangrilli A, et al. Paradoxical Psoriasis Induced by Anti-TNFα Treatment: Evaluation of Disease-Specific Clinical and Genetic Markers. Int J Mol Sci 2020;21(21):7873.

89. Feuerstein JD, Nguyen GC, Kupfer SS, et al. American gastroenterological association institute guideline on therapeutic drug monitoring in inflammatory bowel disease. Gastroenterology 2017;153(3):827–34.

90. Papamichael K, Cheifetz AS, Melmed GY, et al. Appropriate therapeutic drug monitoring of biologic agents for patients with inflammatory bowel diseases. Clin Gastroenterol Hepatol 2019;17(9):1655–68.e1653.

91. Group B. Which biologic drug is your patient on? 2018. 2020. Available at: https://www.bridgeibd.com/biologic-therapy-optimizer. Accessed September 1, 2020.

92. Lega S, Dubinsky MC. What are the targets of inflammatory bowel disease management. Inflamm Bowel Dis 2018;24(8):1670–5.

93. Vande Casteele N, Ferrante M, Van Assche G, et al. Trough concentrations of infliximab guide dosing for patients with inflammatory bowel disease. Gastroenterology 2015;148(7):1320–9.e1323.

94. D'Haens G, Vermeire S, Lambrecht G, et al. Increasing infliximab dose based on symptoms, biomarkers, and serum drug concentrations does not increase clinical, endoscopic, or corticosteroid-free remission in patients with active luminal Crohn's disease. Gastroenterology 2018;154(5). 1343–1351.e1.

95. Dreesen E, Baert F, Laharie D, et al. Monitoring a combination of calprotectin and infliximab identifies patients with mucosal healing of Crohn's disease. Clin Gastroenterol Hepatol 2020;18(3):637–46.e611.

96. Assa A, Matar M, Turner D, et al. OP18 Proactive adalimumab trough measurements increase corticosteroid-free clinical remission in paediatric patients with Crohn's disease: the paediatric Crohn's disease adalimumab-level-based optimisation treatment (PAILOT) trial. J Crohns Colitis 2019;13(Supplement_1): S012–3.

97. Velayos FS, Kahn JG, Sandborn WJ, et al. A test-based strategy is more cost effective than empiric dose escalation for patients with Crohn's disease who lose responsiveness to infliximab. Clin Gastroenterol Hepatol 2013;11(6): 654–66.

98. Guidi L, Pugliese D, Tonucci TP, et al. Therapeutic drug monitoring is more cost-effective than a clinically based approach in the management of loss of response to infliximab in inflammatory bowel disease: an observational multicentre study. J Crohns Colitis 2018;12(9):1079–88.

99. Dubinsky M, Phan B, Tse S, et al. 240 real-world application of an adaptive dosing dashboard reveals accelerated induction dosing of infliximab is necessary in most IBD patients and improves therapuetic outcomes. Gastroenterology 2020;158. S-47.

100. Xiong Y, Mizuno T, Colman R, et al. Real-world infliximab pharmacokinetic study informs an electronic health record-embedded dashboard to guide precision dosing in children with Crohn's disease. Clin Pharmacol Ther 2020;109(6): 1639–47.

101. Strik AS, Löwenberg M, Mould DR, et al. Efficacy of dashboard driven dosing of infliximab in inflammatory bowel disease patients; a randomized controlled trial. Scand J Gastroenterol 2021;56(2):145–54.

102. Clarkston K, Tsai YT, Jackson K, et al. Development of infliximab target concentrations during induction in pediatric Crohn disease patients. J Pediatr Gastroenterol Nutr 2019;69(1):68–74.

103. Walters TD, Kim MO, Denson LA, et al. Increased effectiveness of early therapy with anti-tumor necrosis factor-α vs an immunomodulator in children with Crohn's disease. Gastroenterology 2014;146(2):383–91.

104. Jongsma MME, Aardoom MA, Cozijnsen MA, et al. First-line treatment with infliximab versus conventional treatment in children with newly diagnosed moderate-to-severe Crohn's disease: an open-label multicentre randomised controlled trial. Gut 2020. https://doi.org/10.1136/gutjnl-2020-322339. gutjnl-2020-322339.

105. Colombel J-F, Panaccione R, Bossuyt P, et al. Effect of tight control management on Crohn's disease (CALM): a multicentre, randomised, controlled phase 3 trial. The Lancet 2017;390(10114):2779–89.

106. Ungaro RC, Yzet C, Bossuyt P, et al. Deep remission at 1 year prevents progression of early Crohn's disease. Gastroenterology 2020;159(1):139–47.

107. Peyrin-Biroulet L, Sandborn W, Sands BE, et al. Selecting Therapeutic Targets in Inflammatory Bowel Disease (STRIDE): determining therapeutic goals for treat-to-target. Am J Gastroenterol 2015;110(9):1324–38.

108. Turner D, Ricciuto A, Lewis A, et al. STRIDE-II: an update on the Selecting Therapeutic Targets in Inflammatory Bowel Disease (STRIDE) Initiative of the International Organization for the Study of IBD (IOIBD): determining therapeutic goals for treat-to-target strategies in IBD. Gastroenterology 2020;160(5):1570–83.

109. Maaser C, Petersen F, Helwig U, et al. Intestinal ultrasound for monitoring therapeutic response in patients with ulcerative colitis: results from the TRUST&UC study. Gut 2020;69(9):1629–36.

110. Kucharzik T, Wittig BM, Helwig U, et al. Use of intestinal ultrasound to monitor Crohn's disease activity. Clin Gastroenterol Hepatol 2017;15(4):535–42, e532.

111. Mao R, Xiao YL, Gao X, et al. Fecal calprotectin in predicting relapse of inflammatory bowel diseases: a meta-analysis of prospective studies. Inflamm Bowel Dis 2012;18(10):1894–9.

112. Ordas I, Feagan BG, Sandborn WJ. Therapeutic drug monitoring of tumor necrosis factor antagonists in inflammatory bowel disease. Clin Gastroenterol Hepatol 2012;10(10):1079–87, quiz e1085–e1076.

113. Le Berre C, Peyrin-Biroulet L. Selecting end points for disease-modification trials in inflammatory bowel disease: the SPIRIT consensus from the IOIBD. Gastroenterology 2021;160(5):1452–60.e1421.

114. Ruffle JK, Farmer AD, Aziz Q. Artificial intelligence-assisted gastroenterology-promises and pitfalls. Am J Gastroenterol 2019;114(3):422–8.

115. Wiestler M, Kockelmann F, Kück M, et al. Quality of life is associated with wearable-based physical activity in patients with inflammatory bowel disease: a prospective, observational study. Clin Transl Gastroenterol 2019;10(11): e00094.

116. Choung RS, Princen F, Stockfisch TP, et al. Serologic microbial associated markers can predict Crohn's disease behaviour years before disease diagnosis. Aliment Pharmacol Ther 2016;43(12):1300–10.

117. Turpin W, Lee SH, Raygoza Garay JA, et al. Increased intestinal permeability is associated with later development of Crohn's disease. Gastroenterology 2020; 159(6). 2092–2100.e5.

118. Jacobs JP, Spencer EA, Gettler K, et al. Sa473 risk profiling of unaffected members of families with a history of IBD using serology score, dysbiosis score, polygenic risk score, and fecal calprotectin. Gastroenterology 2021;160(6): S-511-S-512.

119. Agrawal M, Sabino J, Frias-Gomes C, et al. Early life exposures and the risk of inflammatory bowel disease: systematic review and meta-analyses. EClinicalMedicine 2021;36:100884.

Medical Management of Eosinophilic Esophagitis in Pediatric Patients

Melanie A. Ruffner, MD, PhD[a], Linola Juste, BS[b],
Amanda B. Muir, MD[b],*

KEYWORDS

- Eosinophilic esophagitis • Fibrosis • Diet therapy • Endoscopy

KEY POINTS

- Eosinophilic esophagitis is a chronic lifelong disease in which allergic inflammation of the esophagus leads to symptoms such as vomiting, feeding difficulties, dysphagia, and food impaction.
- Therapy for EoE involves medical approaches as well as dietary elimination approaches, and it is important to consider side effects of therapies as well as implications for patient quality of life.
- Decreasing inflammation with medical or dietary therapy is essential to prevent esophageal fibrosis.

INTRODUCTION

Eosinophilic esophagitis (EoE) is a chronic lifelong allergic disorder of the esophagus in which eosinophils infiltrate the esophageal mucosa. EoE was first described in the early 1990s, when 2 groups, Atwood and colleagues[1] and Straumann and colleagues,[2] described adult patients with dysphagia and eosinophilia of the esophagus. In 1995, Kelly and colleagues[3] described the first cohort of pediatric patients with EoE. These 10 children had severe reflux symptoms that were nonresponsive to antacid therapy or surgery, and esophageal eosinophilia. When placed on an exclusively elemental diet (only amino acid-based formula) all 10 children had improved symptoms and histology.

[a] Division of Allergy and Immunology, Department of Pediatrics, Children's Hospital of Philadelphia, University of Pennsylvania Perelman School of Medicine, 34th and Civic Center Boulevard, Wood Building 3rd Floor, Philadelphia, PA 19104, USA; [b] Division of Gastroenterology, Hepatology and Nutrition, Department of Pediatrics, Children's Hospital of Philadelphia, University of Pennsylvania Perelman School of Medicine, Abramson Research Center 902E, 3615 Civic Center Boulevard, Philadelphia, PA 19104, USA
* Corresponding author.
E-mail address: muira@chop.edu

Pediatr Clin N Am 68 (2021) 1191–1204
https://doi.org/10.1016/j.pcl.2021.07.014
0031-3955/21/© 2021 Elsevier Inc. All rights reserved.
pediatric.theclinics.com

Since that time there have been multiple iterations of guidelines and diagnostic criteria.[4–6] However, despite this, there is still no US Food and Drug Administration (FDA)-approved medication for EoE. This lack of medication has led to great variability in practice patterns among pediatricians.[7] Here, we provide a focused review of the pathophysiology and diagnostic criteria of EoE to provide a framework to discuss current medical and dietary approaches for EoE treatment. In this review, we stress the importance of a shared decision-making approach with patients and their families.[8]

EoE is characterized by eosinophil infiltration of the esophagus; however, the disease features mixed immune cell mucosal infiltrate that causes epithelial disruption and fibrosis.[9–11] It is thought that exposure to a food and/or environmental allergen causes infiltration of T helper 2 (Th2)-type lymphocytes, mast cells, basophils, and eosinophils to the esophageal mucosa. Th2 cytokines (interleukin [IL]-4, IL-5, and IL-13) cause loss of barrier function of the esophageal epithelium with dilated intercellular spaces as well as basal cell hyperplasia.[12,13] Furthermore, these cytokines trigger eotaxin-3 expression from the esophageal epithelium, which acts as the major chemoattractant for eosinophils[14] causing granulocyte recruitment and ongoing mucosal damage. Unchecked inflammation over time leads to esophageal fibrosis and narrowing with esophageal narrowing, recurrent food impaction, and stricture as the most severe consequences of the inflammation.[15] Halting inflammation is the best means for reducing dysphagia and swallowing dysfunction.

Several types of studies have demonstrated that there are genetic risks associated with EoE pathogenesis consistent with a multifactorial, complex inheritance. The risk of EoE is increased in persons with first-degree relatives, and the risk of inheritance of EoE and monozygotic twins is increased at 40% compared with the background population.[16] Genome-wide association studies (GWAS) of EoE cohorts have identified several candidate risk loci.[17] Studies identified *CAPN14* variants, which are associated with upregulation of the esophageal epithelial protease calpain 14, which results in loss of desmoglein integrity and poor epithelial barrier function. *TSLP, c11orf30,* and *STAT6* variants were identified,[18,19] which have also been reported in GWAS of patients with asthma and IgE-mediated food allergy, and may represent some common overlap in susceptibility of patients between these atopic disorders. In regard to environmental exposures that may play a role in the development of EoE, epidemiologic studies point to several potential exposures tied to increased risk, including: aeroallergens, cesarean delivery, prematurity, antibiotics, and formula feeding.[20]

PREVALENCE

EoE is now one of the most common causes of dysphagia and is increasingly recognized worldwide. The prevalence and incidence have rapidly increased to as many as 1 case per 1000 people and up to 12.8 per 100,000 new cases per year.[21] EoE is diagnosed in approximately one-half of all patients with food impaction[22] and is one of the most common causes of dysphagia.[23,24]

PATIENT EVALUATION OVERVIEW

Symptoms of EoE can be difficult to assess, especially in pediatrics where symptoms vary with the age of onset. Infants and small children are more likely to present with feeding difficulties, failure to thrive, and vomiting.[25] Older children and adolescents present with dysphagia and food impaction. Symptoms can be subtle because children develop eating strategies to cope with dysphagia. Typical behaviors include increased chewing and lubricating of foods[26] as well as avoidance of tougher-to-swallow foods. In patients with dysphagia, upper gastrointestinal series before endoscopy helps to rule out stricture or motility disorder for which a therapeutic endoscopy would be warranted.[27]

Endoscopy is a requisite for diagnosis of EoE with the most recent guidelines defining EoE as esophageal dysfunction in the setting of 15 or more eosinophils per high-powered field on endoscopic esophageal biopsy.[6] This diagnosis excludes other causes of esophageal eosinophilia including but not limited to achalasia, Crohn disease, and esophageal infections. At least 4 to 6 endoscopic biopsies from multiple levels of the esophagus should be performed in any patient in whom EoE is a possibility.[28] Adequate biopsy evaluation ensures more than 96% sensitivity in diagnosing EoE. Although furrowing, white plaques, edema (loss of vascularity), and circumferential rings are common endoscopic findings,[29] the esophagus can appear normal in approximately 20% of esophagi with EoE, underscoring the importance of adequate esophageal sampling.

APPROACH TO TREATMENT

Treatment failure rates in EoE range from 30% to 50% depending on the treatment. Because there is no therapy that induces likely remission in all patient groups, a full discussion of the pros and cons of pharmacologic versus nonpharmacologic options should be presented to all patients with a discussion of convenience/quality of life, endoscopic follow-up, and remission rates.[30] Furthermore, although the treatment modality may change, treatment is lifelong and therefore requires a long-term commitment from the patient and parent alike. Patient surveys have shown that those undergoing a shared decision-making approach to treatment were more likely to be satisfied with treatment regardless of whether it was pharmacologic or nonpharmocologic therapy.[8,30]

The therapeutic goal of EoE treatment is to achieve symptomatic and histologic remission. The main treatment options for EoE are elimination of causal foods from the diet or pharmacologic therapy with PPIs or topical corticosteroids. Regardless of the therapeutic approach, a follow-up endoscopy in 8 to 12 weeks is recommended following each change in therapy to ensure histologic remission has occurred. If patients do not achieve remission, then we recommend ongoing discussion of the therapeutic options with the patient and parents to achieve remission while respecting the patient's needs.

DIETARY TREATMENT OPTIONS

EoE was initially shown to be driven by food allergens by Kelly and colleagues[3] in the 1990s, establishing that elimination of food allergens on an elemental diet induces remission. Following this, elimination dietary strategies have been shown to be efficacious in both adult and pediatric patients.

Dietary elimination can allow for induction of EoE remission without the use of medication or consideration of medication side effects. Therefore, it is considered a first-line therapy option for many patients. However, when considering dietary therapy several considerations must be discussed fully with patients and their families. Patients with EoE may need to remove multiple food groups to achieve remission. If the patient has concomitant IgE-mediated food allergies or other GI disease requiring dietary restriction, the resultant effect can be multiple significant dietary restrictions that need to be considered. It is important to assess both the family's and patient's willingness to commit as well as potential implications on the child's quality of life if foods are removed.[31]

Dietary elimination can be costly because more expensive substitutes may be needed in lieu of less-expensive staple foods.[32] Patients may also undergo more endoscopies initially, especially if on empirical or step-up dietary approaches. Last, it is critical to consider the nutritional impacts of dietary elimination therapy. Many patients with EoE have concomitant IgE-mediated food allergies, which may also cause dietary restrictions.[33] A multidisciplinary approach involving a gastroenterologist, allergist, and nutritionist can be beneficial to help patients with EoE maximize their dietary options and ensure proper education to manage food elimination and avoid cross-contamination.

Especially in young children, it is important to evaluate their feeding behavior and oromotor skills. Young children are not developmentally able to describe esophageal symptoms and exhibit delayed oromotor skills and food refusal behaviors as a symptom of EoE. It is critical to be mindful of these behaviors while planning dietary therapy, because this can influence if a child will be able to accept substitutes for food that are eliminated from the diet. In children with severe dietary limitations or feeding difficulties, medical therapy may allow for better acquisitions of feeding skills.[34]

Elemental Diet

The initial study of an amino acid formula-based elemental diet for EoE by Kelly and colleagues[3] was validated and shown to be 96% effective at inducing remission in pediatric patients with EoE.[35,36] Based on this, amino acid-based formulas are recommended for the management of EoE over hydrolyzed milk protein therapies.[37,38] In meta-analysis across 12 studies in children and 1 in adults, the pooled efficacy of elemental diet therapy was 90.8% for inducing histologic remission.[39] This form of therapy is most likely to be effective, and if patients were to remain on this diet then there may be relatively few endoscopies. However, many patients may wish to add foods into the diet once remission is achieved, resulting in additional exposure to anesthesia. Difficulty adhering to the diet due to formula taste, degree of diet restriction, cost, and breadth of lifestyle changes required are all a concern in the implementation of this therapy and should be discussed in detail with the patient and family.

Empirical Elimination Diets

Empirical elimination diets for EoE have been designed that target a series of foods that are most likely to cause EoE based on the data derived from case series. Several variations in how this type of diet can be implemented have been studied. These approaches focus on inducing disease remission, but differ in approach. Many empirical diets are more restrictive initially, allowing sequential reintroduction of food to identify the least restrictive diet that maintains remission ("step-down" approach, **Fig. 1**). However, other strategies identify only 1 or 2 restrictions on foods initially and then "step up" the number of restrictions as needed to achieve remission (**Fig. 2**). In both approaches, the long-term goal is to achieve remission on a diet that avoids only the specific food triggers applicable to the individual patient.

Overall, the main advantage of this strategy is that it is less restrictive than an elemental diet because it still permits patients to eat many types of foods. It is recommended that patients work with a clinical nutritionist to ensure that nutritional needs are met and to help answer questions about food substitutions and choices. Especially in younger children, it is important to consider if they eat significant quantities of the foods recommended for elimination in a specific type of diet when determining if the elimination is likely to have a clinical impact. Drawbacks to these approaches include food cost and psychosocial stress associated with maintaining the diet, as well as the need for multiple endoscopies to evaluate the success of dietary intervention.

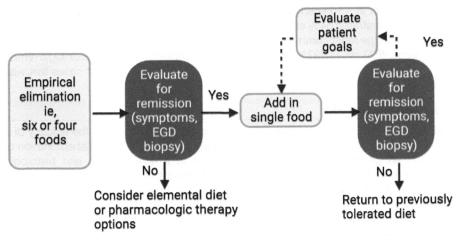

Fig. 1. Step-down approach for diet elimination therapy. EGD, esophogastroduodenoscopy.

Six-food elimination diet

The six-food elimination diet (SFED) was initially studied in children by Kagalwalla and colleagues,[40] who performed a retrospective analysis of the efficacy of a diet excluding cow's milk, soy, wheat, egg, peanut, and seafood, but allowing all other types of table food. In this study, the patients on SFED had a response rate of 74% vs 88% in those children on an elemental diet.[40] Additional studies of SFED have validated this approach in children[36,41] with rates of response ranging from 50% to 81%. Studies in adults have demonstrated similar ranges of efficacy, and meta-analysis combining results from 7 pediatric and adult studies showed a combined efficacy rate of 72.1%.[39]

However, adherence to dietary therapy that requires elimination of multiple foods is difficult, and this has raised the question of if less-restrictive diets could be efficacious for EoE treatment. Fish, shellfish, peanuts, and tree nuts have been shown to be less common triggers of esophageal inflammation than initially thought, leading to studies testing empirical diets that did not include these allergens.

Four-food elimination diet

Subsequent study of food reintroduction in children on SFED identified that the most common dietary triggers were milk, wheat, egg, and soy.[42,43] This combination of 4 foods was studied prospectively in children. This four-food elimination diet (FFED) led to symptomatic improvement in 40% of patients, with histologic response in

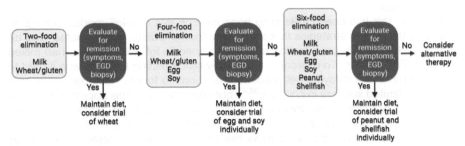

Fig. 2. Step-up approach for diet elimination therapy.

60% of patients at ≤10 eos/hpf and 47% at ≤5 eos/hpf.[44] A later prospective trial in children demonstrated 64% efficacy at inducing histologic remission,[42] and upon food reintroduction the most common food triggers inducing inflammation were cow's milk (85%), egg (35%), wheat (33%), and soy (19%). Of patients achieving histologic remission, 32% were able to reintroduce all but a single food, and in most cases this was milk.

Step-up Elimination Diet

A recent prospective study of Spanish adults and children assessed the efficacy of a combined "step-up" approach to dietary elimination in EoE.[45] The initial elimination of milk and all gluten-containing cereals resulted in a 43% clinical and histologic response rate. If patients continued to have active inflammation then therapy was stepped up to increasingly restrictive diets (4FED (4 Food Elimination Diet by eliminating milk, wheat, soy and egg) and SFED). Subsequent overall remission rates were 54% for patients following 4FED completion, and 79% after SFED completion. One strength of this approach is that it decreases the overall number of endoscopies and may shorten the time to finding a long-term diet. This study noted a relatively high dropout rate of 28% as dietary restrictions increased.

Dairy Elimination

Milk is the most common trigger of EoE, and retrospective study of pediatric patients with EoE undergoing cow's milk elimination reported histologic and clinical remission in 65%.[46] Elimination of cow's milk has been studied prospectively, ranging from 43% to 64% in histologic response rate.[47–49] A recent prospective, multisite, randomized clinical trial comparing cow's milk elimination with FFED elimination in children aged 6 to 17 years reported similar rates of histologic improvement (41% for FFED and 44% for cow's milk elimination).[50] Symptom improvement was marginally better in patients treated with FFED; however, quality of life was significantly improved in patients on cow's milk elimination. A single-site, retrospective comparison of cow's milk elimination and SFED demonstrated similar efficacy between these approaches (57% for cow's milk elimination and 52% for SFED).[51] These studies support milk elimination as the foundation for dietary therapy in EoE.

Targeted Elimination

This approach can also be called a testing-based elimination diet or directed elimination diet. As EoE is an allergen-triggered disorder, there has been great interest in determining if allergy testing can be used to determine the appropriate dietary exclusions for patients. In contrast to empirical approaches, which eliminate foods based on the presumption of their importance from population-level data, a testing-based approach would seek to tie allergens to a patient's pathophysiology before eliminating it from the diet.

However, this has been challenging because EoE is a non-IgE-mediated food allergy and the testing strategies that are helpful for immediate, IgE-mediated food allergies, including skin-prick testing and serum-specific IgE testing, have had mixed results in EoE studies. To overcome this, atopy patch testing to foods was added to attempt to evaluate delayed, cell-mediated reactions to foods. This approaches met with some limited success in children,[36,41] but difficulties with this approach included low negative predictive value for common allergens like cow's milk and lower efficacy of test-directed diet in adult populations. In recent guidelines, a total of 12 testing-based studies was pooled to examine the efficacy of several testing approaches and found that nearly half (49.5%) of all subjects did not achieve histologic remission.[38] Targeted elimination strategies are used infrequently at this time, and the cost of testing must be weighed against the low efficacy. Owing to the low predictive value of testing and high frequency of milk as a causative allergen, empirical milk elimination is still recommended even if testing for other allergens were to be used.

PHARMACOLOGIC TREATMENT OPTIONS
Proton Pump Inhibitors

Until the most recent 2018 guidelines, endoscopy while treated with a PPI was part of the diagnostic algorithm of EoE. However, because of a large amount of clinical and *in vitro* data suggesting that PPIs reduce the inflammation in EoE, PPIs are now considered a therapy for EoE. In fact, there is no difference histologically, clinically, or endoscopically in patients who have EoE responsive to PPI and those who do not,[52] and evaluation of the EoE transcriptome has revealed that treatment with PPI reverses the Th2 inflammatory signature typical of EoE inflammation[53]; this is thought to be due in large part to the ability of PPIs to reduce eotaxin-3 expression in the esophageal epithelium.[54]

Prospective evaluation of children with esophageal eosinophilia revealed high rates (up to 70%) of histologic remission on high-dose (2 mg/kg/d) esomeprazole after 8 weeks of therapy.[55] Furthermore, in a follow-up study, dose reduction to 1 mg/kg/d for 1 year after induction at high dose resulted in maintenance of histologic remission in 70% of children.[56] In a systematic review and meta-analysis of 11 pediatric studies, PPIs were found to have a 54.1% histologic and a 64.9% clinical response rate in pediatric patients with EoE.[57] Recent AGA-JTF (Joint Task Force) meta-analysis found in 23 observational studies that 42% of patients achieved remission of PPI.[38] The efficacy of PPIs compared with other therapies is unknown because most clinical trials to date have excluded subjects with EoE responsive to PPI treatment. In addition, recent concerns have emerged about a wide variety of potentially adverse events with PPI. However, best practices advice from the American Gastroenterologic Association suggests that the quality of the evidence underlying these concerns is low and the absolute increase in risk is modest.[58]

Topical Corticosteroids

Topical corticosteroid therapy involves swallowing off-label preparations of asthma medications. The most common medications used are fluticasone propionate and budesonide. The fluticasone metered-dose inhaler should be used without a spacer so that puffs are administered directly into the mouth and swallowed. For budesonide, vials that historically have been used in nebulizers are opened and mixed with 5 packets of Splenda, or 1 teaspoon of apple sauce or honey, to make a viscous suspension that is swallowed.[59] For both preparations it is essential that there be nothing to eat or drink for the 30 minutes following administration (including brushing teeth or rinsing mouth).

There have been 8 double-blind placebo-controlled studies evaluating the use of some form of topical steroids for EoE. Recent AGA-JTF review found that these preparations induced remission in about 66% of patients in a mix of pediatric and adult trials.[38] Based on these findings the JTF had a strong recommendation for topical steroids over no treatment. There have been recent phase 2 and 3 trials evaluating a standardized preparation (either liquid or tablet) of budesonide that have shown similar efficacy.[60,61]

A randomized controlled trial has shown that in adults 880 µg fluticasone twice daily has similar efficacy to budesonide 1 mg twice daily with 64% and 71% achieving histologic remission (<15 eosinophils per hpf), respectively.[62] Because of similar efficacy, patient age should be considered when prescribing and there should be a discussion about which formulation and administration style is preferable.

The major side effect of topical steroids is esophageal candidiasis. In the trial comparing budesonide with fluticasone, 12% of patients had esophageal candidiasis.[62] Randomized controlled trial evaluating budesonide oral suspension compared with placebo showed the rates of esophageal candidiasis to be 3.8% (8 subjects of 203) compared with 1.9% in the placebo arm (2 subjects of 105).[61] All cases were mild to moderate in severity. Another concern is adrenal insufficiency. Meta-analysis performed in 2017 evaluating rates of adrenal insufficiency with topical steroid use for EoE have shown that 7 randomized trials of topical steroids have shown significantly different rates of adrenal insufficiency over placebo.[63] More recent clinical trial of budesonide oral suspension demonstrated 1.4% of patients in the treatment arm compared with 0.9% of patients in the placebo arm.[61] It is important to consider other steroid preparations, because the effects of concurrent inhaled, nasal, and orally administered steroids may increase the risk of complications.[64]

INTERVENTIONAL TREATMENT: ESOPHAGEAL DILATION

Although dilation does not halt the progression of inflammation, it can improve symptoms in patients with dysphagia.[65,66] Dilation may be seen as an adjunct to therapy, because patients with better resolution of inflammation require less dilation.[67] The rates of dilations for EoE in pediatrics are not well described in the literature. There was a large retrospective review of the practice from a tertiary care center. In this review 68 dilations were performed in patients with EoE with no perforations and only minor (ie, postprocedure pain) adverse events.[68]

COMBINATION THERAPIES

If patients fail to achieve EoE remission using a single therapy, then combinations of pharmacologic and dietary approaches can be used. Although empirical elimination diets are typically prescribed without any additional medication, there is some evidence to suggest that addition of PPI treatment can improve remission rates. A recent randomized controlled trial showed higher rates of histologic remission in children on PPI+4FED (88%) versus PPI alone (45%).[69] Retrospective analyses of pediatric patients suggest that the rate of histologic remission is higher in patients on both a dairy-free diet and PPI (61%) as opposed to a dairy-free diet alone (25%).[51] This finding suggests that a proportion of patients can benefit from the combination of PPI and dietary therapy.

EVALUATION OF OUTCOME AND LONG-TERM RECOMMENDATIONS

Regardless of the type of treatment chosen, all patients require follow-up endoscopy with biopsy to assess therapeutic efficacy. In EoE, esophageal symptoms do not always correlate with active inflammation. Patients may have symptomatic improvement without histologic remission, and vice versa.[70] As histologic remission has been correlated with reduced risk of fibrosis, it is standard practice for patients to return after 8 to 12 weeks of therapy to verify histologic remission.[38] If patients continue to have active inflammation, adjustments in therapy are made and again assessed by endoscopy in 8 to 12 weeks' time (**Fig. 3**).

In addition, therapy is lifelong. There have been 2 retrospective studies describing rare incidence of patients with documented evidence of sustained remission off of

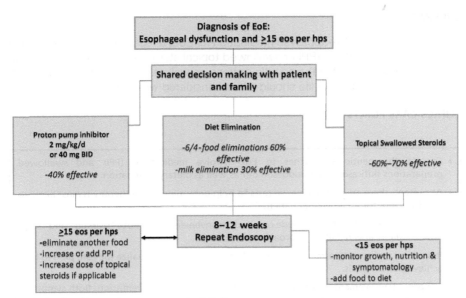

Fig. 3. Evaluation and management of EoE.

treatment, raising the question if sustained tolerance is possible in EoE.[71,72] Therefore, EoE is considered a chronic illness that will require lifetime treatment. There have been studies in which patients in remission on topical budesonide were randomized to dose reduction or placebo. Patients receiving placebo have a rebound in eosinophil count (average eosinophil count was 0.7 before dose reduction and then increased to 64 after 50 weeks of placebo). Furthermore, there was a return of symptoms and a nonsignificant increase in lamina propria fibrosis seen in patients who underwent dose reduction.[73]

NEW DEVELOPMENTS

Recent clinical trials show promise for future biological approach to EoE, with trials for dupilumab (monoclonal antibody directed against the IL-4 receptor-α), cendakimab (a monoclonal antibody against IL-13), benralizumab (a monoclonal antibody against the IL-5 receptor), lirentelimab (a monoclonal antibody directed against eosinophil/mast cell Siglec-8), and mepolizumab (a monoclonal antibody directed against IL-5) all in various stages.[74,75] In addition, standardized formulations of budesonide have been studied with both a dispersible tablet and suspension formulations.[61,76]

Beyond therapeutic developments, evaluating disease activity without endoscopy has been a major goal of the field. Use of transnasal endoscopy with virtual reality goggles to avoid anesthesia has been successfully used in pediatric patients and allows for adequate tissue evaluation.[77] Similarly, the esophageal string test, a capsule containing a nylon string. The capsule is swallowed while holding the string outside of the mouth. Once the capsule dissolves, the string unravels in the esophagus and is able to absorb esophageal secretions. The string is removed, and the eosinophil protein concentration on the string has been shown to positively and significantly correlate with eosinophil count.[78,79] Taken together these recent advances will hopefully decrease the endoscopic burden facing patients with EoE.

SUMMARY

Because there is no FDA-approved medication for EoE, a reasonable first-line therapy could involve medications (PPI or swallowed topical steroids) or dietary therapy. The pros and cons of each the therapeutic options as well as weighing the frequency of endoscopies and quality of life should all be considered when choosing a therapy.

CLINICS CARE POINTS

- Current therapeutic approaches to EoE involve medications (PPIs and swallowed preparations fluticasone and budoesonide) as well as dietary elimination.
- At present, there are no noninvasive tests to help determine which therapy is most likely to be efficacious for an individual patient.
- Barriers to dietary treatment include cost and inconvenience, and both "step-up" and "step-down" empirical elimination approaches have merit.
- It is critical to discuss treatment options with patients and individualize the care plan to help achieve patient goals.
- Symptom improvement is not always correlated with histologic remission. Both symptoms and histology need to be reevaluated after 8 to 12 weeks on therapy to evaluate therapeutic efficacy.

DISCLOSURE

The authors have no commercial or financial conflicts of interest and no funding sources to acknowledge in regard to this article.

REFERENCES

1. Attwood SEA, Smyrk TC, Demeester TR, et al. Esophageal eosinophilia with dysphagia - A distinct clinicopathologic syndrome. Dig Dis Sci 1993;38:109–16.
2. Straumann A, Spichtin H, Bernoulli R, et al. [Idiopathic eosinophilic esophagitis: a frequently overlooked disease with typical clinical aspects and discrete endoscopic findings]. Schweiz Med Wochenschr 1994;124:1419–29.
3. Kelly KJ, et al. Eosinophilic esophagitis attributed to gastroesophageal reflux: improvement with an amino acid-based formula. Gastroenterology 1995;109: 1503–12.
4. Liacouras CA, et al. Eosinophilic esophagitis: updated consensus recommendations for children and adults. J Allergy Clin Immunol 2011;128:3–20.e6 [quiz 21–2].
5. Furuta GT, et al. Eosinophilic esophagitis in children and adults: a systematic review and consensus recommendations for diagnosis and treatment. Sponsored by the American Gastroenterological Association (AGA) Institute and North American Society of Pediatric Gastroenterology, Hepatology, and Nutrition. Gastroenterology 2007;133:1342–63.
6. Lucendo AJ, et al. Guidelines on eosinophilic esophagitis: evidence-based statements and recommendations for diagnosis and management in children and adults. United Eur Gastroenterol J 2017;5 335–358.
7. Miller TL, et al. Drivers of variation in diagnosis and management of eosinophilic esophagitis: a survey of pediatric gastroenterologists. Dig Dis Sci 2021. https://doi.org/10.1007/s10620-021-07039-6.

8. Chang JW, et al. Motivations, barriers, and outcomes of patient-reported shared decision making in eosinophilic esophagitis. Dig Dis Sci 2020. https://doi.org/10.1007/s10620-020-06438-5.

9. Muir AB, Wang JX, Nakagawa H. Epithelial-stromal crosstalk and fibrosis in eosinophilic esophagitis. J Gastroenterol 2019;54:10–8.

10. Noti M, et al. Thymic stromal lymphopoietin-elicited basophil responses promote eosinophilic esophagitis. Nat Med 2013;19:1005–13.

11. Aceves SS. Remodeling and fibrosis in chronic eosinophil inflammation. Dig Dis 2014;32:15–21.

12. Whelan KA, et al. Persistent basal cell hyperplasia is associated with clinical and endoscopic findings in patients with histologically inactive eosinophilic esophagitis. Clin Gastroenterol Hepatol 2020;18:1475–82.e1.

13. Katzka DA, et al. Endoscopic mucosal impedance measurements correlate with eosinophilia and dilation of intercellular spaces in patients with eosinophilic esophagitis. Clin Gastroenterol Hepatol 2015;13:1242–8.e1.

14. Blanchard C, et al. A striking local esophageal cytokine expression profile in eosinophilic esophagitis. J Allergy Clin Immunol 2011;127:208–17, 217.e1-7.

15. Schoepfer AM, et al. Delay in diagnosis of eosinophilic esophagitis increases risk for stricture formation in a time-dependent manner. Gastroenterology 2013;145:1230–6.e2.

16. Alexander ES, et al. Twin and family studies reveal strong environmental and weaker genetic cues explaining heritability of eosinophilic esophagitis. J Allergy Clin Immunol 2014;134:1084–92.e1.

17. Rothenberg ME, et al. Common variants at 5q22 associate with pediatric eosinophilic esophagitis. Nat Genet 2010;42:289–91.

18. Sleiman MA, et al. GWAS identifies four novel eosinophilic esophagitis loci. Nat Commun 2014;5:5593.

19. Kottyan LC, Parameswaran S, Weirauch MT, et al. The genetic etiology of eosinophilic esophagitis. J Allergy Clin Immunol 2020;1459–14515.

20. Jensen ET, Dellon ES. Environmental factors and eosinophilic esophagitis. J Allergy Clin Immunol 2018;142:32–40.

21. Dellon ES, Hirano I. Epidemiology and Natural History of Eosinophilic Esophagitis. Gastroenterology 2018;154:319–32.e3.

22. Hiremath GS, et al. Esophageal food impaction and eosinophilic esophagitis: a retrospective study, systematic review, and meta-analysis. Dig Dis Sci 2015;60:3181–93.

23. Veerappan GR, et al. Prevalence of eosinophilic esophagitis in an adult population undergoing upper endoscopy: a prospective study. Clin Gastroenterol Hepatol 2009;7:420–6, 426.e1-2.

24. Prasad GA, et al. Prevalence and predictive factors of eosinophilic esophagitis in patients presenting with dysphagia: a prospective study. Am J Gastroenterol 2007;102:2627–32.

25. Noel RJ, Putnam E, Rothenberg ME. Eosinophilic Esophagitis. N Engl J Med 2004;351:940–1.

26. Alexander R, et al. Measurement of observed eating behaviors in patients with active and inactive eosinophilic esophagitis. Clin Gastroenterol Hepatol 2019;17:2371–3.

27. Lee J, et al. Esophageal diameter is decreased in some patients with eosinophilic esophagitis and might increase with topical corticosteroid therapy. Clin Gastroenterol Hepatol 2012;10:481–6.

28. Nielsen JA, Lager DJ, Lewin M, et al. The optimal number of biopsy fragments to establish a morphologic diagnosis of eosinophilic esophagitis. Am J Gastroenterol 2014;109:515–20.

29. Hirano I, et al. Endoscopic assessment of the oesophageal features of eosinophilic oesophagitis: validation of a novel classification and grading system. Gut 2013;62:489–95.

30. Safroneeva E, et al. Systematic assessment of adult patients' satisfaction with various eosinophilic esophagitis therapies. Int Arch Allergy Immunol 2020;181:211–20.

31. Klinnert MD, et al. Symptom burden and quality of life over time in pediatric eosinophilic esophagitis. J Pediatr Gastroenterol Nutr 2019;69:682–9.

32. Dellon ES. Cost-effective care in eosinophilic esophagitis. Ann Allergy Asthma Immunol 2019;123:166–72.

33. Capucilli , Hill DA. Allergic comorbidity in eosinophilic esophagitis: mechanistic relevance and clinical implications. Clin Rev Allergy Immunol 2019;57:111–27.

34. Menard-Katcher C, et al. Significance of feeding dysfunction in eosinophilic esophagitis. World J Gastroenterol 2014;20:11019–22.

35. Markowitz JE, Spergel JM, Ruchelli E, et al. Elemental diet is an effective treatment for eosinophilic esophagitis in children and adolescents. Am J Gastroenterol 2003;98:777–82.

36. Spergel JM, et al. Identification of causative foods in children with eosinophilic esophagitis treated with an elimination diet. J Allergy Clin Immunol 2012;130:461–7.e5.

37. Papadopoulou A, et al. Management guidelines of eosinophilic esophagitis in childhood. J Pediatr Gastroenterol Nutr 2014;58:107–18.

38. Hirano I, et al. AGA Institute and the joint task force on allergy-immunology practice parameters clinical guidelines for the management of eosinophilic esophagitis. Gastroenterology 2020;158:1776–86.

39. Arias A, González-Cervera J, Tenias JM, et al. Efficacy of dietary interventions for inducing histologic remission in patients with eosinophilic esophagitis: a systematic review and meta-analysis. Gastroenterology 2014;146:1639–48.

40. Kagalwalla AF, et al. Effect of six-food elimination diet on clinical and histologic outcomes in eosinophilic esophagitis. Clin Gastroenterol Hepatol 2006;4:1097–102.

41. Henderson CJ, et al. Comparative dietary therapy effectiveness in remission of pediatric eosinophilic esophagitis. J Allergy Clin Immunol 2012;129:1570–8.

42. Kagalwalla AF, et al. Efficacy of a 4-food elimination diet for children with eosinophilic esophagitis. Clin Gastroenterol Hepatol 2017;15:1698–707.e7.

43. Kagalwalla AF, et al. Identification of specific foods responsible for inflammation in children with eosinophilic esophagitis successfully treated with empiric elimination diet. J Pediatr Gastroenterol Nutr 2011;53:145–9.

44. Gonsalves N, et al. Elimination diet effectively treats eosinophilic esophagitis in adults; Food reintroduction identifies causative factors. Gastroenterology 2012;142:1451–9.e1.

45. Molina-Infante J, et al. Step-up empiric elimination diet for pediatric and adult eosinophilic esophagitis: the 2-4-6 study. J Allergy Clin Immunol 2018;141:1365–72.

46. Kagalwalla AF, et al. Cow's milk elimination: a novel dietary approach to treat eosinophilic esophagitis. J Pediatr Gastroenterol Nutr 2012;55:711–6.

47. Teoh T, Mill C, Chan E, et al. Liberalized versus strict cow's milk elimination for the treatment of children with eosinophilic esophagitis. J Can Assoc Gastroenterol 2019;2:81–5.
48. Kruszewski G, et al. Prospective, comparative effectiveness trial of cow's milk elimination and swallowed fluticasone for pediatric eosinophilic esophagitis. Dis Esophagus 2016;29:377–84.
49. Wechsler JB, et al. A single food milk elimination diet is effective for treatment of eosinophilic esophagitis in children. Clin Gastroenterol Hepatol 2021. https://doi.org/10.1016/j.cgh.2021.03.049.
50. Kliewer KL, Sun Q, Fei L, et al. Comparing two restrictive diets for treating eosinophilic esophagitis in children. PCORI Final Res Result 2020;1–85.
51. Wong J, et al. Efficacy of dairy free diet and 6-food elimination diet as initial therapy for pediatric eosinophilic esophagitis: a retrospective single-center study. Pediatr Gastroenterol Hepatol Nutr 2020;23:79–88.
52. Molina-Infante J, et al. Proton pump inhibitor-responsive oesophageal eosinophilia: an entity challenging current diagnostic criteria for eosinophilic oesophagitis. Gut 2016;65:521–31.
53. Wen T, et al. Transcriptome analysis of proton pump inhibitor-responsive esophageal eosinophilia reveals proton pump inhibitor-reversible allergic inflammation. J Allergy Clin Immunol 2015;135:187–97.e4.
54. Cheng E, et al. Omeprazole blocks eotaxin-3 expression by oesophageal squamous cells from patients with eosinophilic oesophagitis and GORD. Gut 2013;62:824–32.
55. Gutiérrez-Junquera C, et al. High prevalence of response to proton-pump inhibitor treatment in children with esophageal eosinophilia. J Pediatr Gastroenterol Nutr 2016;62:704–10.
56. Gutiérrez-Junquera C, et al. Long-term treatment with proton pump inhibitors is effective in children with eosinophilic esophagitis. J Pediatr Gastroenterol Nutr 2018;67:210–6.
57. Lucendo AJ, Arias Á, Molina-Infante J. Efficacy of proton pump inhibitor drugs for inducing clinical and histologic remission in patients with symptomatic esophageal eosinophilia: a systematic review and meta-analysis. Clin Gastroenterol Hepatol 2016;14:13–22.e1.
58. Freedberg DE, Kim LS, Yang YX. The risks and benefits of long-term use of proton pump inhibitors: expert review and best practice advice From the American Gastroenterological Association. Gastroenterology 2017;152:706–15.
59. Lee J, et al. Oral viscous budesonide can be successfully delivered through a variety of vehicles to treat eosinophilic esophagitis in children. J Allergy Clin Immunol Pract 2016;4:767–8.
60. Lucendo AJ, et al. Efficacy of budesonide orodispersible tablets as induction therapy for eosinophilic esophagitis in a randomized placebo-controlled trial. Gastroenterology 2019;157:74–86.e15.
61. Hirano I, et al. Budesonide oral suspension improves outcomes in patients with eosinophilic esophagitis: results from a phase 3 trial. Clin Gastroenterol Hepatol 2021. https://doi.org/10.1016/j.cgh.2021.04.022.
62. Dellon ES, et al. Efficacy of budesonide vs fluticasone for initial treatment of eosinophilic esophagitis in a randomized controlled trial. Gastroenterology 2019;157:65–73.e5.
63. Philpott H, et al. Systematic review: adrenal insufficiency secondary to swallowed topical corticosteroids in eosinophilic oesophagitis. Aliment Pharmacol Ther 2018;47:1071–8.

64. Bose , et al. Adrenal insufficiency in children with eosinophilic esophagitis treated with topical corticosteroids. J Pediatr Gastroenterol Nutr 2020;70:324–9.

65. Moawad FJ, et al. Systematic review with meta-analysis: endoscopic dilation is highly effective and safe in children and adults with eosinophilic oesophagitis. Aliment Pharmacol Ther 2017;46:96–105.

66. Safroneeva E, et al. Long-lasting dissociation of esophageal eosinophilia and symptoms following dilation in adults with eosinophilic esophagitis. Clin Gastroenterol Hepatol 2021. https://doi.org/10.1016/j.cgh.2021.05.049.

67. Runge TM, Eluri S, Woosley JT, et al. Control of inflammation decreases the need for subsequent esophageal dilation in patients with eosinophilic esophagitis. Dis Esophagus 2017;30:1–7.

68. Menard-Katcher C, Furuta GT, Kramer RE. Dilation of pediatric eosinophilic esophagitis: adverse events and short-term outcomes. J Pediatr Gastroenterol Nutr 2017;64:701–6.

69. Heine RG, et al. Effect of a 4-food elimination diet and omeprazole in children with eosinophilic esophagitis – a randomized, controlled trial. J Allergy Clin Immunol 2019;143:AB309.

70. Safroneeva E, et al. Symptoms have modest accuracy in detecting endoscopic and histologic remission in adults with eosinophilic esophagitis. Gastroenterology 2016;150:581–90.e4.

71. Ruffner MA, et al. Clinical tolerance in eosinophilic esophagitis. J Allergy Clin Immunol Pract 2018;6:661–3.

72. Hoofien A, et al. Sustained remission of eosinophilic esophagitis following discontinuation of dietary elimination in children. Clin Gastroenterol Hepatol 2020;18:249–51.e1.

73. Straumann A, et al. Long-term budesonide maintenance treatment is partially effective for patients with eosinophilic esophagitis. Clin Gastroenterol Hepatol 2011;9:400–9.e1.

74. Hirano I, et al. Efficacy of dupilumab in a phase 2 randomized trial of adults with active eosinophilic esophagitis. Gastroenterology 2020;158:111–22.e10.

75. Hirano I, et al. RPC4046, a monoclonal antibody against IL13, reduces histologic and endoscopic activity in patients with eosinophilic esophagitis. Gastroenterology 2019;156:592–603.e10.

76. Straumann A, et al. Budesonide orodispersible tablets maintain remission in a randomized, placebo-controlled trial of patients with eosinophilic esophagitis. Gastroenterology 2020;159:1672–85.e5.

77. Nguyen N, et al. Transnasal endoscopy in unsedated children with eosinophilic esophagitis using virtual reality video goggles. Clin Gastroenterol Hepatol 2019;17:2455–62.

78. Ackerman SJ, et al. One-hour esophageal string test: a nonendoscopic minimally invasive test that accurately detects disease activity in eosinophilic esophagitis. Am J Gastroenterol 2019;114:1614–25.

79. Furuta GT, et al. The oesophageal string test: a novel, minimally invasive method measures mucosal inflammation in eosinophilic oesophagitis. Gut 2013;62:1395–405.

Celiac Disease in Children

Jennifer Jimenez, MD[a], Beth Loveridge-Lenza, MD[a],
Karoly Horvath, MD, PhD[b],*

KEYWORDS

- Celiac disease • Symptoms of celiac disease • Tissue transglutaminase-2 test
- Gluten-free diet • Other gluten-related conditions

KEY POINTS

- Celiac disease is an autoimmune small intestinal disease developing in genetically predisposed individuals who ingest gluten (wheat, barley, rye).
- Celiac disease has protean clinical manifestations and it is important for all pediatricians to be aware of its various clinical presentations.
- Celiac disease is treated successfully by a lifelong exclusion of gluten from the diet.
- A complete nutritional assessment and a detailed gluten-free diet education is recommended at diagnosis of celiac disease.
- In children, ongoing medical follow-ups and support system are key for dietary compliance.

INTRODUCTION

Celiac disease (CD) is an autoimmune enteropathy triggered by the ingestion of gluten in genetically susceptible individuals carrying the HLA class II haplotypes (DQ2 or DQ8 or both). The word "gluten" describes the alcohol soluble proteins, known as prolamins, in wheat (gliadin), rye (secalin), and barley (hordein), which are the triggers of the immune response resulting in small intestinal damage.

The clinical manifestation of CD is protean with a spectrum from latent to classical symptoms. An Italian epidemiologic study reported that the classical manifestation was present only 1 out of 7 children diagnosed with CD (called the "tip of the iceberg").[1]

Conflicts of interest and source of Funding: The authors have no conflicts of interest and have not received any funding for the study. All authors equally contributed to the manuscript writing.
[a] Division of Pediatric Gastroenterology and Nutrition, Jersey Shore University Medical Center, K. Hovnanian Children's Hospital, Hackensack Meridian Health, 19 Davis Avenue, 5th Floor, Neptune, NJ 07753, USA; [b] Florida State University, Center for Digestive Health and Nutrition, Arnold Palmer Hospital for Children, Orlando Health, 60 W Gore Street, Orlando, FL 32806, USA
* Corresponding author.
E-mail address: karoly.horvath@orlandohealth.com

Pediatr Clin N Am 68 (2021) 1205–1219
https://doi.org/10.1016/j.pcl.2021.07.007
0031-3955/21/© 2021 Elsevier Inc. All rights reserved.

The discovery of gluten as a trigger for CD was made by the observation of a pediatrician, Dr Dicke, who noticed significant decrease in the prevalence of CD cases during World War II when the wheat was rarely harvested and an increase when it became widely available.[2] This important discovery simplified the treatment of celiac patients with a gluten-free diet.

The intestinal histopathology on CD became known after the 1960s, when the small intestinal capsule biopsy technique was introduced. Another significant milestone was the discovery of sensitive and specific serum antibody tests in the 1980s. It allowed to collect important epidemiologic data on the prevalence of CD worldwide and the recognition of the risk groups for CD.

In this article, we aimed to provide a thorough review on the epidemiology, pathogenesis, symptoms, diagnosis and the management of CD to help general practitioners in their clinical practice.

PATHOGENESIS

The 3 components of celiac pathogenesis include the triad of gluten ingestion, genetic susceptibility, and loss of immune tolerance to gluten (**Fig. 1**).

Gluten consists of the ethanol-soluble prolamines and the ethanol-insoluble glutenins. The prolamins trigger the immune response and they have a very high glutamine (>30%) and proline (>15%) content.[3] The gluten is not completely digestible by human intestinal enzymes and its partially digested peptides can trigger the host responses including intestinal permeability and innate and adaptive immune responses.[4]

In individuals having HLA DQ2 and DQ8-positive antigen-presenting cells, the gluten peptides deamidated by tissue transglutaminase-2 (tTG2) trigger T-cell activation in the by lamina propria[5] that ultimately results in a loss of tolerance to gluten.[4] The CD4+ T cells activation leads to the production of proinflammatory cytokines, metalloproteases, and keratinocyte growth factor, which induce crypt hyperplasia and villous blunting secondary to intestinal epithelial cell death.[6,7] Many studies showed that IL-15 in the epithelium and the lamina propria plays a central role in the development of villous atrophy that was further confirmed in a mouse model.[8]

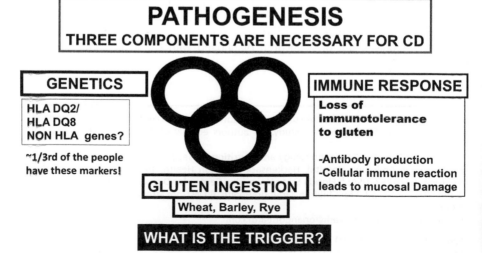

Fig. 1. The triad of the CD pathogenesis.

Although CD has a strong genetic component, concordance rates in monozygotic twins are only about 50%,[9] indicating that environmental factors play a role for disease etiology.

It is not known what triggers the loss of the immune tolerance to gluten. Studies examined the age of introduction of gluten to the diet and the amount of gluten consumption, among many other factors. A large-scale study in India included 23,331 healthy adults in 3 regions with similar HLA DQ2/8 background, but different mean daily wheat intake (355 g in the northern part, 37 g in the northeastern part, and 25 g in the southern part) and found that the prevalence of CD correlated with wheat intake and did not reflect differences in the genetic background.[10] In a pediatric study in the Netherlands, high intake of vegetables, vegetable oils, pasta, and grains and low consumption of refined cereals and sweet beverages at 1 year of age significantly decreased the odds of having CD at 6 years of age.[11]

In the past, it was thought that the duration of breastfeeding and the age at gluten introduction are important. However, 2 randomized clinical trials published in 2014 failed to find an effect on various infant feeding strategies on the risk of CD.[12,13] To clearly prove the role of amount and time of gluten ingestion, future randomized prospective clinical trials would be warranted.[14]

Refractory CD manifests with persistent small intestinal villous atrophy with symptoms despite 12 months or more of a strict gluten-free diet, in the absence of an overt lymphoma or another condition that causes villous atrophy.[15] It is characterized by the absence (type I) or presence (type II) of an aberrant population of intraepithelial lymphocytes that lack lineage differentiation surface markers (eg, CD4, CD8, or the IL-2 receptor) but are positive for cytoplasmic CD3, indicating a T-cell phenotype.[16] Refractory CD occurs in 1% to 2% of adult patients with CD.[17] In pediatric practice, true refractory CD is uncommon, and usually due to unrecognized exposure to gluten. Only 1 pediatric case of refractory CD is reported in the pediatric literature.[18]

Other Gluten-Related Diseases and Their Pathogenesis

There are 3 other gluten related diseases: wheat allergy, nonceliac gluten sensitivity and dermatitis herpetiformis.

The estimated prevalence of wheat allergy in children is between 2% and 9% and between 0.5% and 3.0% in adults.[19] In wheat allergy, gluten peptides and nongluten proteins in wheat induce the release of immune mediators from basophils and mast cells.[20] Wheat allergy can be determined by IgE radioallergosorbent testing or skin prick testing by an allergist.

The exact pathogenesis of nonceliac gluten sensitivity is not known. Patients with nonceliac gluten sensitivity have normal levels of intestinal permeability and expression of tight junction proteins, with the exception of overexpression of claudin-4.[20] Interestingly, compared with patients with CD or controls, intestinal tissues from patients with nonceliac gluten sensitivity have increased levels of the Toll-like receptor-2 and -4 increased numbers of α and β intraepithelial lymphocytes.[21] The diagnosis of nonceliac gluten sensitivity can be established after screening tests ruled out CD and IgE-mediated wheat allergy, and there is symptomatic improvement if a patient is adhering to a gluten-free diet for at least 1 week.[20]

Dermatitis herpetiformis is a chronic, recurrent skin disease that manifests with a papulovesicular, usually symmetric pruriginous rash, mainly on the extensor surface of limbs, buttocks, and scapular area.[22] It is diagnosed by the presence of granular IgA deposits on top of the dermal papillae. Patients with dermatitis herpetiformis have HLA DQ2 or HLA DQ8 alleles and abnormal CD serology tests. In addition to a gluten-free diet, the initial treatment includes medical therapy.

SYMPTOMS

In 2011, the Oslo classification of CD identified the following clinical presentations: classic, nonclassic, subclinical, potential and refractory.[15] Classical CD is usually detected in children younger than 2 years of age and is characterized by diarrhea, loss of appetite, abdominal distention, weight loss and failure to thrive,[23] whereas in older children and adults bloating, constipation, abdominal pain, or irritable bowel syndrome–like symptoms are more typical.

Nonclassical CD cases represent the majority of pediatric cases owing to serology screening and they have no apparent malabsorption symptoms. The presenting symptoms may include abdominal pain, constipation, and gassiness. CD is associated with many nongastrointestinal signs and symptoms, such as osteoporosis, iron deficiency anemia, transaminitis, arthritis, myalgia, headaches, fatigue, recurrent oral ulcers, and dental enamel defects of the permanent teeth of children, as well as adverse pregnancy outcomes or infertility in adults. Children can present with behavioral disturbances and hindered educational performance.[24]

In a recent systematic review and meta-analysis including 3759 patients with short stature, 1 in 9 patients with idiopathic short stature had biopsy-confirmed CD. Therefore, children with short stature need screening for CD.[25] Children with poor growth and anemia tend to have more severe histologic damage at diagnosis compared with screen-detected cases.[26]

It is important to emphasize that many patients with CD have a body mass index that is greater than the 50th percentile for age and the possibility of CD in these cases should not be overlooked, because overweight children can have CD[27] (**Fig. 2**).

Subclinical cases are those patients undergoing antibody screening owing to being relatives of patients with CD or at-risk for CD but do not have symptoms.[15] However, previously unrecognized symptoms such as fatigue may improve after diagnosis on a gluten-free diet. Children with potential CD have positive tTG2 and anti-endomysium

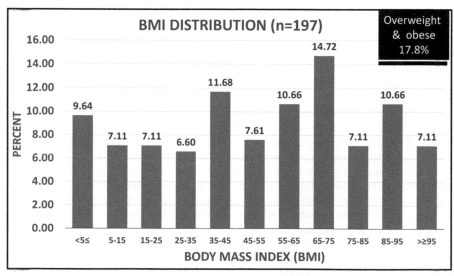

*over 55th percentile: 50.25%

Fig. 2. Body mass index of 197 children diagnosed with CD (Karoly Horvath, unpublished data, 2021).

antibody IgA tests with normal duodenal histology. It is important to ensure that adequate biopsies were taken, including in the duodenal bulb. Children with such a diagnosis require long-term follow-up. In a large study including 280 cases followed for 12 years, 43% of these patients developed CD.[28]

Celiac Disease and Autoimmune and Genetic Disorders

A large Danish population study revealed that the prevalence of autoimmune diseases was 16.4% among patients with CD compared with 5.3% in the general population in 2016.[29] It remains unclear whether CD directly leads to other autoimmune disease and whether early diagnosis and treatment with a gluten-free diet alters this risk.[30] Children with autoimmune diseases including Hashimoto's thyroiditis, Graves' disease, and type 1 diabetes,[29,31] need to be screened for CD because they are the most common autoimmune diseases that occur with CD.

Patients with chromosomal abnormalities such as trisomy 21, Williams syndrome, and Turner syndrome also have a high risk of CD and should also be screened regularly.[32]

EPIDEMIOLOGY

The prevalence of CD in the general population worldwide is approximately 1%, with regional differences,[15] and it is even higher in certain Northern European countries.[33] CD became a common disorder in North Africa,[34] the Middle East,[35] and India.[10] It is thought that the increase in prevalence is attributed to the adaptation of Western gluten-rich diet. Worldwide, many CD cases may remain undetected owing to the absence of serologic screening, heterogeneous symptoms, and/or poor disease awareness.

We have learned that the prevalence of CD is increasing in Western countries. CD prevalence increased by 4.5 times since the 1950s based on a large-scale study that used sera of young soldiers from 1950s for comparison.[36] The reasons for the increase are unknown. Similar increases are reported for other autoimmune diseases in the Western hemisphere.[37]

DIAGNOSIS

In adults, because of the various presentations and the lack of awareness among health care professionals, diagnostic delays reached up to 11 years in the United States.[38] In a study from Spain, the average time to diagnosis after the appearance of symptoms was 7.6 months for children and 90.0 months for adults.[23] The diagnosis of CD is based on the presence of mucosal damage in small intestinal biopsies in patients having circulating CD-specific antibodies on serologic testing.

The average age of diagnosis changed significantly since the introduction of screening blood tests and most of the cases are diagnosed in elementary school age.[39] Socioeconomically deprived children are more likely to be underdiagnosed based on a study performed in South-West England and it was estimated that 83% to 91% of children with CD were still being missed there.[40]

Histologic Findings

Intestinal biopsies should be considered in patients who consume gluten. We learned in the 1960s that the histologic features of CD are more pronounced in the proximal intestine, and mild or absent distally. It is important to get biopsies from the duodenal bulb because approximately 5% of cases present with damage isolated to the duodenal bulb alone.[41] It is recommended to obtain 5 or more duodenal biopsy specimens, including duodenal bulb biopsies labeled and submitted in a separate container. The location, number, and quality (size and orientation) of biopsy specimen can affect diagnostic yield. As many as 76.1% of children had variability of histologic lesions among the multiple biopsies[42]

The characteristic histologic findings include villous blunting, increased number of intraepithelial lymphocytes (>25 per 100 enterocytes), infiltration of the lamina propria by mononuclear cells, and elongation of the crypts with increased mitoses.[32,43,44] The individual histologic changes, including increased numbers of intraepithelial lympho-cytes and villous atrophy alone, are not pathognomonic for CD; they also are associ-ated with other disorders such as seronegative enteropathies.[45] However, the combination of these features is highly suggestive of CD. The classification of histo-logic changes were made by Marsh,[46] starting from 0 (normal) to flat mucosa (Marsh I, II, III). Later the Marsh III lesion was subdivided into a, b, and c categories by Ober-huber[47] (**Fig. 3**).

During the 1980s, it became clear that CD was associated with dermatitis herpeti-formis, a gluten-induced dermatopathy.[48] However, although the skin lesions are the basis of the diagnosis, intestinal damage was found in approximately 72% of the cases.[49]

Serologic Testing

In patients with suspected CD, measurement of serum IgA antibodies to tTG2 (anti-tTG2) (or IgG class in patients with IgA deficiency) has a high sensitivity and specificity and is the first screening test that should be ordered. Although the anti-endomysium IgA antibody is 98% specific for active CD, it serves best as a confirmatory screening tool.[50] Deamidated gliadin peptides, which include antibodies of the IgG class, have a sensitivity and specificity close to IgA and anti-tTG antibodies and should be used for patients with IgA deficiency.

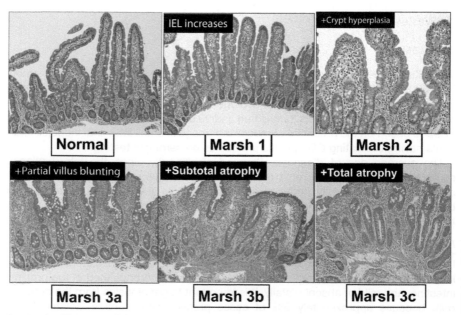

Fig. 3. Classification of the histologic small intestinal damage.

Children with diabetes may have a falsely positive elevation in the tTG2 antibodies. Some diabetics who were anti-tTG2 positive were endomysium antibody (EMA) negative and had normal histology on intestinal biopsy[51]; therefore, some experts recommend that a positive tTG should be followed by a positive EMA before biopsy is considered in patients with type 1 diabetes.

A study in infants showed that high concentrations of deamidated gliadin peptide antibodies more accurately detect CD in children than tests for anti-tTG2.[52] However, another study concluded that anti-tTG2 IgA could be used as an initial screening assay for CD in all subjects from 6 months of age because there was a substantial agreement between anti-tTGA and deamidated gliadin peptide IgA antibodies.[53]

Genetic Testing

HLA-DQ2 and -DQ8 analysis has a high negative predictive value (>99%). When there is a discrepancy between the serologic studies and histologic findings, HLA-DQ2 and HLA-DQ8 determination may be helpful as individuals who are negative for both cannot develop CD.[50] This test is valuable with an equivocal diagnosis (ie, seronegative for anti-tTG with enteropathy) or those already on gluten-free diet because CD can be excluded in patients who are negative for both entities. The class II HLA types DQ2 and/or DQ8 are found in almost all patients with CD, but also in 30% to 40% of the Western Caucasian population; only approximately 3% of individuals with these haplotypes develop CD.[52] It is likely that other genetic and/or environmental factors play a role in the disease onset.

Is Diagnosis Possible Without Biopsy?

A consensus guideline produced by the European Society of Pediatric Gastroenterology, Hepatology, and Nutrition proposed a strategy to avoid intestinal biopsies.[54] In children who have symptoms suggestive of CD, a strongly positive tTG2 antibody titer (10 times above the laboratory cut-off value), and positive anti-EmA test and the presence of CD-associated HLA genotypes, the diagnosis of CD can be made without the need for small intestinal biopsies. Recently, the modified guidelines stated that the confirmation of the greater than 10× tTG2 elevation by anti-endomysium antibody test is sufficient to start children on a gluten-free diet and HLA analysis is not required for the diagnosis.[55] **Fig. 4** shows an algorithm for the diagnosis of CD.

Who Should be Screened for Celiac Disease in Pediatric Practice?

It is important to emphasize that a gluten-free diet should not be initiated before the confirmation of CD. Unfortunately, it is not uncommon that pediatricians recommend starting a gluten-free diet based on the less sensitive and specific antigliadin IgG antibody tests. Patients who started a gluten-free diet for a few months without confirmatory testing may need to undergo a medically supervised exposure to gluten.[56] In a recent small study after 14 days of 10-g gluten exposure, IL-2 levels appeared the earliest, and were the most sensitive, marker of acute gluten exposure[57] Based on the previous information, **Tables 1** and **2** list the symptoms and diseases associated with CD that should prompt screening.

TREATMENT

Since the 1950s, when gluten was identified as the causative trigger of CD, a strict and lifelong gluten-free diet with the elimination of wheat, barley, rye, and their hybrids containing these grains has been the mainstay of treatment. Oats are considered safe for consumption by most people with CD, although adverse immune and clinical

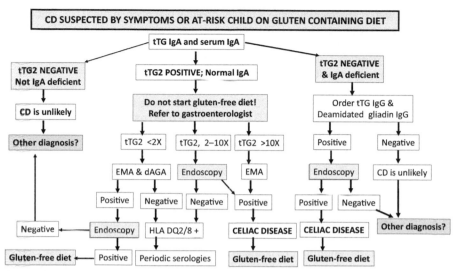

Fig. 4. Flow chart for the diagnosis of CD.

effects have been reported owing to cross-contamination with gluten.[58] Strict adherence to a gluten-free diet results in a recovery of the mucosal damage, and there is an observation that the recovery is faster in younger children. It is likely that early treatment with a gluten-free diet might also prevent the development of complications associated with CD.[59,60]

A National Institutes of Health consensus conference in 2004 developed a mnemonic with the 6-key elements of CD management corresponding with the 6 letters of *CELIAC*: Consultation with a skilled dietitian, Education about the disease, Lifelong adherence to a gluten-free diet, Identification and treatment of nutritional deficiencies, Access to an advocacy group and Continuous long-term follow-up.[61] **Fig. 5** outlines the typical follow-up schedule for CD.

It is important for the family to have a visit with an experienced dietician to get accurate education on the gluten-free diet. The North American Society for Pediatric Gastroenterology, Hepatology and Nutrition published a *Gluten-free Diet Guide for*

Table 1
Who needs to be screened for CD?

Symptoms		
Gastrointestinal	**Extraintestinal**	**Associated Conditions**
Chronic diarrhea	Short stature	First-degree relatives with CD
Chronic abdominal pain	Delayed puberty	Type 1 diabetes
Bloating	Iron deficiency anemia	Autoimmune thyroid disease
Failure to thrive	Recurrent aphthous stomatitis	Autoimmune liver disease
Weight loss	Dental enamel hypoplasia	Selective IgA deficiency
Constipation (>2 y of age)	Transaminitis	Sjogren syndrome
Anorexia	Dermatitis herpetiformis	Down syndrome
Vomiting	Osteopenia and osteoporosis	Turner syndrome
Malabsorption	Peripheral neuropathy	Williams syndrome
	Fatigue	

Table 2 Nutritional management	
Initial Counseling	**Follow-Up Visits**
Definition of gluten	Diet compliance
Gluten-containing products	Importance of strict compliance
Gluten-free labeling	Growth parameters
Hidden sources of gluten	Balanced nutrition
Causes of cross-contamination	Support systems
Gluten-free resources	
Gluten-free product information	
Eating out instructions	
Gluten-free drug information	
Importance of strict compliance	
Local and national support groups	
Access to nutritionist if there is any question	

Families that is available freely on the internet. In 2013, the US Food and Drug Administration introduced a rule for the labeling of gluten-free products. However, eating out can be an obstacle to being compliant with diet, although most popular restaurant chains are offering a gluten-free menu.

At the first visit after the diagnosis, the physician should discuss the degree of intestinal damage, the expected time of mucosal recovery, the disaccharidase test results (if performed), the beneficial effect of the diet to prevent complications, the typical follow-up schedule, and recommendation for family screening and also give information on how to connect to local support groups. A study evaluated children with CD after they spent a week in a gluten-free camp and demonstrated improvement in well-being, self-perception, and emotional outlook. The positive effects of the camp

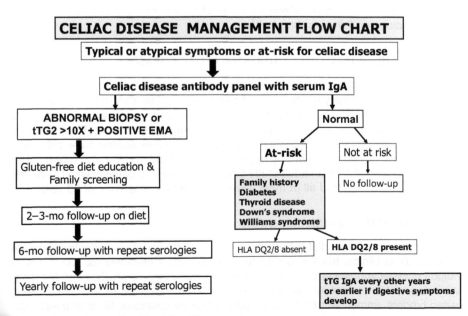

Fig. 5. Management flowchart for CD.

were more apparent among the campers who had been on a gluten-free diet for less than 4 years.[62]

The typical follow-up schedule after the initial diagnosis includes visits within the first 2 to 3 months after starting the gluten-free diet and then at 6 and 12 months, and then yearly, if the patient is asymptomatic and compliant. The role of the 2- to 3-month visit is to assess the symptomatic changes and provide further counseling to families who started practicing a gluten-free diet. The first follow-up visit after post-biopsy counseling and dietary teaching is important because it allows for an assessment of the emotional status of children and parents, which can be predictive for future compliance with the diet.

The medical management of CD includes the assessment of changes in clinical symptoms, improvement in the celiac serology tests, treating nutritional deficiencies, checking growth parameters of children on a gluten-free diet, and screening for well-known complications (eg, associated autoimmune conditions). Approximately two-thirds of children diagnosed with CD who had been vaccinated against hepatitis B virus as an infant have no hepatitis B surface antibody[63,64]; therefore, it is recommended to screen the newly diagnosed cases for it.

In an Italian study, adolescents diagnosed through mass screening had lower compliance in comparison with age-matched patients diagnosed with classic symptoms.[65] Compliance with gluten-free diet is important to achieve a good quality of life. Psychosocial and educational support should be provided for teenagers having difficulties in strictly adhering to gluten-free diet. The gluten-free diet can be challenging psychologically and socially, because they may have a difficult time accommodating to occasions such as parties, eating out, and snack time at school.

Nonresponsive CD is when symptoms persist despite attempted adherence to a gluten-free diet. The most common cause of persistent symptoms is being inadvertently exposed to gluten. A serologic test alone is not always helpful in determining if contamination has occurred and repeat endoscopy maybe necessary to look for signs of ongoing inflammation.[66] Although the tTG2 is considered normal if it is less than 4, in adults, only an undetectable value of less than 1.2 was associated with normal histology on follow-up biopsy.[67]

MORBIDITY AND MORTALITY OF UNTREATED CELIAC DISEASE

Symptomatic and untreated disease is associated with increased morbidity and mortality and impaired quality of life[36,68] and a considerable burden to health care systems.[59,69] Complications associated with untreated disease are intestinal lymphoma, small bowel adenocarcinoma, and ulcerative jejunoileitis. The frequency of malignant complications of CD is much lower than earlier studies have indicated, with lymphoma having increased by approximately fivefold and the absolute number of tumors were small.[70] In an adult study 5 (0.65%) of our 770 patients with CD developed adenocarcinoma and all of them were female with a mean age of 53 years.[71]

NONDIET THERAPIES IN RESEARCH STAGE

At this time, a gluten-free diet is the safest therapy and without side effects. There are many ongoing clinical trials in adults to find alternative therapies for CD.[72] These include enzyme supplementation to break down immunogenic gliadin peptides, zonulin antagonist to restore intestinal permeability, tTG2 inhibitors, HLA-DQ2 blockers, gluten binders, immunosuppressants, and peptide vaccinations. Most of these substances are in the research stage and not ready to replace the gluten-free diet.

SUMMARY

CD is a worldwide disease and a high index of clinical suspicion is needed to make an early diagnosis. The initial step for diagnosis includes serologic tests (tTG2 IgA, anti-endomysium IgA, deamidated antigliadin antibodies) followed by confirmatory testing with biopsies of the duodenum and duodenal bulb in adults. In the pediatric population a tTG2 is more than 10× over the cut-off and abnormal anti-endomysium test is considered sufficient to make the diagnosis of CD. Starting a gluten-free diet prevents further damage and results in symptom resolution. Lifelong adherence to a gluten-free diet is the only proven method for successful treatment of CD.

Children with CD need regular clinical follow-up visits. Compliance with a gluten-free diet can be a problem more commonly in teenagers. Pediatric nutritionists play a critical role in clinical follow-ups. Clinical trials have been ongoing to offer possible nondietary treatment of CD in the future. Ultimately, the definitive resolution would be a gluten-free world.

CLINICS CARE POINTS

- Pediatric practitioners should be aware of the various clinical manifestations of CD.

- When there is discrepancy between serologic studies and histologic findings, HLA-DQ2 and HLA-DQ8 determination may be helpful as individuals who are negative for both unlikely develop CD.

- Experts recommend that a positive tTG2 IgA antibody test to be followed by a positive EMA before biopsy is considered in patients with Type 1 diabetes, as these patients have a high rate of false positive elevation in the tTG2 antibodies.

- In children who have symptoms suggestive of CD, a strongly positive tTG2 antibody titer (10 times greater than the laboratory cut-off value), and positive anti-EmA test and/or the presence of CD-associated HLA genotypes, the diagnosis of CD can be made without the need for small intestinal biopsies.

- Many patients with CD have a body mass index that is greater than the 50th percentile for age and the possibility of CD in these cases should not be overlooked, because overweight children can have CD.

- Approximately two-thirds of children diagnosed with CD who had been vaccinated against hepatitis B virus as an infant have no hepatitis B surface antibody; therefore, it is recommended to screen the newly diagnosed cases for it.

- It is recommended to obtain 5 or more duodenal biopsy specimens including duodenal bulb biopsies labeled and submitted in a separate container during upper endoscopy to make a diagnosis of CD.

REFERENCES

1. Catassi C, Fabiani E, Ratsch IM, et al. The coeliac iceberg in Italy. A multicentre antigliadin antibodies screening for coeliac disease in school-age subjects. Acta Paediatr Suppl 1996;412:29–35.
2. van Berge-Henegouwen GP, Mulder CJ. Pioneer in the gluten free diet: Willem-Karel Dicke 1905-1962, over 50 years of gluten free diet. Gut 1993;34(11):1473–5.
3. Wieser H. Chemistry of gluten proteins. Food Microbiol 2007;24(2):115–9.
4. Leonard MM, Sapone A, Catassi C, et al. Celiac disease and nonceliac gluten sensitivity: a review. JAMA 2017;318(7):647–56.

5. Schuppan D. Current concepts of celiac disease pathogenesis. Gastroenterology 2000;119(1):234–42.
6. Pagliari D, Urgesi R, Frosali S, et al. The interaction among microbiota, immunity, and genetic and dietary factors is the condicio sine qua non celiac disease can develop. J Immunol Res 2015;2015:123653.
7. Hue S, Mention J, Montoiro R, et al. A direct role for NKG2D/MICA interaction in villous atrophy during celiac disease. Immunity 2004;21(3):367–77.
8. Abadie V, Kim SM, Lejeune T, et al. IL-15, gluten and HLA-DQ8 drive tissue destruction in coeliac disease. Nature 2020;578(7796):600–4.
9. Kuja-Halkola R, Lebwohl B, Halfvarson J, et al. Heritability of non-HLA genetics in coeliac disease: a population-based study in 107 000 twins. Gut 2016;65(11): 1793–8.
10. Ramakrishna BS, Makharia GK, Chetri K, et al. Prevalence of adult celiac disease in India: regional variations and associations. Am J Gastroenterol 2016;111(1): 115–23.
11. Barroso M, Beth SA, Voortman T, et al. Dietary patterns after the weaning and lactation period are associated with celiac disease autoimmunity in children. Gastroenterology 2018;154(8):2087–96.e7.
12. Vriezinga SL, Auricchio R, Bravi E, et al. Randomized feeding intervention in infants at high risk for celiac disease. N Engl J Med 2014;371(14):1304–15.
13. Lionetti E, Castellaneta S, Francavilla R, et al. Introduction of gluten, HLA status, and the risk of celiac disease in children. N Engl J Med 2014;371(14):1295–303.
14. Ludvigsson JF, Lebwohl B. Three papers indicate that amount of gluten play a role for celiac disease - But only a minor role. Acta Paediatr 2020;109(1):8–10.
15. Ludvigsson JF, Leffler DA, Bai JC, et al. The Oslo definitions for coeliac disease and related terms. Gut 2013;62(1):43–52.
16. Arguelles-Grande C, Brar P, Green PH, et al. Immunohistochemical and T-cell receptor gene rearrangement analyses as predictors of morbidity and mortality in refractory celiac disease. J Clin Gastroenterol 2013;47(7):593–601.
17. Roshan B, Leffler DA, Jamma S, et al. The incidence and clinical spectrum of refractory celiac disease in a north American referral center. Am J Gastroenterol 2011;106(5):923–8.
18. Mubarak A, Oudshoorn JH, Kneepkens CM, et al. A child with refractory coeliac disease. J Pediatr Gastroenterol Nutr 2011;53(2):216–8.
19. Sapone A, Bai JC, Ciacci C, et al. Spectrum of gluten-related disorders: consensus on new nomenclature and classification. BMC Med 2012;10(1):13.
20. Fasano A, Sapone A, Zevallos V, et al. Nonceliac gluten sensitivity. Gastroenterology 2015;148(6):1195–204.
21. Mansueto P, Seidita A, D'Alcamo A, et al. Non-celiac gluten sensitivity: literature review. J Am Coll Nutr 2014;33(1):39–54.
22. Clarindo MV, Possebon AT, Soligo EM, et al. Dermatitis herpetiformis: pathophysiology, clinical presentation, diagnosis and treatment. An Bras Dermatolog 2014; 89(6):865–75 [quiz: 876–7].
23. Vivas S, Ruiz de Morales JM, Fernandez M, et al. Age-related clinical, serological, and histopathological features of celiac disease. Am J Gastroenterol 2008; 103(9):2360–5 [quiz: 2366].
24. Smith LB, Lynch KF, Kurppa K, et al. Psychological manifestations of celiac disease autoimmunity in young children. Pediatrics 2017;139(3):e20162848.
25. Singh AD, Singh P, Farooqui N, et al. Prevalence of celiac disease in patients with short stature: a systematic review and meta-analysis. J Gastroenterol Hepatol 2021;36(1):44–54.

26. Laurikka P, Nurminen S, Kivela L, et al. Extraintestinal manifestations of celiac disease: early detection for better long-term outcomes. Nutrients 2018;10(8):1015.
27. Capriati T, Francavilla R, Ferretti F, et al. The overweight: a rare presentation of celiac disease. Eur J Clin Nutr 2016;70(2):282–4.
28. Auricchio R, Mandile R, Del Vecchio MR, et al. Progression of celiac disease in children with antibodies against tissue transglutaminase and normal duodenal architecture. Gastroenterology 2019;157(2):413–20.e3.
29. Canova C, Pitter G, Ludvigsson JF, et al. Celiac disease and risk of autoimmune disorders: a population-based matched birth cohort study. J Pediatr 2016;174: 146–52.e1.
30. Lundin KE, Wijmenga C. Coeliac disease and autoimmune disease-genetic overlap and screening. Nat Rev Gastroenterol Hepatol 2015;12(9):507–15.
31. Hagopian W, Lee HS, Liu E, et al. Co-occurrence of type 1 diabetes and celiac disease autoimmunity. Pediatrics 2017;140(5).
32. Hill ID, Dirks MH, Liptak GS, et al. Guideline for the diagnosis and treatment of celiac disease in children: recommendations of the North American Society for Pediatric Gastroenterology, Hepatology and Nutrition. J Pediatr Gastroenterol Nutr 2005;40(1):1–19.
33. Barton SH, Murray JA. Celiac disease and autoimmunity in the gut and elsewhere. Gastroenterol Clin North Am 2008;37(2):411–28, vii.
34. Catassi C, Ratsch IM, Gandolfi L, et al. Why is coeliac disease endemic in the people of the Sahara? [letter]. Lancet 1999;354(9179):647–8.
35. Shamir R, Lerner A, Shinar E, et al. The use of a single serological marker underestimates the prevalence of celiac disease in Israel: a study of blood donors. Am J Gastroenterol 2002;97(10):2589–94.
36. Rubio-Tapia A, Kyle RA, Kaplan EL, et al. Increased prevalence and mortality in undiagnosed celiac disease. Gastroenterology 2009;137(1):88–93.
37. Bach JF. The hygiene hypothesis in autoimmunity: the role of pathogens and commensals. Nat Rev Immunol 2018;18(2):105–20.
38. Green P, Stavropoulos S, Panagi S, et al. Characteristics of adult celiac disease in the USA: results of a national survey. Am J Gastroenterol 2001;96(1):126–31.
39. Kori M, Goldstein S, Hofi L, et al. Adherence to gluten-free diet and follow-up of pediatric celiac disease patients, during childhood and after transition to adult care. Eur J Pediatr 2021;180(6):1817–23.
40. Whitburn J, Rao SR, Paul SP, et al. Diagnosis of celiac disease is being missed in over 80% of children particularly in those from socioeconomically deprived backgrounds. Eur J Pediatr 2021;180(6):1941–6.
41. McCarty TR, O'Brien CR, Gremida A, et al. Efficacy of duodenal bulb biopsy for diagnosis of celiac disease: a systematic review and meta-analysis. Endosc Int open 2018;6(11):E1369–78.
42. Prasad KK, Thapa BR, Nain CK, et al. The frequency of histologic lesion variability of the duodenal mucosa in children with celiac disease. World J Pediatr 2010; 6(1):60–4.
43. Rubio-Tapia A, Hill ID, Kelly CP, et al. ACG clinical guidelines: diagnosis and management of celiac disease. Am J Gastroenterol 2013;108(5):656–76 [quiz: 677].
44. Hill PG, Holmes GK. Coeliac disease: a biopsy is not always necessary for diagnosis. Aliment Pharmacol Ther 2008;27(7):572–7.
45. Leonard MM, Lebwohl B, Rubio-Tapia A, et al. AGA clinical practice update on the evaluation and management of seronegative enteropathies: expert review. Gastroenterology 2021;160(1):437–44.

46. Marsh MN. Gluten, major histocompatibility complex, and the small intestine. A molecular and immunobiologic approach to the spectrum of gluten sensitivity ('celiac sprue'). Gastroenterology 1992;102(1):330–54.

47. Oberhuber G. Histopathology of celiac disease. Biomed Pharmacother 2000; 54(7):368–72.

48. Accetta P, Kumar V, Beutner EH, et al. Anti-endomysial antibodies. A serologic marker of dermatitis herpetiformis. Arch Dermatol 1986;122(4):459–62.

49. Mansikka E, Hervonen K, Kaukinen K, et al. Prognosis of dermatitis herpetiformis patients with and without villous atrophy at diagnosis. Nutrients 2018;10(5).

50. Giersiepen K, Lelgemann M, Stuhldreher N, et al. Accuracy of diagnostic antibody tests for coeliac disease in children: summary of an evidence report. J Pediatr Gastroenterol Nutr 2012;54(2):229–41.

51. Bao F, Yu L, Babu S, et al. One third of HLA DQ2 homozygous patients with type 1 diabetes express celiac disease-associated transglutaminase autoantibodies. J Autoimmun 1999;13(1):143–8.

52. Kelly CP, Bai JC, Liu E, et al. Advances in diagnosis and management of celiac disease. Gastroenterology 2015;148(6):1175–86.

53. Frulio G, Polimeno A, Palmieri D, et al. Evaluating diagnostic accuracy of anti-tissue transglutaminase IgA antibodies as first screening for celiac disease in very young children. Clin Chim Acta 2015;446:237–40.

54. Husby S, Koletzko S, Korponay-Szabo IR, et al. European Society for Pediatric Gastroenterology, Hepatology, and Nutrition guidelines for the diagnosis of coeliac disease. J Pediatr Gastroenterol Nutr 2012;54(1):136–60.

55. Werkstetter KJ, Korponay-Szabo IR, Popp A, et al. Accuracy in diagnosis of celiac disease without biopsies in clinical practice. Gastroenterology 2017;153(4): 924–35.

56. Oxentenko AS, Rubio-Tapia A. Celiac disease. Mayo Clin Proc 2019;94(12): 2556–71.

57. Leonard MM, Silvester JA, Leffler D, et al. Evaluating responses to gluten challenge: a randomized, double-blind, 2-dose gluten challenge trial. Gastroenterology 2021;160(3):720–33.e8.

58. Hardy MY, Tye-Din JA, Stewart JA, et al. Ingestion of oats and barley in patients with celiac disease mobilizes cross-reactive T cells activated by avenin peptides and immuno-dominant hordein peptides. J Autoimmun 2015;56:56–65.

59. Tio M, Cox MR, Eslick GD. Meta-analysis: coeliac disease and the risk of all-cause mortality, any malignancy and lymphoid malignancy. Aliment Pharmacol Ther 2012;35(5):540–51.

60. Vilppula A, Kaukinen K, Luostarinen L, et al. Clinical benefit of gluten-free diet in screen-detected older celiac disease patients. BMC Gastroenterol 2011;11:136.

61. National Institutes of Health Consensus Development Conference Statement on Celiac Disease, June 28-30, 2004. Gastroenterology 2005;128(4 Suppl 1):S1–9.

62. Bongiovanni TR, Clark AL, Garnett EA, et al. Impact of gluten-free camp on quality of life of children and adolescents with celiac disease. Pediatrics 2010;125(3): e525–9.

63. Park SD, Markowitz J, Pettei M, et al. Failure to respond to hepatitis B vaccine in children with celiac disease. J Pediatr Gastroenterol Nutr 2007;44(4):431–5.

64. Noh KW, Poland GA, Murray JA. Hepatitis B vaccine nonresponse and celiac disease. Am J Gastroenterol 2003;98(10):2289–92.

65. Fabiani E, Taccari L, Ratsch I, et al. Compliance with gluten-free diet in adolescents with screening-detected celiac disease: a 5-year follow-up study. J Pediatr 2000;136(6):841–3.

66. Leonard MM, Weir DC, DeGroote M, et al. Value of IgA tTG in predicting mucosal recovery in children with celiac disease on a gluten-free diet. J Pediatr Gastroenterol Nutr 2017;64(2):286–91.
67. Fang H, King KS, Larson JJ, et al. Undetectable negative tissue transglutaminase IgA antibodies predict mucosal healing in treated coeliac disease patients. Aliment Pharmacol Ther 2017;46(7):681–7.
68. Godfrey JD, Brantner TL, Brinjikji W, et al. Morbidity and mortality among older individuals with undiagnosed celiac disease. Gastroenterology 2010;139(3): 763–9.
69. Fuchs V, Kurppa K, Huhtala H, et al. Delayed celiac disease diagnosis predisposes to reduced quality of life and incremental use of health care services and medicines: A prospective nationwide study. United Eur Gastroenterol J 2018;6(4):567–75.
70. Lewis NR, Holmes GK. Risk of morbidity in contemporary celiac disease. Expert Rev Gastroenterol Hepatol 2010;4(6):767–80.
71. Caio G, Volta U, Ursini F, et al. Small bowel adenocarcinoma as a complication of celiac disease: clinical and diagnostic features. BMC Gastroenterol 2019; 19(1):45.
72. Serena G, Kelly CP, Fasano A. Nondietary therapies for celiac disease. Gastroenterol Clin North Am 2019;48(1):145–63.

Advances in Endoscopic Procedures in Pediatric Patients

Amornluck Krasaelap, MD[a],*, Diana G. Lerner, MD[b]

KEYWORDS

- Advanced endoscopy • Transnasal endoscopy • FLIP • Mucosal impedance
- Endoscopic vacuum • Chromoendoscopy • Artificial intelligence

KEY POINTS

- Following their adoption in the adult population, new diagnostic and therapeutic modalities are making their way into pediatrics.
- New technologies such as transnasal endoscopy, functional luminal imaging probe, mucosal impedance, chromoendoscopy, artificial intelligence, and machine learning enable more accurate and faster diagnosis of GI diseases in children.
- New therapeutic procedures, such as peroral endoscopic myotomy for achalasia and endoscopic vacuum-assisted closure system for esophageal perforations, demonstrate encouraging and safe results in children.

INTRODUCTION

Pediatric endoscopy has been performed over several decades and continues to be an integral part of the diagnostic and therapeutic modality in managing gastrointestinal (GI) disorders in children. Despite limitations in pediatric-specific devices, remarkable advances have been made in pediatric GI endoscopy in the past several years. This article highlights recent advances in state-of-the-art diagnostic and therapeutic GI endoscopic procedures in the pediatric population.

TRANSNASAL ENDOSCOPY

Unsedated transnasal endoscopy (TNE) has been an established technique in pediatric pulmonary and otolaryngology specialties and has gained attention over the past several years. In Asia, particularly Japan, nearly half of all endoscopies are performed by the transnasal route and in clinic settings.[1,2] Early studies on unsedated TNE

ª Division of Pediatric Gastroenterology, Hepatology and Nutrition, Children's Mercy Hospital, 2401 Gillham Road, Kansas City, MO 64108, USA; ᵇ Division of Pediatric Gastroenterology, Hepatology and Nutrition, Department of Pediatrics, Medical College of Wisconsin, 8701 Watertown Plank Road, Milwaukee, WI 53226, USA
* Corresponding author.
E-mail address: akrasaelap@cmh.edu

Pediatr Clin N Am 68 (2021) 1221–1235
https://doi.org/10.1016/j.pcl.2021.07.005
0031-3955/21/© 2021 Elsevier Inc. All rights reserved.

demonstrated its utility in esophageal diseases, mainly for Barrett's esophagus screening in patients with chronic gastroesophageal reflux[3] or variceal screening in patients with cirrhosis.[4] Recently, TNE has become a promising alternative to a conventional esophagogastroduodenoscopy (EGD) in pediatric patients with eosinophilic esophagitis (EoE) who typically require serial EGDs. Advantages of TNE over EGD are the lack of anesthesia, parents' presence during the procedure, the procedure's shorter duration, and rapid recovery. During TNE, the endoscope or bronchoscope is passed through the nose and the procedure can be completed with a local anesthetic spray within 5 to 15 minutes. The use of virtual reality and video goggles can improve patient experience during the procedure.[5] (**Fig. 1**) According to Friedlander and colleagues,[6] visual findings from TNE correlated with histologic findings in 85% of subjects. The epithelial surface area of the samples obtained by TNE with 2-mm or 1.2-mm biopsy forceps was not significantly different from that obtained by EGD with 2.8-mm biopsy forceps.[6] TNE is currently being used mostly to assess pathologic condition in the esophagus.

Studies have demonstrated TNE to be a safe, effective, and well-tolerated option. Self-reported symptoms associated with TNE included gagging and sore throat. However, no adverse event has been associated with the need for emergency department evaluation.[6] Overall perception of TNE among families was positive, and most families preferred TNE to EGD and would reelect to have TNE if needed.[7] For some families, total billed charges for TNE were reduced by 50% to 70% when compared with EGD.[5]

FUNCTIONAL LUMEN IMAGING PROBE

Functional lumen imaging probe (FLIP) is a novel endoscopic tool that uses high-resolution impedance planimetry to measure pressure-geometry relationships of GI luminal space during volume-controlled distension.[8] A cylinder-shaped balloon with a 16-sensor catheter inside measures the electrical voltage between neighboring sensors. FLIP provides many luminal parameters, including diameter, compliance, cross-sectional area (CSA), pressure, and disability index. FLIP is considered a complementary tool to assess the esophageal wall's mechanical properties

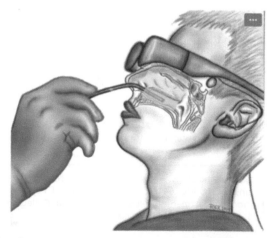

Fig. 1. *Transnasal endoscopy* insertion between the inferior turbinate (green) and middle turbinate (yellow). (*From* Koo S., Leinwand K., Panter S., Friedlander JA. Transnasal Gastrointestinal Endoscopy. Practical Pediatric Gastrointestinal Endoscopy. 3rd ed. Wiley Blackwell; n.d. p. 377–84, with permission.)

and the dynamics of the upper esophageal sphincter and lower esophageal sphincter (LES) in various esophageal diseases.[8] Although promising data focused primarily on esophagogastric junction (EGJ) obstruction and EoE, FLIP has also been used in esophageal stenosis, gastroparesis, sphincter of Oddi, and anal sphincter disease.[9]

There are 2 versions of the FLIP: EndoFLIP and EsoFLIP (Medtronic, Minneapolis, MN, USA). EndoFLIP is a soft balloon tool used solely for geographic measurements. EsoFLIP uses a stiffer balloon, similar to a controlled radial expansion dilation balloon. In contrast to EndoFLIP, EsoFLIP can dilate the narrowing while providing the exact diameter and CSA changes in real time[10] (**Fig. 2**).

The utility of EndoFLIP in pediatric EoE was reported in a few recent pediatric studies. Menard-Katcher and colleagues[11] reported decreased distensibility in subjects with EoE compared with controls. In contrast, a study from Hassan and colleagues[12] showed a significant difference in compliance but not distensibility between the 2 groups. There was a strong correlation between compliance and both epithelial remodeling and eosinophilic density in the esophagus. These findings differ from adult data that showed no association between esophageal eosinophilia, decreased distensibility,[13] and food impaction risk.[14]

Taylor and colleagues[15] reported the first pediatric case using EsoFLIP to dilate esophageal anastomotic stricture in 2018. Ng and colleagues[10] described a cohort of 18 pediatric patients with esophageal stenosis undergoing either EndoFLIP with traditional balloon dilation or EsoFLIP procedure. Although both techniques were effective, esophageal dilation using EsoFLIP may yield a larger diameter change and potentially reduce procedure time compared with traditional balloon dilation. No complication was observed.[10]

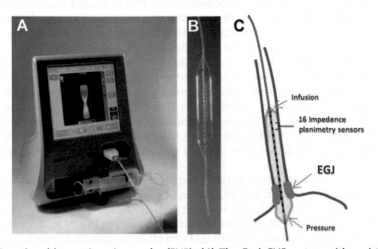

Fig. 2. Functional lumen imaging probe (FLIP). (*A*) The EndoFLIP system with real-time 3D imaging of the EGJ. The blue color on the screen represents the narrowest portion at the EGJ. (*B*) The EndoFLIP balloon. (*C*) Positioning of the distal portion of the EndoFLIP balloon through the EGJ and 10 recording segments in the body of the esophagus. The paired impedance planimetry rings (black) provide the measure of diameter and cross-sectional area. The pressure sensor (blue circle) is located in the distal aspect of the catheter and the infusion port (red circle) in the balloon's proximal aspect. (*From* Hirano I., Pandolfino JE., Boeckxstaens GE. Functional Lumen Imaging Probe for the Management of Esophageal Disorders: Expert Review From the Clinical Practice Updates Committee of the AGA Institute. Clin Gastroenterol Hepatol 2017;15(3):325–34, with permission.)

The use of FLIP in children is still limited to a few pediatric GI centers due to the lack of standardized protocol for children, cost, and invasiveness, particularly compared with conventional manometric testing with additional provocative studies.[16] Future studies should focus on obtaining normative data in children, investigating the utility of FLIP in pediatric dysphagia, and intraoperative assessment of the EGJ, upper esophageal sphincter, pylorus, and anal sphincter.[17]

PERORAL ENDOSCOPIC MYOTOMY PROCEDURE

Peroral endoscopic myotomy (POEM) was first described in an animal model in 2007 by Pasricha and colleagues[18] and introduced to clinical practice in Japan in 2010 by Inoue and colleagues.[19] POEM is performed by creating a submucosal tunnel endoscopically to reach the LES and dissect the muscle fibers (**Fig. 3**). POEM has emerged as a promising treatment modality for achalasia in adults, with good short- and long-term outcomes.[20] POEM is less invasive and cheaper and offers faster recovery when compared with conventional Heller myotomy (HM).

The steps of the POEM procedure in children are mainly similar to those in adults, and only slight modifications are required to accommodate the structural anatomic size differences in children. The length of myotomy is usually shorter than that of adults.

The most recent systematic review, comprising 11 studies with 389 children, showed a pooled technical success rate of 97%.[21] The pooled clinical success rate was achieved in 92% of children (94% success rate in <1-year, 97% in 1- to 3-year, and 96% in >3-year follow-up). After POEM, the Eckardt score was significantly decreased by 6.7 points (*P*<.00001) and the LES pressure was significantly reduced by 19.4 mm Hg (*P*<.00001). The pooled major POEM-related adverse event rate was 13%. Common adverse events were pneumoperitoneum, mucosal injury, pneumonitis, subcutaneous emphysema, mediastinal emphysema, and pneumothorax, which were mainly self-limited. The postoperative gastroesophageal reflux rate was 18%. POEM is an effective and safe technique for treating pediatric achalasia.[21]

The most recent guidelines in 2021 from the Society of American Gastrointestinal and Endoscopic Surgeons strongly recommended the use of either POEM or HM with fundoplication for achalasia subtypes 1 and 2 based on surgeon and patient shared decision making.[22] This recommendation was also generalized to the pediatric population, given the lack of contradictory data in children. The panel also favored POEM over HM for type III adult or pediatric achalasia based on expert opinion.[22]

In 2019, a survey of 44 pediatric gastrologists from 38 centers (95% being secondary referral centers) showed that POEM was considered the treatment of choice by only 29% compared with 58% for HM and 46% for pneumatic dilation[23]; this could be in part due to the lack of available specialists to perform POEM in children. Further randomized comparative studies of POEM and other therapeutic methods for managing pediatric achalasia are needed to measure long-term outcomes and postoperative reflux.

MUCOSAL IMPEDANCE

Another novel technology that was developed to identify the degree of esophageal mucosal integrity is multichannel intraluminal impedance (MII). Baseline impedance was originally determined by obtaining measurements during a nocturnal fast when the esophagus was in constant contact with the probe. Mean nocturnal baseline

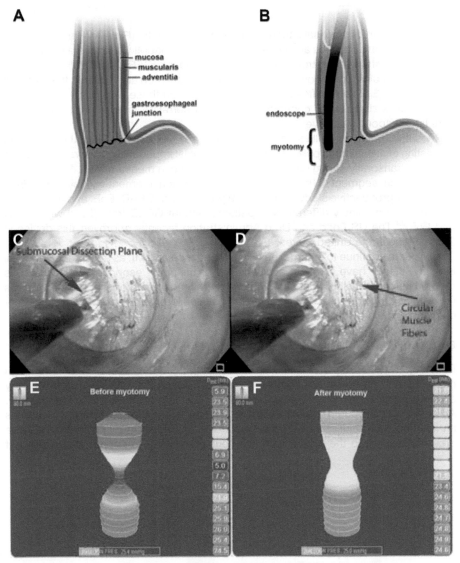

Fig. 3. Peroral endoscopic myotomy procedure. (*A*) Diagram demonstrating premyotomy esophageal anatomy. (*B*) Anatomy after myotomy with endoscope within the methylene blue submucosal dissection plane and remaining longitudinal muscle after incising the LES's circular muscle. (*C, D*) Endoscopic images demonstrating submucosal dissection plane and circular muscle fibers. (*E, F*) EndoFLIP screenshots with esophageal diameters at the LES before and after myotomy. (*From* Wood LS., Chandler JM., Portelli KE., Taylor JS., Kethman WC., Wall JK. Treating children with achalasia using per-oral endoscopic myotomy (POEM): Twenty-one cases in review. Journal of Pediatric Surgery 2020;55(6):1006–12, with permission.)

impedance has been shown to correlate with acid exposure time and potentially distinguish patients with pathologic reflux from those with functional heartburn.[24,25]

The newest development is a 2-mm, through-the-scope catheter that can detect changes in electrical impedance to compromised epithelial barrier integrity at the time of endoscopy. This mucosal impedance (MI) catheter can decrease potential artifacts, eliminating discomfort from the transnasal catheter, and prove the ability to the target evaluation of mucosal integrity in regions of interest[26] (**Fig. 4**). A large prospective study in adults by Ates and colleagues[27] showed that MI values were significantly lower in patients with gastroesophageal reflux disease (GERD) and EoE than in patients with achalasia or in controls. The first study in children also showed that patients with active EoE have significantly lower MI values than those with inactive EoE, nonerosive reflux disease, or controls.[28] MI values correlate inversely with eosinophil counts and spongiosis severity.[28]

Recently, Patel and colleagues[29] developed a novel balloon MI catheter system consisting of an inflatable balloon with radial and axial impedance sensors. This device is placed transorally during sedated endoscopy and can measure MI at 180° intervals along a 10-cm segment of the esophagus, reducing measurement variability (**Fig. 5**). A multicenter prospective study evaluated 69 patients with GERD, EoE, and non-GERD. The MI pattern reliably differentiated patients without GERD from those with GERD and EoE.[29] The US Food and Drug Administration recently approved this device in 2019 for use in the United States.

While data continue to emerge, baseline impedance and MI, as a marker of mucosal integrity, clearly have a role in evaluating and managing esophageal disease. This method can potentially obviate ambulatory pH/MII monitoring or esophageal biopsies for histology in the future. Prospective studies in children are needed to evaluate efficacy in pediatric disorders.

ENDOSCOPIC VACUUM-ASSISTED CLOSURE SYSTEM

Esophageal perforations and leakage after esophagogastrostomy can cause high morbidity and mortality. For primary endoscopic management, self-expanding fully covered metallic stent (SEMS) placement is typically considered first-line therapy. An endoscopic vacuum-assisted closure system (E-VAC) has recently emerged as an alternative or adjunct for leak therapy. E-VAC is based on a continuous negative pressure applied to the wound with a porous material. E-VAC promotes healing of

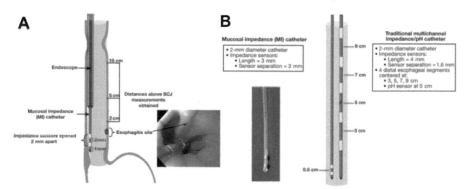

Fig. 4. Mucosal impedance (MI) catheter. (*A*) Two 2-mm-long impedance sensing electrodes positioned 1 mm from the tip of a 2-mm soft catheter were advanced through an upper endoscope. MI measurements were obtained by direct mucosal contact of sensors at the site of esophagitis (if present) and 2, 5, and 10 cm above the squamocolumnar junction (SCJ). (*B*) MI catheter (*inset*) and schematic comparison of the MI catheter with the traditional multichannel impedance pH catheter along the esophageal lumen. Measurements represent distances from the SCJ. (*From* Ates F., Yuksel ES., Higginbotham T., et al. Mucosal impedance discriminates GERD from non-GERD conditions. Gastroenterology 2015;148(2):334–43, with permission.)

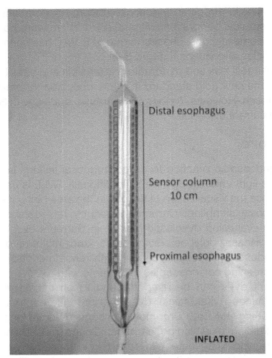

Fig. 5. A mucosal impedance balloon catheter with 36 channels measuring impedance axially and radially along a 10 cm length of the esophagus. (*From* Patel DA., Higginbotham T., Slaughter JC., et al. Development and Validation of a Mucosal Impedance Contour Analysis System to Distinguish Esophageal Disorders. Gastroenterology 2019;156(6):1617-1626.e1, with permission.)

leaks/perforations by maintaining source control, debriding wounds, and encouraging tissue reperfusion.

Several adult cohorts demonstrated the effectiveness of E-VAC as a sole therapy or as part of a multimodality approach for anastomotic leaks and iatrogenic perforations of the esophagus. Studies showed that E-VAC had an excellent healing rate of 83% to 100%, with a median treatment duration between 5 and 14 days.[30–35] Possible complications of E-VAC include stricture formation and acute bleeding during E-VAC placement, which is rare but potentially life threatening. A more extensive study of 366 patients by Schniewind and colleagues[36] showed that E-VAC is superior to other modalities. E-VAC has a lower mortality rate when compared with surgery (12% vs 50%, $P = .01$) and SEMS (12% vs 83%, $P = .0014$).[36]

A recent systematic review and meta-analysis by do Monte Junior and colleagues[37] included five studies with a total of 279 adult patients who underwent SEMS or E-VAC for treatment of upper GI transmural defects. In this study, E-VAC was reported to have a 21% higher fistula closure rate ($P = .0003$); a 12% decrease in mortality ($P = .006$), with a shorter duration of treatment by 14 days ($P<.00001$); and a 24% decrease in adverse events ($P = .0001$) when compared with SEMS.[37]

Manfredi and colleagues[38] reported the first pediatric study in 17 patients with esophageal atresia undergoing esophageal perforation for surgical and endoscopic therapy perforation. The success rates for E-VAC and stent placement were 88% (7 of 8) and 63% (15 of 24), respectively. The study showed that E-VAC was comparable to esophageal stenting in iatrogenic endoscopic therapy perforations (P = .36) and superior to stenting surgical perforations (P = .032).[38] There were no technical failures with placement or complications. The technique of E-VAC has been illustrated in multiple published articles and videos[39] (**Figs. 6–8**).

E-VAC for esophageal leak and perforations is feasible and safe. E-VAC has the potential to become the new gold standard in the endoscopic treatment of esophageal leaks and perforations. However, further comparative studies with SEMS are needed to strengthen the current evidence.

CHROMOENDOSCOPY

Current clinical endoscopic practice to detect mucosal lesions in the GI tract uses conventional white-light endoscopy (WLE). Traditionally, WLE is used in combination with dyes to enhance the visualization of tissues in the area being inspected and facilitate optimal mucosal sampling. Chromoendoscopy has demonstrated improved diagnostic yield in evaluating dysplastic lesions in Barrett's esophagus and related disorders, celiac disease, polyposis syndromes, and inflammatory bowel disease (IBD).[40] Chromoendoscopy with dye is the currently recommended method for detecting dysplasia in screening colonoscopies in patients with IBD.[41]

Different types of dyes can be used depending on indications, such as dyes absorbed by the mucosa (vital stains), dyes that produce contrast (reactive stains), and dyes for tattooing mucosa. Chromoendoscopy dyes include methylene blue, Lugol solution, toluidine blue, indigo carmine, Congo red, phenol red, and India ink.[42] Despite its significant advantage in detecting lesions, dye-based chromoendoscopy is not widely used because it is time consuming, not readily available, and may cause side effects in some patients.[43]

Virtual chromoendoscopy (VCE) is a new technology that can provide visualization of tissues without dyes, enabling the endoscopist to identify abnormal tissues in real time during endoscopy. In optical VCE, optic filters, which are integrated into the endoscope's light source, selectively filter white light, as in narrow-band imaging technology (NBI, Olympus, Tokyo, Japan). In digital VCE, further systems digitally

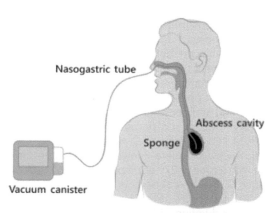

Fig. 6. Diagram of the basic endoscopic vacuum-assisted closure system setup. A black wound sponge is attached to the end of a 14F nasogastric tube and placed endoscopically into the abscess cavity or luminal defect. The nasogastric tube is then attached to a negative pressure wound vacuum therapy system. (*From* Watkins JR., Farivar AS. Endoluminal Therapies for Esophageal Perforations and Leaks. Thorac Surg Clin 2018;28(4):541–54, with permission.)

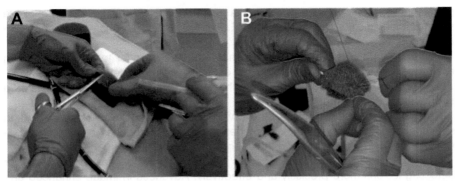

Fig. 7. Endoscopic vacuum-assisted closure system assembly. (*A*) Preparing the sponge in the operating room by trimming it to size. (*B*) Securing the sponge to the end of a nasogastric tube after placing it through the nares. (*From* Watkins JR., Farivar AS. Endoluminal Therapies for Esophageal Perforations and Leaks. Thorac Surg Clin 2018;28(4):541–54, with permission.)

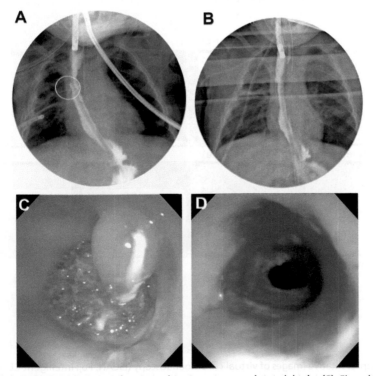

Fig. 8. (*A*) Before E-VAC, esophagram showing an esophageal leak. (*B*) Five days after E-VAC, esophagram showing the resolution of esophageal leak. (*C*) E-VAC is placed inside the esophagus. (*D*) Five days after E-VAC, endoscopic inspection showing the resolution of esophageal leak.

process endoscopic images to provide a series of light wavelengths, as in flexible spectral imaging color enhancement (FICE, FujiFilm, Willich, Germany) or i-scan (Pentax, Tokyo, Japan).

Recent meta-analyses demonstrated that VCE was superior to WLE in detecting esophageal squamous cell carcinoma[44,45] or similar to WLE in detecting neoplastic lesions in patients with IBD.[46,47] VCE was, however, technically easier and required a shorter examination time.

Other emerging technologies that allow microscopic visualization of surface and subsurface tissues include confocal laser endomicroscopy, optical coherence tomography, Raman spectroscopy, and multiphoton tomography[48] (**Fig. 9**).

New technologies in endoscopic imaging provide vast potential for detecting lesions more precisely and effectively. Advances in image-enhanced and new-generation endoscopic imaging may allow near-histologic assessment of tissue during endoscopy and may replace the need for tissue biopsy in the future.

ARTIFICIAL INTELLIGENCE AND MACHINE LEARNING

The quality of endoscopic imaging in gastroenterology has increased significantly in recent years through high-definition WLE and preprocessing optical chromoendoscopy. As a result, the endoscopy challenge has shifted from diagnostic visualization to interpretation using artificial intelligence (AI) or machine learning (ML).[49]

AI is commonly used interchangeably with ML, but it is generally a broader term. AI refers to an algorithm that performs tasks usually requiring human intelligence. ML is a

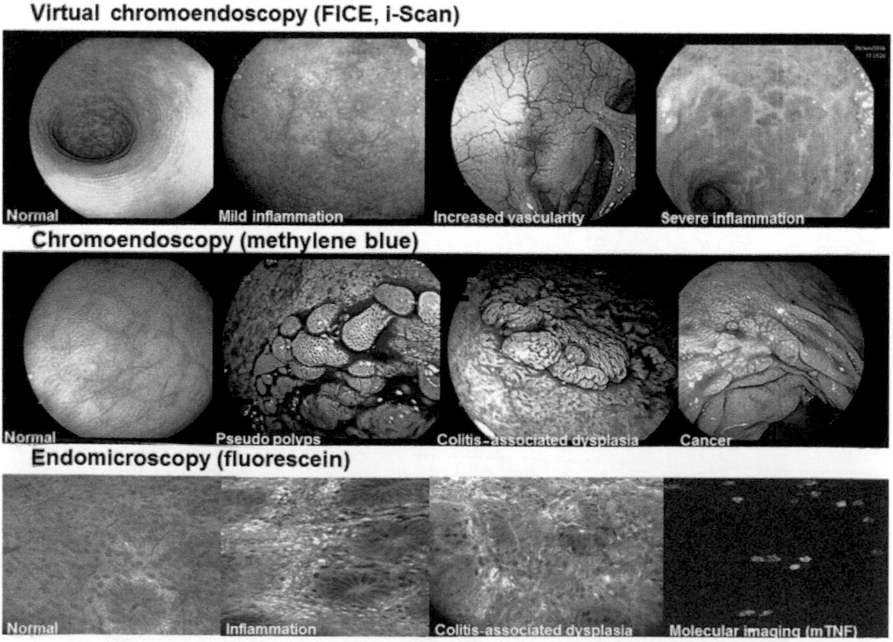

Fig. 9. Representative images of virtual chromoendoscopy (iSCAN, Fuji intelligent CE [FujiFilm, Willich, Germany]), dye-based chromoendoscopy (*methylene blue*), and confocal laser endomicroscopy for the detection of mucosal inflammation and neoplasias in patients with inflammatory bowel disease. (*From* Kiesslich R., Neurath MF. Advanced endoscopy imaging in inflammatory bowel diseases. Gastrointestinal Endoscopy 2017;85(3):496–508, with permission.)

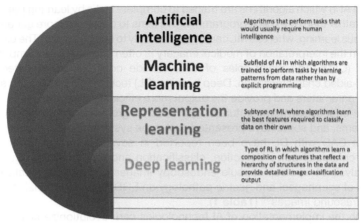

Fig. 10. Hierarchy of artificial intelligence domains. RL, representation learning. (*From* Pannala R., Krishnan K., Melson J., et al. Emerging role of artificial intelligence in GI endoscopy. Gastrointestinal Endoscopy 2020;92(6):1151–2, with permission.)

Table 1	
Reported applications of computer-aided diagnosis and artificial intelligence in various endoscopic procedures	
Procedure	**Applications**
Colon	• Detection of polyps (real time and on still images and video) • Classification of polyps (neoplastic vs hyperplastic) Detection of malignancy within polyps (depth of invasion on endocytoscopic images) • Presence of mucosal inflammation on endocytoscopic images • Assessment of disease activity in inflammatory bowel disease • Evaluation of quality metrics in colonoscopy
Wireless capsule endoscopy	• Lesion detection and classification (bleeding, ulcers, polyps) • Assessment of intestinal motility • Celiac disease (assessment of villous atrophy, intestinal motility) • Improve the efficiency of image review • Deletion of duplicate images and uninformative image frames (eg, images with debris)
Upper endoscopy	• Identify anatomic location • Diagnosis of *Helicobacter pylori* infection • Gastric cancer detection and assessing depth of invasion • Esophageal squamous dysplasia • Detection and delineation of early dysplasia in Barrett's esophagus • Real-time image segmentation in volumetric laser endomicroscopy in Barrett's esophagus
Endoscopic ultrasonography	• Differentiation of pancreatic cancer from chronic pancreatitis and normal pancreas • Differentiation of autoimmune pancreatitis from chronic pancreatitis • Endoscopic ultrasonographic elastography

From Pannala R., Krishnan K., Melson J., et al. Emerging role of artificial intelligence in GI endoscopy. Gastrointest Endosc 2020;92(6):1151–2; with permission.

subfield of AI in which algorithms are trained to complete tasks by learning patterns from raw data rather than by explicit programming. AI aims to develop a more generic form of autonomous learning, whereas ML can be applied only to specific tasks. The use of ML in assisting in the interpretation of medical imagery is often referred to as computer-aided diagnosis (CAD). The major roles of CAD include computer-aided detection and computer-aided characterization. Deep learning (DL) technology enables the system to adapt the parameters and provide the output more efficiently (**Fig. 10**).

Multiple endoscopy manufacturers and research groups are currently developing CAD systems, and some have presented prototype systems. So far, numerous applications of CAD with DL have been reported in several areas of GI endoscopy, including colorectal polyp detection, classification and real-time histologic assessment, analysis of wireless capsule endoscopy images and videos, localization and diagnosis of esophageal and gastric pathology on EGD, and image analysis of endoscopic ultrasound images[50] (**Table 1**).

Although the implementation of AI technologies can revolutionize clinical practice and are introduced as "game-changers" in endoscopy, studies reporting results of CAD implementation during real-time procedures are still scarce. An AI system that can be used in clinical practice is not currently commercially available.

CLINICS CARE POINTS

- Endoscopy is a crucial part of the diagnosis and therapy in pediatric GI disorders.
- New modalities are transitioning to pediatrics after adoption in the adult population
- Advancements in current technologies provide accurate and more rapid diagnosis and offer an alternative treatment of multiple GI conditions.

SUMMARY

In recent years, new imaging technologies and advanced therapeutic procedures have transformed endoscopy. Most of the new modalities are often used initially in adult patients and gradually applied to the pediatric field. Advancements in current technologies do not only generate excitement among gastroenterologists but also benefit patients' care by providing an accurate and faster diagnosis and offering alternative treatment in multiple GI conditions.

ACKNOWLEDGMENTS

The authors thank the Medical Writing Center at Children's Mercy Kansas City for editing this article.

DISCLOSURE

A. Krasaelap has nothing to disclose. D. Lerner is the founder of Lerner Media Inc.

REFERENCES

1. Tatsumi Y, Harada A, Matsumoto T, et al. Current Status and Evaluation of Transnasal Esophagogastroduodenoscopy. Dig Endosc 2009;21(3):141–6.
2. Tanuma T, Morita Y, Doyama H. Current status of transnasal endoscopy worldwide using ultrathin videoscope for upper gastrointestinal tract. Dig Endosc 2016;28(Suppl 1):25–31.

3. Saeian K, Staff DM, Vasilopoulos S, et al. Unsedated transnasal endoscopy accurately detects Barrett's metaplasia and dysplasia. Gastrointest Endosc 2002; 56(4):472–8.
4. Saeian K, Staff D, Knox J, et al. Unsedated transnasal endoscopy: a new technique for accurately detecting and grading esophageal varices in cirrhotic patients. Am J Gastroenterol 2002;97(9):2246–9.
5. Nguyen N, Lavery WJ, Capocelli KE, et al. Transnasal Endoscopy in Unsedated Children With Eosinophilic Esophagitis Using Virtual Reality Video Goggles. Clin Gastroenterol Hepatol 2019;17(12):2455-62.
6. Friedlander JA, DeBoer EM, Soden JS, et al. Unsedated transnasal esophagoscopy for monitoring therapy in pediatric eosinophilic esophagitis. Gastrointest Endosc 2016;83(2):299–306.e1.
7. Scherer C, Sosensky P, Schulman-Green D, et al. Pediatric Patients' and Parents' Perspectives of Unsedated Transnasal Endoscopy in Eosinophilic Esophagitis: A Qualitative Descriptive Study. J Pediatr Gastroenterol Nutr 2020;72(4):558–62.
8. Hirano I, Pandolfino JE, Boeckxstaens GE. Functional Lumen Imaging Probe for the Management of Esophageal Disorders: Expert Review From the Clinical Practice Updates Committee of the AGA Institute. Clin Gastroenterol Hepatol 2017; 15(3):325–34.
9. Desprez C, Roman S, Leroi AM, et al. The use of impedance planimetry (Endoscopic Functional Lumen Imaging Probe, EndoFLIP®) in the gastrointestinal tract: A systematic review. Neurogastroenterol Motil 2020;32(9):e13980.
10. Ng K, Mogul D, Hollier J, et al. Utility of functional lumen imaging probe in esophageal measurements and dilations: a single pediatric center experience. Surg Endosc 2020;34(3):1294–9.
11. Menard-Katcher C, Benitez AJ, Pan Z, et al. Influence of age and eosinophilic esophagitis on esophageal distensibility in a pediatric cohort. Am J Gastroenterol 2017;112(9):1466–73.
12. Hassan M, Aceves S, Dohil R, et al. Esophageal compliance quantifies epithelial remodeling in pediatric patients with eosinophilic esophagitis. J Pediatr Gastroenterol Nutr 2019;68(4):559–65.
13. Kwiatek MA, Hirano I, Kahrilas PJ, et al. Mechanical Properties of the Esophagus in Eosinophilic Esophagitis. Gastroenterology 2011;140(1):82–90.
14. Carlson D, Lin Z, Hirano I, et al. Evaluation of esophageal distensibility in eosinophilic esophagitis: An update and comparison of functional lumen imaging probe analytic methods. Neurogastroenterol Motil 2016;28(12):1844–53.
15. Taylor JS, Danzer E, Berquist WE, et al. Dilation of Esophageal Stricture in a Pediatric Patient Using Functional Lumen Imaging Probe Technology Without the Use of Fluoroscopy. J Pediatr Gastroenterol Nutr 2018;67(2):e20–1.
16. Massey BT. Clinical Functional Lumen Imaging Probe Testing in Esophageal Disorders: A Need for Better Quality Evidence. Am J Gastroenterol 2020;115(11): 1799–801.
17. Savarino E, Pietro M di, Bredenoord A, et al. Use of the Functional Lumen Imaging Probe in Clinical Esophagology. Am J Gastroenterol 2020;115(11):1786–96.
18. Pasricha PJ, Hawari R, Ahmed I, et al. Submucosal endoscopic esophageal myotomy: a novel experimental approach for the treatment of achalasia. Endoscopy 2007;39(09):761–4.
19. Inoue H, Minami H, Kobayashi Y, et al. Peroral endoscopic myotomy (POEM) for esophageal achalasia. Endoscopy 2010;42(04):265–71.
20. Shiwaku H, Inoue H, Onimaru M, et al. Multicenter collaborative retrospective evaluation of peroral endoscopic myotomy for esophageal achalasia: analysis

of data from more than 1300 patients at eight facilities in Japan. Surg Endosc 2020;34(1):464–8.

21. Zhong C, Tan S, Huang S, et al. Clinical outcomes of peroral endoscopic myotomy for achalasia in children: a systematic review and meta-analysis. Dis Esophagus 2020;34(4):doaa112.

22. Kohn GP, Dirks RC, Ansari MT, et al. SAGES guidelines for the use of peroral endoscopic myotomy (POEM) for the treatment of achalasia. Surg Endosc 2021;35(5):1931–48.

23. van Lennep M, van Wijk MP, Omari TIM, et al. Clinical Management of Pediatric Achalasia: A Survey of Current Practice. J Pediatr Gastroenterol Nutr 2019;68(4): 521–6.

24. Frazzoni M, Savarino E, de Bortoli N, et al. Analyses of the Post-reflux Swallow-induced Peristaltic Wave Index and Nocturnal Baseline Impedance Parameters Increase the Diagnostic Yield of Impedance-pH Monitoring of Patients With Reflux Disease. Clin Gastroenterol Hepatol 2016;14(1):40 -6.

25. Frazzoni L, Frazzoni M, Bortoli N de, et al. Postreflux swallow-induced peristaltic wave index and nocturnal baseline impedance can link PPI-responsive heartburn to reflux better than acid exposure time. Neurogastroenterol Motil 2017;29(11): e13116.

26. Clarke JO, Ahuja NK, Chan WW, et al. Mucosal impedance for esophageal disease: evaluating the evidence. Ann N Y Acad Sci 2020;1481(1):247–57.

27. Ates F, Yuksel ES, Higginbotham T, et al. Mucosal impedance discriminates GERD from non-GERD conditions. Gastroenterology 2015;148(2):334–43.

28. Lowry MA, Vaezi MF, Correa H, et al. Mucosal Impedance Measurements Differentiate Pediatric Patients with Active vs Inactive Eosinophilic Esophagitis. J Pediatr Gastroenterol Nutr 2018;67(2):198–203.

29. Patel DA, Higginbotham T, Slaughter JC, et al. Development and Validation of a Mucosal Impedance Contour Analysis System to Distinguish Esophageal Disorders. Gastroenterology 2019;156(6):1617–26.e1.

30. Schorsch T, Müller C, Loske G. [Endoscopic vacuum therapy of perforations and anastomotic insufficiency of the esophagus]. Chirurg 2014;85(12):1081–93.

31. Laukoetter MG, Mennigen R, Neumann PA, et al. Successful closure of defects in the upper gastrointestinal tract by endoscopic vacuum therapy (EVT): a prospective cohort study. Surg Endosc 2017;31(6):2687–96.

32. Wedemeyer J, Brangewitz M, Kubicka S, et al. Management of major postsurgical gastroesophageal intrathoracic leaks with an endoscopic vacuum-assisted closure system. Gastrointest Endosc 2010;71(2):382–6.

33. Jung CFM, Müller-Dornieden A, Gaedcke J, et al. Impact of Endoscopic Vacuum Therapy with Low Negative Pressure for Esophageal Perforations and Postoperative Anastomotic Esophageal Leaks. Digestion 2020;102(3):469–79.

34. Zhang CC, Liesenfeld L, Klotz R, et al. Feasibility, effectiveness, and safety of endoscopic vacuum therapy for intrathoracic anastomotic leakage following transthoracic esophageal resection. BMC Gastroenterol 2021;21(1):72.

35. Bludau M, Fuchs HF, Herbold T, et al. Results of endoscopic vacuum-assisted closure device for treatment of upper GI leaks. Surg Endosc 2018;32(4):1906–14.

36. Schniewind B, Schafmayer C, Voehrs G, et al. Endoscopic endoluminal vacuum therapy is superior to other regimens in managing anastomotic leakage after esophagectomy: a comparative retrospective study. Surg Endosc 2013;27(10): 3883–90.

37. do Monte Junior ES, de Moura DTH, Ribeiro IB, et al. Endoscopic vacuum therapy versus endoscopic stenting for upper gastrointestinal transmural defects:

Systematic review and meta-analysis. Dig Endosc 2020. https://doi.org/10.1111/den.13813.

38. Manfredi MA, Clark SJ, Staffa SJ, et al. Endoscopic Esophageal Vacuum Therapy: A Novel Therapy for Esophageal Perforations in Pediatric Patients. J Pediatr Gastroenterol Nutr 2018;67(6):706–12.
39. Wong J, Lal D, Schneider J, et al. Novel placement of an esophageal wound vacuum for a persistent anastomotic leak. Endoscopy 2020. https://doi.org/10.1055/a-1308-1007.
40. Coletta M, Sami SS, Nachiappan A, et al. Acetic acid chromoendoscopy for the diagnosis of early neoplasia and specialized intestinal metaplasia in Barrett's esophagus: a meta-analysis. Gastrointest Endosc 2016;83(1):57–67.e1.
41. Laine L, Kaltenbach T, Barkun A, et al. SCENIC international consensus statement on surveillance and management of dysplasia in inflammatory bowel disease. Gastroenterology 2015;148(3):639–51.e28.
42. Thomson M, Hurlstone P. Chromoendoscopy. Practical pediatric gastrointestinal endoscopy. Hoboken, New Jersey: John Wiley & Sons, Ltd; 2021. p. 157–66.
43. Ho S-H, Uedo N, Aso A, et al. Development of Image-enhanced Endoscopy of the Gastrointestinal Tract: A Review of History and Current Evidences. J Clin Gastroenterol 2018;52(4):295–306.
44. Morita FHA, Bernardo WM, Ide E, et al. Narrow band imaging versus lugol chromoendoscopy to diagnose squamous cell carcinoma of the esophagus: a systematic review and meta-analysis. BMC Cancer 2017;17(1):54.
45. Chung C-S, Lo W-C, Lee Y-C, et al. Image-enhanced endoscopy for detection of second primary neoplasm in patients with esophageal and head and neck cancer: A systematic review and meta-analysis. Head Neck 2016;38(Suppl 1): E2343–9.
46. Bessissow T, Dulai PS, Restellini S, et al. Comparison of Endoscopic Dysplasia Detection Techniques in Patients With Ulcerative Colitis: A Systematic Review and Network Meta-analysis. Inflamm Bowel Dis 2018;24(12):2518–26.
47. El-Dallal M, Chen Y, Lin Q, et al. Meta-analysis of Virtual-based Chromoendoscopy Compared With Dye-spraying Chromoendoscopy Standard and High-definition White Light Endoscopy in Patients With Inflammatory Bowel Disease at Increased Risk of Colon Cancer. Inflamm Bowel Dis 2020;26(9):1319–29.
48. Glover B, Teare J, Patel N. A Review of New and Emerging Techniques For Optical Diagnosis of Colonic Polyps. J Clin Gastroenterol 2019;53(7):495–506.
49. van der Sommen F, Groof J de, Struyvenberg M, et al. Machine learning in GI endoscopy: practical guidance in how to interpret a novel field. Gut 2020; 69(11):2035–45.
50. Pannala R, Krishnan K, Melson J, et al. Emerging role of artificial intelligence in GI endoscopy. Gastrointest Endosc 2020;92(6):1151–2.

Upper Gastrointestinal Functional and Motility Disorders in Children

Jonathan Miller, MD[a], Julie Khlevner, MD[a],
Leonel Rodriguez, MD, MS[b],*

KEYWORDS

- Functional • Motility • Children • Cricopharyngeal achalasia • Esophageal achalasia
- Gastroesophageal reflux • Gastroparesis • Functional dyspepsia

KEY POINTS

- Upper gastrointestinal (UGI) motility disorders are common in children and often have nonspecific presentations requiring careful evaluation.
- Guidelines for diagnosis and management of pediatric UGI motility disorders are largely adapted from adults, necessitating thoughtful interpretation of test results and expert understanding of the benefits and risks of therapeutic options for the pediatric patient.
- Novel diagnostic and new therapeutic approaches provide better insight into understanding and treating UGI motor disorders in children.

CRICOPHARYNGEAL ACHALASIA

The upper esophageal sphincter (UES), consisting of the cricopharyngeus muscle among others, remains tonically contracted to prevent air entry into the esophagus or reflux of enteric contents. Dysfunction of the UES in children primarily manifests as dyscoordination between pharyngeal contraction and UES relaxation, and also as increased UES tone and/or absent or incomplete UES relaxation in response to swallows, the latter first described as cricopharyngeal achalasia (CPA) in pediatrics in 1969.[1]

---

[a] Division of Pediatric Gastroenterology, Hepatology and Nutrition, Morgan Stanley Children's Hospital, Columbia University Irving Medical Center, 3959 Braodway CHN7, New York, NY 10032, USA; [b] Section of Pediatric Gastroenterology, Hepatology and Nutrition, Yale New Haven Children's Hospital, Yale University School of Medicine, 333 Cedar Street, LMP 4093, New Haven, CT 06510, USA
* Corresponding author.
E-mail address: leonel.rodriguez@yale.edu

Pediatr Clin N Am 68 (2021) 1237–1253
https://doi.org/10.1016/j.pcl.2021.07.009   **pediatric.theclinics.com**

Diagnosis

CPA often presents as dysphagia, also nonspecifically in infancy (salivation, regurgitation, nasal reflux, cough, or choking), resulting in delayed diagnosis, with a history of cyanotic episodes or brief resolved unexplained events, recurrent aspiration pneumonia, failure to thrive, or even sudden infant death.[2]

Although CPA refers to primary cricopharyngeal dysfunction, known neurologic insults such as hypoxic ischemic encephalopathy, cerebral palsy, hypotonia, muscular dystrophies, or Chiari malformation have been implicated.[3,4]

A thorough history should guide evaluation to rule out other disorders (esophageal stenosis, web or rings, dysphagia lusoria, trachea-esophageal fistula, or laryngeal cleft). In most cases, imaging and/or manometry are required for diagnosis, whereas endoscopy is unlikely to add diagnostic information.

Videofluoroscopic Swallow Study (VFSS), the primary mode of diagnosis, allows for swallow evaluation in real time, slow motion, and frame-by-frame. The finding of posterior filling defect or cricopharyngeal bar suggests failure of UES relaxation and supports the diagnosis of CPA.[5] However, concerns exist regarding interobserver interpretation of VFSS for diagnoses other than aspiration.[6]

UES Manometry complements VFSS[7] by measuring UES function. One may observe discoordination between pharyngeal contraction and UES relaxation, but classic is absent or incomplete UES relaxation. The residual UES pressure drops to less than 15 mm Hg in healthy adults, with similar values extrapolated to children, although specific criteria are not defined.[8]

Treatment

Historically, CPA required surgical management; however, less invasive modalities may offer nonpermanent symptomatic relief before considering myotomy. Calcium channel blockers and nitrates have poor efficacy, and accompanying side effects limit their utility in children. Injections with botulinum toxin-A (BTX-A) in adult patients with stroke demonstrated a significant improvement in aspiration and VFSS.[9] The pediatric literature is limited to small case series,[10,11] with 1 prospective survey of 6 children after BTX-A injections reporting all eventually tolerated regular diet and 2 underwent myotomy.[12]

A pediatric study evaluated 1 to 6 monthly dilations (balloon, bougie, or both) reporting 19 of 30 patients had complete symptom resolution, whereas 3 had persistent symptoms despite improvement on VFSS. Complications included 2 perforations and 1 death.[13] Prospective trials in adult patients with stroke demonstrated dilations improved UES relaxation compared with controls,[14] and a retrospective study in adults reported balloon dilation produced similar clinical improvement compared with myotomy (57% required repeat dilations, 17% eventually underwent myotomy).[15] There is no consensus protocol for dilations with varied inflation times of 30 to 60 seconds up to 5 minutes,[16,17] frequency and number of pneumatic dilations (PDs) often tailored to patient's symptoms.

The expectation of immediate symptomatic relief and minimal recurrence risk have led some investigators to recommend cricopharyngeal myotomy (CPM) as an early therapeutic consideration.[18,19] The risks of CPM (hemorrhage, infection, pharyngocutaneous fistula, and esophageal or recurrent laryngeal nerve damage) have long been recognized, although an endoscopic approach may alleviate some risk. A systematic review found significantly higher success rate with endoscopic (84%) versus open CPM (71%) with fewer complications (2% vs 11%, respectively).[20] Although patient-size constraints might deter against endoscopic CPM, success is reported in infants as young as 6 months.[21]

ACHALASIA

Pediatric achalasia, a rare esophageal motor disorder, is characterized by degeneration of the inhibitory myenteric neurons in the esophageal body and lower esophageal sphincter (LES), resulting in loss of peristalsis and incomplete or absent LES relaxation on deglutition. The precise etiology is unclear, but autoimmune, genetic, and infectious causes have been implicated.[22] Achalasia is mostly diagnosed between 7 and 15 years of age, with a slight male predominance. It has been associated with Trisomy 21, congenital hypoventilation syndrome, familial dysautonomia, Triple A syndrome (achalasia, alacrima, and adenocorticotropic hormone insensitivity),[23] and Alport syndrome.[24] Children with achalasia usually present with progressive dysphagia, regurgitation, vomiting, and weight loss. Chest pain and recurrent food impaction also have been reported.[25] Younger children often present atypically (recurrent pneumonia, nocturnal cough, aspiration, hoarseness, feeding difficulties, food refusal, and failure to thrive).[25] Given its rarity, achalasia should be managed where access to appropriate diagnostic and treatment modalities exist.

Diagnosis

Diagnosis is suspected by clinical history, but often delayed and symptoms are often attributed to gastroesophageal reflux disease (GERD), asthma, or an eating disorder.[23] The Eckardt score (sum of symptom scores for dysphagia, regurgitation, chest pain, and weight loss, success defined as score ≤3) was developed to objectify achalasia symptoms in adults.[26]

Contrast esophagram typically demonstrates a dilated esophagus with "bird-beak"-like tapering of the distal esophagus (**Fig. 1**). The timed barium esophagram (TBE) and esophageal scintigraphy (**Fig. 2**) are used to evaluate esophageal bolus transit and clearance, but their interpretation lacks standardization and clinical utility is not well

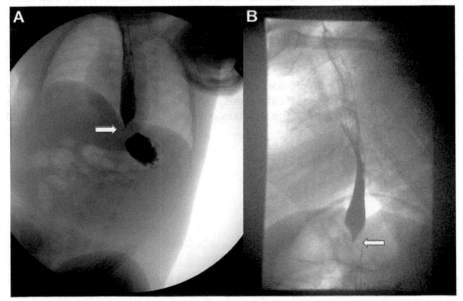

Fig. 1. Contrast esophagram demonstrating classic "bird's beak" sign (*arrow*) in achalasia in an infant (*A*) and in an adolescent with persistent symptoms pos-operatively (*B*).

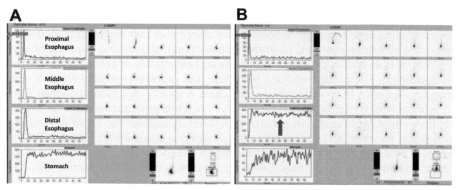

Fig. 2. Esophageal scintigraphy demonstrating normal esophageal transit (*A*) and delayed transit (*B*) in distal esophagus (*arrow*) in esophageal achalasia.

defined. Esophagogastroduodenoscopy (EGD) is not routinely indicated in children but can rule out other diagnoses; that is, eosinophilic esophagitis.

High-Resolution Esophageal Manometry (HRM) is the gold standard for diagnosing and subtyping achalasia. Elevated resting LES pressure, absent peristalsis, and incomplete or non-relaxing LES upon swallowing are diagnostic on HRM. However, absence of the LES findings does not exclude the diagnosis because LES function in children with achalasia is often heterogeneous. Parameters to define motor abnormalities using HRM have resulted in the adult-based algorithm, the Chicago Classification (CC), focusing on disorders of esophagogastric junction (EGJ) outflow and peristalsis.[27] The CC has defined 3 subtypes of achalasia, differentiated by the patterns of nonperistaltic esophageal pressurization[27] (**Fig. 3**). All 3 subtypes are observed in children. Applying CC to pediatric patients can be problematic, as it relies on adult-derived criteria. Small pediatric studies showing CC metrics (integrated relaxation pressure [IRP] and distal latency) are age and size dependent. One study showed younger age significantly correlated with higher IRP, potentially leading to overdiagnosis of achalasia and other IRP-driven CC diagnoses.[28] Studies in children showed excellent reliability of differentiating achalasia from nonachalasia based on application of the CC to HRM recordings. However, differentiating subtypes in adults appears less reliable,[29] with provider experience influencing the diagnosis of motility disorders.[30] Because of these differences, the CC diagnostic criteria should be used with caution in children. The addition of intraluminal impedance to the HRM

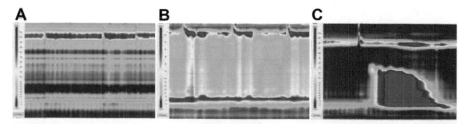

Fig. 3. Achalasia subtypes. (*A*) Type I: IRP >15 mm Hg and 100% failed peristalsis. (*B*) Type II: IRP >15 mm Hg, absent peristalsis, and panesophageal pressurization in >20% of swallows. (*C*) Type III: IRP >15 mm Hg, absent peristalsis, spastic contractions with distal contractile integral >450 mm Hg/s/cm in ≥20% of swallows.[27]

(HRIM) is a valuable objective parameter to evaluate the effect of peristalsis on bolus transit. The HRIM variables, bolus presence time (BPT) and trans-EGJ-bolus flow time (BFT) estimate the duration of EGJ opening and trans-EGJ bolus flow. In adults, these measurements correlate with dysphagia severity, achalasia subtype, and efficacies of therapies in treating EGJ obstruction.[31,32] Similar findings have been described in children with achalasia having significantly reduced BPT and BFT.[33] Furthermore, HRIM promises to be a more comprehensive evaluation of EGJ function than the IRP alone.

Despite wider availability of contrast studies over HRM, it is recommended to confirm diagnosis with HRM before any therapeutic intervention.

The novel functional lumen imaging probe (EndoFLIP) allows the measurement of EGJ distensibility in real time and has been recommended in the assessment and management of adult patients with achalasia.[34] EndoFLIP improves characterization of achalasia subtypes by detecting nonocclusive esophageal contractions not observed with HRM in adults[35] and a recent study in children showed increased EGJ distensibility and immediate treatment effect with intraoperative EndoFLIP.[36] Robust pediatric studies are needed before recommending its routine use.

Treatment

The goal is reduction of LES pressure to minimize outflow functional obstruction. Calcium channel blockers and nitrates are rarely used due to short-term effectiveness and side effects. BTX-A should be used only as a diagnostic tool in equivocal cases and for temporary relief in children who are poor candidates for more definitive therapy. To date, PD and laparoscopic/open Heller myotomy ([L]HM) with or without fundoplication are considered the most effective therapeutic options in children.

Pneumatic dilation and Heller myotomy

Pediatric cohort studies have reported successful surgical outcomes; however, HM has not been universally successful with inadequate length of myotomy and persistence of residual high-pressure zones at the gastroesophageal junction as causes for treatment failure. Intraoperative HRM confirming the adequacy of myotomy has improved surgical outcomes in children.[37] Overall, short-term and long-term success is similar for PD and laparoscopic HM (LHM).[38] In one pediatric prospective study, patients who underwent PD (6-year follow-up) had a 67% success rate and overall success rate after a maximum of 3 PDs was 87%.[39] A pediatric retrospective study showed that both PD and myotomy were effective.[40] Another study looking at long-term outcomes of HM and PD showed a higher asymptomatic rate at median 3-year follow-up among those treated with HM compared with PD (HM 53.6% PD 30%, $P<.05$) and all children who underwent PD required HM due to symptom recurrence.[41] Thoracoscopic HM (THM) is a minimally invasive surgical approach offered to children with achalasia. A retrospective cohort study of 31 children undergoing THM without fundoplication reported that 97% had symptom relief, although 26% required postoperative PD for recurrent symptoms (odds ratio 8.5 if they had a preoperative dilation) and 2 patients experienced mucosal injury.[42]

Per oral endoscopic myotomy

Per oral endoscopic myotomy (POEM), a newer technique in which a myotomy is performed via an endoscopically created submucosal tunnel, is showing encouraging results in adults and pediatrics although long-term follow-up data in children are lacking. POEM was associated with shorter operative time, longer myotomy, fewer complications, faster time to feeding, and shorter hospital stay with equivalent outcomes to

LHM.[43] A study of 10 children reported improved Eckardt score, TBE, and HRM after POEM, and previous procedures (LHM or PD) did not preclude the success to POEM.[44] Limited by provider expertise, POEM holds tremendous promise for pediatric patients with achalasia.

Post Intervention Complications

The primary postoperative complications in children are GERD and recurrence of dysphagia. A systematic review of 21 pediatric case series concluded that LHM is effective in 85% of children, with 7% requiring revision, and no difference in GERD or dysphagia with and without fundoplication.[45] Patients should be monitored clinically with periodic endoscopy for esophagitis as needed. For recurrent dysphagia, the recommendation is to repeat the barium esophagram (assess for incomplete myotomy or dilation, see **Fig. 1**B), if abnormal then repeat the HRM, and if IRP >10 to consider changing treatment modality (HM to PD or vice versa).[46]

GASTROESOPHAGEAL REFLUX DISEASE

GERD, retrograde passage of gastric contents into the esophagus leading to bothersome symptoms, is highly prevalent in children.[47] Pediatric guidelines extrapolate from adult terminology and data[48,49] aiming to limit unnecessary and invasive evaluation and guide therapy. Although empiric therapy is often warranted (nutritional or pharmacologic), response to treatment depends on accurate diagnosis. Not all GERD signifies esophagitis or other subclass of disease. Nonerosive reflux disease (NERD), esophageal hypersensitivity (EH), and functional heartburn (FH) may require further exploration if patients are not responding to therapy. In fact, a retrospective review of children with nonerosive disease who underwent endoscopy and pH-impedance testing found that the most common diagnosis was FH.[50]

Presentation

GERD symptoms are often nonspecific, although older children are more likely to report classic heartburn. Nonverbal children and infants often prove difficult to diagnose owing to the high prevalence of reflux as well as commonality of regurgitation, fussiness, and crying in both affected and nonaffected infants. Cough or aspiration concerns may be related to dysphagia and are known extra-esophageal manifestations of GERD.

Diagnosis

For most children, a diagnosis can be made clinically and in the absence of red-flag symptoms many children can be treated empirically. Initial choice of treatment is often dietary in infants or various anti-acid therapies in older children. A thorough interview should probe for the time course of symptoms, dietary history, and objective data, such as growth charts and prior interventions, to limit unnecessary testing.

EGD is helpful but is not required in making the diagnosis, and normal endoscopy may not definitively exclude the diagnosis. Endoscopy can distinguish GERD from NERD, EH, and FH, which may be managed differently.[50] Adult guidelines recommend endoscopy off of proton-pump inhibitor (PPI) therapy so as not to miss PPI-responsive eosinophilic esophagitis or 1 of the 3 diagnoses mentioned previously.[51] The flow chart in **Fig. 4** depicts the evaluation algorithm for GERD symptoms, esophagitis distinguishes GERD from NERD, and pH-impedance aids in differentiating NERD, EH, and FH. Adding pH-impedance enables detection of refluxate with pH greater than 4 to distinguish patients with non-acid reflux, including also those on PPI therapy.

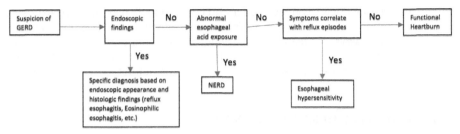

Fig. 4. Flow diagram showing classification of GERD disorders.

Although consensus is lacking on normative values for impedance studies, Mousa and colleagues[52] used a multicenter database to provide ranges of values for impedance testing parameters in 117 infants and children with symptoms deemed unrelated to reflux following impedance testing.

Although other modalities (contrast imaging studies and scintigraphy) may demonstrate either direct or indirect evidence of reflux, those lack utility for routine use in diagnosis or assessing treatment response.

HRM is infrequently part of the GERD diagnostic algorithm, as its ability to identify transient LES relaxations (TLESR) or hypotensive LES does not correlate well with GERD.[48] It may, however, play a role in predicting complications of antireflux surgery.[53]

Nonsurgical Management

Empiric therapeutic options are age-dependent. In infants, first-line dietary options include thickening feeds or formula changes. Thickening may provide some benefit with regurgitation, but the impact on other symptoms is debated.[54,55] Similarly, best practices for positioning a feeding infant lack consensus. PPIs are not superior to placebo in infants.[56]

In adults, a trial of PPI to aid in diagnosing GERD may be justified, and this likely applies to older children as well. Several studies have shown the symptomatic relief and mucosal healing of an 8-week to 12-week course of a PPI.[57,58] Histamine antagonists and other antacid therapies are used commonly, although few good head-to-head trials exist among the different medication classes, and these fall outside the scope of this article. Prokinetic agents offer indirect aid in preventing reflux symptoms by primarily promoting gastric emptying. These are discussed further under gastroparesis and functional dyspepsia.

Due to the positive correlation between reflux and symptoms, patients with EH may respond to typical antireflux therapies,[48] and neuromodulators (selective antidepressants) have been trialed in adults to target the heightened visceral response.[59,60]

For FH, in which there is absence of observable trigger on impedance testing, as many as half of adults respond to PPIs, whereas there has been varying success with melatonin, antidepressants, biofeedback, and multiple complementary or alternative therapies,[61] although data are lacking in pediatrics.

Surgical Management

In some refractory cases, surgery becomes necessary. EGD and pH-impedance are typically necessary in the evaluation before surgery, specifically in confirming that GERD is responsible for the symptoms being targeted. Fundoplication, which reduces GERD primarily by increasing LES pressure, has median success of 86% in children.[62] A prospective study of 25 children undergoing pH-impedance monitoring 3 months before and after fundoplication reported a significant reduction in total acid exposure time and number of reflux episodes.[63] Known side effects to consider include new-onset dysphagia, aspiration risk due to esophageal stasis, early satiety, pain, bloating, dumping syndrome, retching, or unwrapping of the fundoplication requiring repeat intervention. It is currently recommended only for refractory cases and life-threatening GERD complications.

GASTROPARESIS AND FUNCTIONAL DYSPEPSIA

Gastroparesis (GP) is defined as dyspeptic symptoms associated with delayed passage of gastric contents into the small intestine in the absence of mechanical obstruction. Inadequate coordination of complex neuromuscular activities leads to delayed emptying of gastric contents and the resultant symptoms. The prevalence is largely unknown but likely increasing.[64]

Although many cases are idiopathic, approximately 20% have identifiable etiology (eg, post-viral, medication-induced, genetic, or metabolic).[65–67] Often, inherited or acquired risk factors; neuromuscular, connective tissue, and mitochondrial diseases; diabetes; and malnutrition are associated with abnormal gastric motility.[68] The symptoms of GP are common in patients with autonomic dysfunction and specifically postural orthostatic tachycardia syndrome (POTS), but the association between POTS and rates of gastric emptying are not uniform.[69,70] The relatively high prevalence of these symptoms was demonstrated in a recent cross-sectional study, with 7.6% of children meeting Rome IV criteria for 1 of the 2 functional dyspepsia (FD) subtypes.[71] GP and FD exist on ends of the same spectrum of disease rather than as discreet entities.

Presentation

Most patients have nausea and abdominal pain with vomiting.[67,72] Vomiting is not a requisite for diagnosis, although delayed postprandial emesis, especially with food contents, may raise suspicion for GP.[67,72] Although younger children may have feeding difficulties, older children are more likely to articulate early satiety or postprandial fullness. GP may be difficult to distinguish clinically from FD, and imaging may help differentiate the two. This is because FD is defined by the presence of specific symptoms that overlap with GP. Although separating these diagnoses clinically is challenging, more severe abdominal symptoms were associated with true delayed gastric emptying in one pediatric cohort.[73]

Diagnosis

The gold standard for diagnosis of GP remains solid-meal 4-hour nuclear gastric emptying scintigraphy (GES)[74]; EGD and contrast studies are useful to rule out mucosal diseases and a gastro-duodenal obstructive process.[75] Consistently, greater than 10% retention of radiolabeled food contents at 4 hours outperformed normative cutoffs at earlier timepoints. Recently, Ng and colleagues[76] reported using adult normative values on more than 1000 GESs, finding no statistically significant difference in normative values in children consuming at least 50% of the standard meal when compared with the full meal and a predefined cheese-based alternative meal adhered to the same normative values. Patients with FD may have accelerated or delayed gastric emptying despite similar symptoms. GES is recommended before starting prokinetic therapies.[77]

An alternative to the radiolabeled GES is gastric emptying breath test (GEBT), which uses a nonradioactive ^{13}Carbon isotope, with overall similar sensitivity and specificity to GES between symptomatic children and controls.[78] Similarly, the wireless motility capsule (Medtronic, Dublin, Ireland) evaluates transit and contractility and has been validated with GES in adults,[79] recently showing utility in children.[80,81]

Antroduodenal manometry is a more invasive modality indicated only in refractory cases to assess intestinal involvement of a more generalized motility disorder.

No specific diagnostic tests are required to diagnose FD if a patient meets Rome IV criteria.[82] The utility of all diagnostic studies is summarized in **Table 1**.

Dietary and Pharmacologic Therapies

Treatment of GP, like other disorders leading to inadequate nutrition, may require correction of any vitamin or mineral deficiencies and caloric support by using frequent, smaller meals and avoidance of high fat/fiber foods that prolong gastric transit. Post-pyloric feeds are preferred to parenteral nutrition, which carries significant risks.

Although antiemetics may alleviate symptoms, prokinetics improve gastric transit time. Macrolide antibiotics (erythromycin and azithromycin) activate motilin receptors, improving antral contractility.[83,84] In adults with FD, erythromycin improved gastric emptying time (by GEBT) but not symptoms.[85] Metoclopramide, a dopamine 2-receptor antagonist, is effective in adults for improving gastric emptying and associated symptoms,[86] but in a retrospective study, 80% of children were nonresponsive, with frequent side effects, including tardive dyskinesia.[67] Other effective prokinetics like cisapride and domperidone are not approved by the Food and Drug Administration in the United States because of concerns for fatal arrhythmias. In a subset of patients failing first-line pharmacologic therapies for GP, 74% had clinical improvement with domperidone and fewer adverse effects than metoclopramide.[67] Recently, prucalopride, a 5-HT$_4$ agonist, significantly improved symptoms, quality-of-life scores, and gastric emptying on GEBT.[87] Although not a prokinetic, cyproheptadine improves gastric accommodation, which may improve some symptoms of GP and FD.

Limited data exist for specific medical therapies for FD in children. Omeprazole seems superior to H2-receptor antagonists in relieving abdominal symptoms over 4 weeks,[88] possibly by treating low-grade duodenal inflammation; however, long-term PPI use is not recommended.[48] Famotidine also seems to be effective in children compared with placebo.[89] Mirtazapine, a tricyclic antidepressant, amitriptyline, and buspirone (serotonin partial agonist) improved symptoms in adults,[90–92] but no pediatric trials exist. Complementary and alternative medicines have been used with varying success, including peppermint oil.[93]

Endoscopic and Surgical Management of Gastroparesis

In medically refractory cases, endoscopic and surgical interventions may be required. BTX-A pyloric injections offer potential temporary relief in two-thirds of children for a median duration of 3 months.[94] BTX-A injections are not routinely recommended in adults because of lack of improvement in 2 double blind placebo controlled (DBPC) trials[77,95] despite multiple uncontrolled studies showing efficacy. In a retrospective review, 20 of 23 children undergoing pyloroplasty reported symptomatic improvement, 8 of whom underwent fluoroscopically guided balloon dilation (FGBD) of the pylorus, with all reporting improvement.[96] One potential benefit of FGBD may be in assessing response before surgical pyloromyotomy.

Finally, percutaneous or implanted gastric electrical stimulation has been found safe and effective in children and adults.[97] In adolescents, gastric electrical stimulation significantly improved symptom scores beyond 1 year and improved nausea and vomiting in children with FD.[98,99]

Table 1
Diagnostic utility of various test in esophageal and gastric functional and motility disorders

	Cricopharyngeal Achalasia	Esophageal Achalasia	Gastroesophageal Reflux Disease	Gastroparesis	Functional Dyspepsia
Upper gastrointestinal series	X	X	X	X	(−)
Videofluoroscopic swallow study	+++	(−)	(−)	(−)	(−)
Esophagram	(−)	++	+	(−)	(−)
Gastric scintigraphy	(−)	(−)	(−)	+++	+
Esophageal scintigraphy	(−)	++	(−)	(−)	(−)
Gastric emptying breath test	(−)	(−)	(−)	++	(−)
Esophagogastroduodenoscopy	X	X	++	X	X
High-resolution manometry	++	+++	+	+ (Antroduodenal Manometry)	(−)
Impedance	(−)	++ (EndoFlip)	++ (pH-impedance)	(−)	(−)
Empiric therapy	(−)	(−)	++	+	++

+++, gold standard; ++, useful adjunct; +, may provide supporting evidence; X, role in ruling out alternative diagnoses; (−), not useful.

CLINICS CARE POINTS

- In infants with dysphagia, contrast imaging with videofluoroscopic swallow study and/or upper gastrointestinal series can help identify an anatomic etiology, and is typically accessible in most health care settings.

- Manometry and scintigraphy can help differentiate an upper gastrointestinal motility disorder from a functional disorder.

- Esophagogastroduodenoscopy is rarely diagnostic in pediatric upper gastrointestinal motility disorders but may help identify alternative diagnoses.

- Accurate diagnosis and management of some motility disorders, specifically achalasia, are best managed in centers with experience in performing high-resolution manometry and where surgical and/or endoscopic therapeutic options exist.

- For CPA and delayed gastric emptying, Botulinum toxin-A injections have shown temporary success, which may provide relief or help confirm a diagnosis before more definitive surgical therapy.

- When concerned for GERD in the absence of any "red-flag" symptoms, empiric course of antacid medications may be trialed in older children or empiric dietary change in infants. However, the long-term use of anti-acid medications, specifically PPIs, are not recommended, and failure to respond to an appropriate course of medication should prompt further evaluation.

- Functional disorders are common in children and often present similarly to gastrointestinal motility disorders; however, if Rome IV criteria are met for a functional gastrointestinal disorder, unnecessary evaluation can be avoided.

- Whenever possible, a full 4-hour gastric emptying study provides the most accurate diagnosis for delayed gastric emptying, whereas ability to consume the entire prescribed meal may be less critical.

- Motility disorders in children may be secondary to underlying illness or medication side effect, which must be considered as the treatment will likely differ from children with primary motility disorder.

DISCLOSURE

The authors have nothing to disclose.

REFERENCES

1. Utian HL, Thomas RG. Cricopharyngeal incoordination in infancy. Pediatrics 1969;43(3):402–6.
2. Huoh KC, Messner AH. Cricopharyngeal achalasia in children: indications for treatment and management options. Curr Opin Otolaryngol Head Neck Surg 2013;21(6):576–80.
3. Putnam PE, Orenstein SR, Pang D, et al. Cricopharyngeal dysfunction associated with Chiari malformations. Pediatrics 1992;89(5 Pt 1):871–6.
4. Jensen PS, Gulati IK, Shubert TR, et al. Pharyngeal stimulus-induced reflexes are impaired in infants with perinatal asphyxia: does maturation modify? Neurogastroenterol Motil 2017;29(7):10.1111/nmo.13039. https://doi.org/10.1111/nmo.13039.
5. Samanci C, Onal Y, Korman U. Videofluoroscopic and manometric evaluation of oropharyngeal and esophageal motility disorders. Curr Med Imaging Rev 2020;16(1):65–9.

6. Stoeckli SJ, Huisman TA, Seifert B, et al. Interrater reliability of videofluoroscopic swallow evaluation. Dysphagia 2003;18(1):53–7.
7. Türer Ö B, Demir N, Ciecieraga T, et al. Assessment of pediatric cricopharyngeal achalasia with high resolution manometry. Turk J Pediatr 2019;61(5):804–9.
8. Bhatia SJ, Shah C. How to perform and interpret upper esophageal sphincter manometry. J Neurogastroenterol Motil 2013;19(1):99–103.
9. Terré R, Panadés A, Mearin F. Botulinum toxin treatment for oropharyngeal dysphagia in patients with stroke. Neurogastroenterol Motil 2013;25(11):896.
10. Barnes MA, Ho AS, Malhotra PS, et al. The use of botulinum toxin for pediatric cricopharyngeal achalasia. Int J Pediatr Otorhinolaryngol 2011;75(9):1210–4.
11. Sewell RK, Bauman NM. Congenital cricopharyngeal achalasia: management with botulinum toxin before myotomy. Arch Otolaryngol Head Neck Surg 2005; 131(5):451–3.
12. Scholes MA, McEvoy T, Mousa H, et al. Cricopharyngeal achalasia in children: botulinum toxin injection as a tool for diagnosis and treatment. Laryngoscope 2014;124(6):1475–80.
13. Gollu G, Demir N, Ates U, et al. Effective management of cricopharyngeal achalasia in infants and children with dilatation alone. J Pediatr Surg 2016;51(11): 1751–4.
14. Lan Y, Xu GQ, Dou ZL, et al. [Effect of balloon dilatation on upper esophageal sphincter in brainstem stroke patients with dysphagia: an investigation using high-resolution solid-state manometry]. Zhonghua Yi Xue Za Zhi 2013;93(33): 2631–6.
15. Marston AP, Maldonado FJ, Ravi K, et al. Treatment of oropharyngeal dysphagia secondary to idiopathic cricopharyngeal bar: surgical cricopharyngeal muscle myotomy versus dilation. Am J Otolaryngol 2016;37(6):507–12.
16. Lew RJ, Kochman ML. A review of endoscopic methods of esophageal dilation. J Clin Gastroenterol 2002;35(2):117–26.
17. Cakmak M, Boybeyi O, Gollu G, et al. Endoscopic balloon dilatation of benign esophageal strictures in childhood: a 15-year experience. Dis Esophagus 2016;29(2):179–84.
18. Brooks A, Millar AJ, Rode H. The surgical management of cricopharyngeal achalasia in children. Int J Pediatr Otorhinolaryngol 2000;56(1):1–7.
19. Muraji T, Takamizawa S, Satoh S, et al. Congenital cricopharyngeal achalasia: diagnosis and surgical management. J Pediatr Surg 2002;37(5):E12.
20. Kocdor P, Siegel ER, Tulunay-Ugur OE. Cricopharyngeal dysfunction: a systematic review comparing outcomes of dilatation, botulinum toxin injection, and myotomy. Laryngoscope 2016;126(1):135–41.
21. Basler KJ, Swanson C, Andreoli SM. Endoscopic cricopharyngeal myotomy in infants. Int J Pediatr Otorhinolaryngol 2019;116:15–7.
22. Ruiz-de-Leon A, Mendoza J, Sevilla-Mantilla C, et al. Myenteric antiplexus antibodies and class II HLA in achalasia. Dig Dis Sci 2002;47(1):15–9.
23. Hallal C, Kieling CO, Nunes DL, et al. Diagnosis, misdiagnosis, and associated diseases of achalasia in children and adolescents: a twelve-year single center experience. Pediatr Surg Int 2012;28(12):1211–7.
24. Boeckxstaens GE, Jonge WD, van den Wijngaard RM, et al. Achalasia: from new insights in pathophysiology to treatment. J Pediatr Gastroenterol Nutr 2005; 41(Suppl 1):S36–7.
25. Franklin AL, Petrosyan M, Kane TD. Childhood achalasia: a comprehensive review of disease, diagnosis and therapeutic management. World J Gastrointest Endosc 2014;6(4):105–11.

26. Taft TH, Carlson DA, Triggs J, et al. Evaluating the reliability and construct validity of the Eckardt symptom score as a measure of achalasia severity. Neurogastroenterol Motil 2018;30(6):e13287.

27. Kahrilas PJ, Bredenoord AJ, Fox M, et al. The Chicago Classification of esophageal motility disorders, v3.0. Neurogastroenterol Motil 2015;27(2):160–74.

28. Singendonk MM, Kritas S, Cock C, et al. Applying the Chicago Classification criteria of esophageal motility to a pediatric cohort: effects of patient age and size. Neurogastroenterol Motil 2014;26(9):1333–41.

29. Hernandez JC, Ratuapli SK, Burdick GE, et al. Interrater and intrarater agreement of the chicago classification of achalasia subtypes using high-resolution esophageal manometry. Am J Gastroenterol 2012;107(2):207–14.

30. Singendonk MM, Smits MJ, Heijting IE, et al. Inter- and intrarater reliability of the Chicago Classification in pediatric high-resolution esophageal manometry recordings. Neurogastroenterol Motil 2015;27(2):269–76.

31. Lin Z, Carlson DA, Dykstra K, et al. High-resolution impedance manometry measurement of bolus flow time in achalasia and its correlation with dysphagia. Neurogastroenterol Motil 2015;27(9):1232–8.

32. Lin Z, Imam H, Nicodeme F, et al. Flow time through esophagogastric junction derived during high-resolution impedance-manometry studies: a novel parameter for assessing esophageal bolus transit. Am J Physiol Gastrointest Liver Physiol 2014;307(2):G158–63.

33. Singendonk MMJ, Omari TI, Rommel N, et al. Novel pressure-impedance parameters for evaluating esophageal function in pediatric achalasia. J Pediatr Gastroenterol Nutr 2018;66(1):37–42.

34. Hirano I, Pandolfino JE, Boeckxstaens GE. Functional lumen imaging probe for the management of esophageal disorders: expert review from the clinical practice updates committee of the AGA institute. Clin Gastroenterol Hepatol 2017;15(3):325–34.

35. Carlson DA, Lin Z, Kahrilas PJ, et al. The functional lumen imaging probe detects esophageal contractility not observed with manometry in patients with achalasia. Gastroenterology 2015;149(7):1742–51.

36. Yeung F, Wong IYH, Chung PHY, et al. Peroral endoscopic myotomy with Endo-FLIP and double-endoscope: novel techniques for achalasia in pediatric population. J Laparoendosc Adv Surg Tech A 2018;28(3):343–7.

37. Jafri M, Alonso M, Kaul A, et al. Intraoperative manometry during laparoscopic Heller myotomy improves outcome in pediatric achalasia. J Pediatr Surg 2008;43(1):66–70 [discussion 70].

38. Moonen A, Annese V, Belmans A, et al. Long-term results of the European achalasia trial: a multicentre randomised controlled trial comparing pneumatic dilation versus laparoscopic Heller myotomy. Gut 2016;65(5):732–9.

39. Di Nardo G, Rossi P, Oliva S, et al. Pneumatic balloon dilation in pediatric achalasia: efficacy and factors predicting outcome at a single tertiary pediatric gastroenterology center. Gastrointest Endosc 2012;76(5):927–32.

40. Pastor AC, Mills J, Marcon MA, et al. A single center 26-year experience with treatment of esophageal achalasia: is there an optimal method? J Pediatr Surg 2009;44(7):1349–54.

41. Saliakellis E, Thapar N, Roebuck D, et al. Long-term outcomes of Heller's myotomy and balloon dilatation in childhood achalasia. Eur J Pediatr 2017;176(7):899–907.

42. Duggan EM, Nurko S, Smithers CJ, et al. Thoracoscopic esophagomyotomy for achalasia in the pediatric population: a retrospective cohort study. J Pediatr Surg 2019;54(3):572–6.

43. Caldaro T, Familiari P, Romeo EF, et al. Treatment of esophageal achalasia in children: today and tomorrow. J Pediatr Surg 2015;50(5):726–30.

44. Nabi Z, Ramchandani M, Reddy DN, et al. Per oral endoscopic myotomy in children with Achalasia Cardia. J Neurogastroenterol Motil 2016;22(4):613–9.

45. Pacilli M, Davenport M. Results of laparoscopic Heller's myotomy for achalasia in children: a systematic review of the literature. J Laparoendosc Adv Surg Tech Part A 2017;27(1):82–90.

46. Pensabene L, Nurko S. Approach to the child who has persistent dysphagia after surgical treatment for esophageal achalasia. J Pediatr Gastroenterol Nutr 2008; 47(1):92–7.

47. Singendonk M, Goudswaard E, Langendam M, et al. Prevalence of gastroesophageal reflux disease symptoms in infants and children: a systematic review. J Pediatr Gastroenterol Nutr 2019;68(6):811–7.

48. Rosen R, Vandenplas Y, Singendonk M, et al. Pediatric gastroesophageal reflux clinical practice guidelines: joint recommendations of the North American Society for pediatric gastroenterology, hepatology, and nutrition and the European Society for Pediatric Gastroenterology, Hepatology, and Nutrition. J Pediatr Gastroenterol Nutr 2018;66(3):516–54.

49. Vakil N, van Zanten SV, Kahrilas P, et al. The Montreal definition and classification of gastroesophageal reflux disease: a global evidence-based consensus. Am J Gastroenterol 2006;101(8):1900–20 [quiz 1943].

50. Mahoney LB, Nurko S, Rosen R. The prevalence of rome IV nonerosive esophageal phenotypes in children. J Pediatr 2017;189:86–91.

51. Katz PO, Gerson LB, Vela MF. Guidelines for the diagnosis and management of gastroesophageal reflux disease. Am J Gastroenterol 2013;108(3):308–28 [quiz 329].

52. Mousa H, Machado R, Orsi M, et al. Combined multichannel intraluminal impedance-pH (MII-pH): multicenter report of normal values from 117 children. Curr Gastroenterol Rep 2014;16(8):400.

53. Loots C, van Herwaarden MY, Benninga MA, et al. Gastroesophageal reflux, esophageal function, gastric emptying, and the relationship to dysphagia before and after antireflux surgery in children. J Pediatr 2013;162(3):566–73.e2.

54. Wenzl TG, Schneider S, Scheele F, et al. Effects of thickened feeding on gastroesophageal reflux in infants: a placebo-controlled crossover study using intraluminal impedance. Pediatrics 2003;111(4 Pt 1):e355–9.

55. Corvaglia L, Ferlini M, Rotatori R, et al. Starch thickening of human milk is ineffective in reducing the gastroesophageal reflux in preterm infants: a crossover study using intraluminal impedance. J Pediatr 2006;148(2):265–8.

56. van der Pol RJ, Smits MJ, van Wijk MP, et al. Efficacy of proton-pump inhibitors in children with gastroesophageal reflux disease: a systematic review. Pediatrics 2011;127(5):925–35.

57. Baker R, Tsou VM, Tung J, et al. Clinical results from a randomized, double-blind, dose-ranging study of pantoprazole in children aged 1 through 5 years with symptomatic histologic or erosive esophagitis. Clin Pediatr (Phila) 2010;49(9): 852–65.

58. Fiedorek S, Tolia V, Gold BD, et al. Efficacy and safety of lansoprazole in adolescents with symptomatic erosive and non-erosive gastroesophageal reflux disease. J Pediatr Gastroenterol Nutr 2005;40(3):319–27.

59. Limsrivilai J, Charatcharoenwitthaya P, Pausawasdi N, et al. Imipramine for treatment of esophageal hypersensitivity and functional heartburn: a randomized placebo-controlled trial. Am J Gastroenterol 2016;111(2):217–24.
60. Viazis N, Karamanolis G, Vienna E, et al. Selective-serotonin reuptake inhibitors for the treatment of hypersensitive esophagus. Therap Adv Gastroenterol 2011; 4(5):295–300.
61. Hachem C, Shaheen NJ. Diagnosis and management of functional heartburn. Am J Gastroenterol 2016;111(1):53–61 [quiz 62].
62. Mauritz FA, van Herwaarden-Lindeboom MY, Stomp W, et al. The effects and efficacy of antireflux surgery in children with gastroesophageal reflux disease: a systematic review. J Gastrointest Surg 2011;15(10):1872–8.
63. Mauritz FA, Conchillo JM, van Heurn LWE, et al. Effects and efficacy of laparoscopic fundoplication in children with GERD: a prospective, multicenter study. Surg Endosc 2017;31(3):1101–10.
64. Lu PL, Moore-Clingenpeel M, Yacob D, et al. The rising cost of hospital care for children with gastroparesis: 2004-2013. Neurogastroenterol Motil 2016;28(11): 1698–704.
65. Nurko S. Motility disorders in children. Pediatr Clin North Am 2017;64(3):593–612.
66. Chumpitazi B, Nurko S. Pediatric gastrointestinal motility disorders: challenges and a clinical update. Gastroenterol Hepatol (N Y) 2008;4(2):140–8.
67. Rodriguez L, Irani K, Jiang H, et al. Clinical presentation, response to therapy, and outcome of gastroparesis in children. J Pediatr Gastroenterol Nutr 2012; 55(2):185–90.
68. Kovacic K, Elfar W, Rosen JM, et al. Update on pediatric gastroparesis: a review of the published literature and recommendations for future research. Neurogastroenterol Motil 2020;32(3):e13780.
69. Antiel RM, Risma JM, Grothe RM, et al. Orthostatic intolerance and gastrointestinal motility in adolescents with nausea and abdominal pain. J Pediatr Gastroenterol Nutr 2008;46(3):285–8.
70. Park KJ, Singer W, Sletten DM, et al. Gastric emptying in postural tachycardia syndrome: a preliminary report. Clin Auton Res 2013;23(4):163–7.
71. Robin SG, Keller C, Zwiener R, et al. Prevalence of pediatric functional gastrointestinal disorders utilizing the rome IV criteria. J Pediatr 2018;195:134–9.
72. Waseem S, Islam S, Kahn G, et al. Spectrum of gastroparesis in children. J Pediatr Gastroenterol Nutr 2012;55(2):166–72.
73. Chitkara DK, Camilleri M, Zinsmeister AR, et al. Gastric sensory and motor dysfunction in adolescents with functional dyspepsia. J Pediatr 2005;146(4): 500–5.
74. Chogle A, Saps M. Gastroparesis in children: the benefit of conducting 4-hour scintigraphic gastric-emptying studies. J Pediatr Gastroenterol Nutr 2013;56(4): 439–42.
75. Fukami N, Anderson MA, Khan K, et al. The role of endoscopy in gastroduodenal obstruction and gastroparesis. Gastrointest Endosc 2011;74(1):13–21.
76. Ng TSC, Putta N, Kwatra NS, et al. Pediatric solid gastric emptying scintigraphy: normative value guidelines and nonstandard meal alternatives. Am J Gastroenterol 2020;115(11):1830–9.
77. Camilleri M, Parkman HP, Shafi MA, et al. Clinical guideline: management of gastroparesis. Am J Gastroenterol 2013;108(1):18–37 [quiz 38].
78. Hauser B, Roelants M, De Schepper J, et al. Gastric emptying of solids in children: reference values for the (13) C-octanoic acid breath test. Neurogastroenterol Motil 2016;28(10):1480–7.

79. Kuo B, McCallum RW, Koch KL, et al. Comparison of gastric emptying of a non-digestible capsule to a radio-labelled meal in healthy and gastroparetic subjects. Aliment Pharmacol Ther 2008;27(2):186–96.

80. Green AD, Belkind-Gerson J, Surjanhata BC, et al. Wireless motility capsule test in children with upper gastrointestinal symptoms. J Pediatr 2013;162(6):1181–7.

81. Rodriguez L, Heinz N, Colliard K, et al. Diagnostic and clinical utility of the wireless motility capsule in children: a study in patients with functional gastrointestinal disorders. Neurogastroenterol Motil 2021;33(4):e14032.

82. Hyams JS, Di Lorenzo C, Saps M, et al. Childhood functional gastrointestinal disorders: child/adolescent. Gastroenterology 2016;150(6):1456–68.

83. Peeters T, Matthijs G, Depoortere I, et al. Erythromycin is a motilin receptor agonist. Am J Physiol 1989;257(3 Pt 1):G470–4.

84. Cucchiara S, Minella R, Scoppa A, et al. Antroduodenal motor effects of intravenous erythromycin in children with abnormalities of gastrointestinal motility. J Pediatr Gastroenterol Nutr 1997;24(4):411–8.

85. Arts J, Caenepeel P, Verbeke K, et al. Influence of erythromycin on gastric emptying and meal related symptoms in functional dyspepsia with delayed gastric emptying. Gut 2005;54(4):455–60.

86. Perkel MS, Moore C, Hersh T, et al. Metoclopramide therapy in patients with delayed gastric emptying: a randomized, double-blind study. Dig Dis Sci 1979; 24(9):662–6.

87. Carbone F, Van den Houte K, Clevers E, et al. Prucalopride in gastroparesis: a randomized placebo-controlled crossover study. Am J Gastroenterol 2019; 114(8):1265–74.

88. Dehghani SM, Imanieh MH, Oboodi R, et al. The comparative study of the effectiveness of cimetidine, ranitidine, famotidine, and omeprazole in treatment of children with dyspepsia. ISRN Pediatr 2011;2011:219287.

89. See MC, Birnbaum AH, Schechter CB, et al. Double-blind, placebo-controlled trial of famotidine in children with abdominal pain and dyspepsia: global and quantitative assessment. Dig Dis Sci 2001;46(5):985–92.

90. Tack J, Janssen P, Masaoka T, et al. Efficacy of buspirone, a fundus-relaxing drug, in patients with functional dyspepsia. Clin Gastroenterol Hepatol 2012; 10(11):1239–45.

91. Tack J, Ly HG, Carbone F, et al. Efficacy of mirtazapine in patients with functional dyspepsia and weight loss. Clin Gastroenterol Hepatol 2016;14(3):385–92.e4.

92. Talley NJ, Locke GR, Saito YA, et al. Effect of amitriptyline and escitalopram on functional dyspepsia: a multicenter, randomized controlled study. Gastroenterology 2015;149(2):340–9.e2.

93. Fifi AC, Axelrod CH, Chakraborty P, et al. Herbs and spices in the treatment of functional gastrointestinal disorders: a review of clinical trials. Nutrients 2018; 10(11):1715. https://doi.org/10.3390/nu10111715.

94. Rodriguez L, Rosen R, Manfredi M, et al. Endoscopic intrapyloric injection of botulinum toxin A in the treatment of children with gastroparesis: a retrospective, open-label study. Gastrointest Endosc 2012;75(2):302–9.

95. Bai Y, Xu MJ, Yang X, et al. A systematic review on intrapyloric botulinum toxin injection for gastroparesis. Digestion 2010;81(1):27–34.

96. Jawaid W, Abdalwahab A, Blair G, et al. Outcomes of pyloroplasty and pyloric dilatation in children diagnosed with nonobstructive delayed gastric emptying. J Pediatr Surg 2006;41(12):2059–61.

97. Andersson S, Ringström G, Elfvin A, et al. Temporary percutaneous gastric electrical stimulation: a novel technique tested in patients with non-established indications for gastric electrical stimulation. Digestion 2011;83(1–2):3–12.
98. Islam S, McLaughlin J, Pierson J, et al. Long-term outcomes of gastric electrical stimulation in children with gastroparesis. J Pediatr Surg 2016;51(1):67–71.
99. Teich S, Mousa HM, Punati J, et al. Efficacy of permanent gastric electrical stimulation for the treatment of gastroparesis and functional dyspepsia in children and adolescents. J Pediatr Surg 2013;48(1):178–83.

Lower Gastrointestinal Functional and Motility Disorders in Children

Ricardo Arbizu, MD, MS, Ben Freiberg, MD,
Leonel Rodriguez, MD, MS*

KEYWORDS

- Colon • Anorectum • Dysmotility • Manometry • Pseudo-obstruction
- Hirschsprung's • Constipation • Incontinence

KEY POINTS

- Motility disorders involving the midgut and hindgut can be primary or secondary to an underlying systemic disease affecting the enteric nervous system.
- Supplemental testing, including manometry studies, can further clarify the pathophysiology and guide treatment in patients with a suspected motility disorder.
- Management aims to restore bowel function thereby improving symptomatology, nutrition, and quality of life.

MOTILITY DISORDERS INVOLVING SMALL BOWEL
Chronic Intestinal Pseudo-obstruction

Chronic intestinal pseudo-obstruction (CIPO) is a rare disorder characterized by recurrent episodes of symptoms resembling mechanical obstruction in the absence of a luminal occlusion.[1,2] There is no diagnostic criteria for CIPO, and diagnosis is based on clinical features supported by radiographic and manometry findings.[1-4] The prevalence and incidence of CIPO is largely unknown. A US nationwide survey estimates that approximately 100 infants are born with a congenital form of CIPO each year,[5] with 65% to 76% of children developing symptoms during the first year and 43% to 67% by the first month of life.[6-9] Prenatal signs are detected in 16% to 17% of cases.[6,7]

Section of Pediatric Gastroenterology, Hepatology and Nutrition, Pediatric Gastroenterology and Hepatology, Neurogastroenterology and Motility Center, Yale School of Medicine, Yale University School of Medicine, Yale New Haven Children's Hospital, 333 Cedar Street, LMP 4093, PO Box 208064, New Haven, CT 06520, USA
* Corresponding author.
E-mail address: leonel.rodriguez@yale.edu

Pediatr Clin N Am 68 (2021) 1255–1271
https://doi.org/10.1016/j.pcl.2021.07.010
0031-3955/21/© 2021 Elsevier Inc. All rights reserved.

pediatric.theclinics.com

Abnormalities of smooth muscle cells, interstitial cells of Cajal (ICC), intrinsic and extrinsic nerves, and the central nervous system lead to abnormalities in gastrointestinal motor function and symptoms of CIPO.[10–14] These may be idiopathic or secondary to a specific disease.[5,12,14] Common manifestations include abdominal pain, distension, nausea, vomiting, and constipation.[1,3,5,15,16] In 2018, the European Society for Pediatric Gastroenterology, Hepatology, and Nutrition developed guidelines for the definition, evaluation, and management of CIPO in children.[2]

Diagnostic investigation should be geared toward excluding mechanical bowel obstruction, identifying potential causes of secondary CIPO, and finding pathophysiologic features that may help direct management. Imaging studies typically demonstrate bowel distention without luminal occlusion (**Fig. 1**). Antroduodenal manometry (ADM) is indicated in those unresponsive to medical therapy. The presence of phase III of the migrating motor complex (MMC) excludes CIPO (**Fig. 2**) and should warrant further investigation.[17,18] ADM can be used to predict enteral tolerance in those with intestinal phase III of the MMC[19] and response to cisapride.[20] Full-thickness biopsies can help detect neuropathy, myopathy, or ICC abnormalities.[5] However, our understanding of the histopathology is limited due to lack of site-specific and age-specific tissue controls. Tissue sampling should be obtained only when another surgical intervention is planned.

A multidisciplinary approach is recommended to manage patients with CIPO.[1,2] Treatment aims in restoring fluid and electrolyte balance, maintaining adequate caloric intake, promoting intestinal motility, and treating complications. Small, frequent meals with liquid or homogenized foods should be encouraged in those with adequate intestinal absorption. Enteral feeds should be considered when oral intake is insufficient to

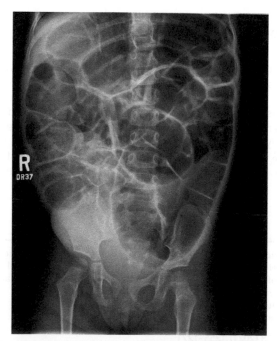

Fig. 1. Abdominal radiograph in a patient with CIPO depicting significant intestinal distension with no evidence of obstruction.

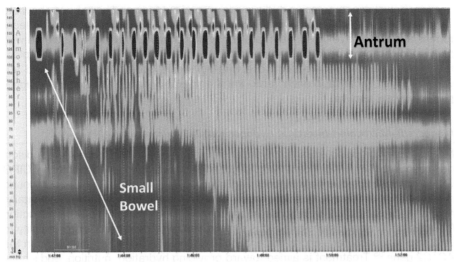

Fig. 2. High-resolution ADM demonstrating phase III of the MMC migrating from antrum to small bowel.

meet nutritional needs. Perform a trial of feeds via a nasogastric or nasojejunal feeding tube before a permanent feeding tube is placed.[21] Continuous feeds are better tolerated than bolus feeds, and should be started at a slow rate and progressively increased as a way to challenge the functional absorptive capacity of the gut. Parenteral nutrition (PN) is reserved for severe cases in which the enteral route cannot maintain caloric needs or hydration[21] given its long-term complications.[22] Survival rates in children on PN are 87%, 79%, 76%, and 73% at 1, 3, 5, and 10 years, respectively with an overall survival of 75%.[6,7,9,23–26] Better outcomes are reported in those able to tolerate oral feeds.[22] Factors associated with increased mortality in children with PN include CIPO at birth, acute onset, malrotation, myopathic origin, urinary involvement and repeated surgery.[6,7,9,25]

The goal of medical therapy is to promote motility, thereby improving oral intake and decreasing symptoms. Erythromycin, a macrolide and motilin receptor agonist, may be effective in some patients with CIPO.[27] Metoclopramide and domperidone exert their prokinetic effect by increasing acetylcholine release, but clinical data for their use in CIPO are lacking. Further, metoclopramide has a black box warning from the Food and Drug Administration (FDA) for risk of tardive dyskinesia, and domperidone is not FDA approved. Octreotide is a long-acting somatostatin analogue that induces phase III of the MMC and has been shown to be effective in children.[28] Prucalopride, a highly selective serotonin 5-HT$_4$ receptor agonist, has shown efficacy on symptom improvement and decreased use of analgesic drugs.[29] Pain control can be challenging, opiates should be used with caution because they decrease smooth muscle contractions and increase tone. potentially worsening symptoms of CIPO. Non-narcotic neuromodulators (tricyclic antidepressants, serotonin-norepinephrine reuptake inhibitors) can be used but should be monitored for their side effects. Transdermal buprenorphine, a µ-partial agonist and κ-opioid and δ-opioid receptor antagonist, was found to be effective in relieving pain in a small group of children.[30]

Surgical interventions may be necessary but should be limited, as they may worsen dysmotility or create adhesions. Gastrostomy or jejunostomy tubes can be used for bowel decompression and provide enteral nutrition and have been shown to improve abdominal distention, vomiting, and number of hospitalizations.[4,6,7,31] Ileostomies appear to have the highest rates of symptom relief,[7] but are associated with high rates of stomal prolapse and necrosis.[7,32] Intestinal or multivisceral transplantation should be considered in those with severe PN complications[1,3,5] and advances in surgical approach and immunotherapy have resulted on higher posttransplant survival.[33]

Megacystis-Microcolon-Intestinal Hypoperistalsis Syndrome

Megacystis-microcolon-intestinal hypoperistalsis syndrome (MMIHS) is a rare disorder associated with significant morbidity and mortality clinically resembling CIPO with a nonobstructed urinary bladder and microcolon (**Fig. 3**).[34] Prenatal ultrasound demonstrating a distended bladder should raise the suspicion of MMIHS. Postnatally, neonates present with symptoms secondary to bladder and bowel obstruction (massive abdominal distension, bilious emesis, failure to pass meconium, inability to void spontaneously requiring catheterization). MMIHS is caused by mutations in the *ACTG2* gene.[35] Treatment is aimed toward providing hydration, nutrition, and symptom relief. A systematic review (n = 227) demonstrated that most patients were female (70.6%), one or more surgical interventions were required (51%), most survivors were on PN and 12 underwent multivisceral transplants, and persistent bladder dysfunction requiring catheterization remained a morbidity. Survival rate was low (19.7%) and the most frequent causes of death were sepsis, multiorgan failure, and malnutrition.[36] However, specialized centers with multidisciplinary care have been credited for improved survival rates.[37]

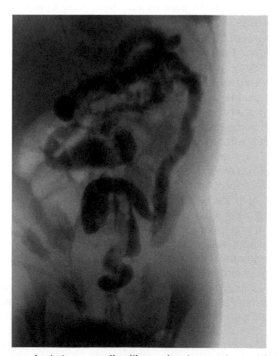

Fig. 3. Contrast enema depicting a small-caliber colon in a patient with MMIHS.

MOTILITY DISORDERS INVOLVING THE LARGE BOWEL
Medical Refractory Functional Constipation

Functional constipation (FC) is a symptoms-based diagnosis that centers around frequency and consistency of bowel movements. Most children with FC do not have an underlying organic condition. History and physical examination are key to diagnosis, and in the absence of alarming symptoms, there is no need for additional screening. In 2014, the North American Society of Pediatric Gastroenterology, Hepatology, and Nutrition (NASPGHAN) published its most recent guidelines for the management of children with constipation beginning with treatment of fecal impaction and establishing maintenance therapy.[38] Currently there seems to be no debate in the treatment of fecal impaction, with 2 randomized trials showing no difference in final outcome between oral polyethylene glycol or rectal enemas. Both should be recommended, and choice determined by parental and physician preferences.[39,40] Osmotic in combination with simulant laxatives are used for maintenance. Daily use of sennosides is the initial step and, in nonresponders, the regular use of bisacodyl has been found safe and effective for long-term use with most successfully weaned off.[41] Secretagogues, such as linaclotide, a guanylate cyclase-C agonist, lubiprostone, a type-2 chloride channel agonist, and prucalopride, have been shown to be safe and effective in adults but none are approved for use in pediatrics. Recent data demonstrated that linaclotide is safe and effective in children.[42] Lubiprostone was also shown to be effective and well tolerated in children.[43] The only data available for prucalopride are conflictive.[44,45]

Supplementary testing is indicated in patients refractory to medical therapy. Evaluation of colon transit by radiopaque markers (ROM) is an effective initial method to assess the need for more advanced and invasive testing.[46] Recently, the wireless motility capsule that simultaneously evaluates intestinal transit time and contractility has been proven useful to assess colon transit in children.[47] The most important indication to perform anorectal manometry in children is to assess the presence and quality of the recto-anal inhibitory reflex[48] (RAIR; **Fig. 4**), making it a useful screening modality in patients with suspected Hirschsprung disease (HSCR; see later in this article). Lower external anal squeeze pressure, blunted sensation, anal spasms, and prolonged RAIR with sustained rectal distension can be seen with spinal anomalies.[49] Colon manometry (CM) is used to assess the gastro-colonic response to a meal, and presence and quality of high-amplitude propagating contractions (**Fig. 5**). CM can help differentiate constipation from colonic motor dysfunction,[50] help guide surgical interventions,[51] determine if a diverted colon may be re-anastomosed,[52] and assess improvement of colonic dysmotility after long-term use of antegrade continence enemas (ACE).[51]

Surgical interventions should be considered only when all available medical therapies have failed and symptoms are significantly affecting quality of life.[38] ACE via percutaneous cecostomy or appendicostomy can be used to successfully achieve colonic emptying and continence.[53–55] In more severe cases or those not responsive to ACE, ostomies or colectomy can be considered with CM guidance.[52]

Hirschsprung Disease

HSCR is a congenital disorder caused by defective craniocaudal migration, proliferation, differentiation, and survival of neural crest cells, leading to the absence of ganglion cells of the hindgut submucosal and myenteric plexuses. The aganglionic segment starts distally in rectum and extends proximally throughout different lengths, most commonly limited to the rectosigmoid colon (short-segment HSCR, 80%), but

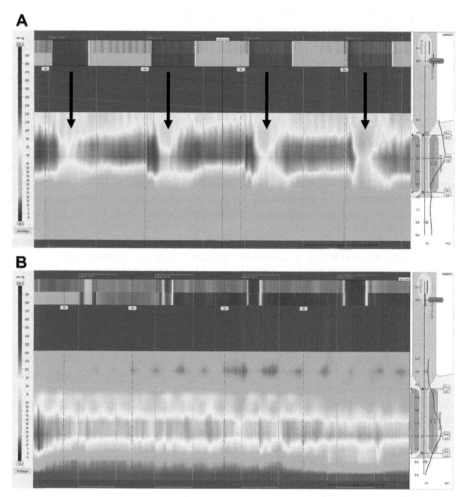

Fig. 4. High-resolution anorectal manometry demonstrating presence (*A, arrows*) and absence (*B*) of the RAIR in a patient with constipation and HSCR, respectively.

also proximal to the sigmoid colon (long-segment HSCR, 15%–20%) and rarely affecting the entire colon (5%) and extending to the small intestine.[56] HSCR affecting a small portion of the rectum (very short-segment HSCR, ≤2 cm) has been reported.[57] Skip segment HSCR is a rare entity, characterized by an area of ganglionated intestine surrounded proximally and distally by aganglionosis. Most cases describe skip areas affecting the colon in total colonic aganglionosis,[58] and one reported case involving the small bowel.[59]

The worldwide incidence of HSCR is 1 to 2 in 10,000 live births[60,61] varying by race and ethnicity,[62–64] with an overall 3:1 to 4:1 male predominance that becomes nearly 1:1 in total colonic aganglionosis.[65] Affected families carry a 200 times higher risk of recurrence,[66] and in siblings (nonsyndromic HSCR) the recurrence risk is approximately 3% and 17% for short-segment and long-segment disease, respectively.[56] Approximately 30% of patients have an associated chromosomal or genetic defect (syndromic HSCR),[67] with trisomy 21 being the most common (∼7%).[68] Other associated syndromes include Waardenburg type 4, Mowat-Wilson, multiple endocrine

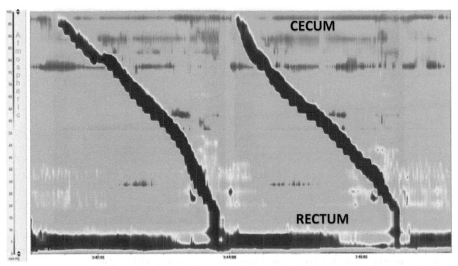

Fig. 5. High-resolution CM demonstrating high-amplitude propagating contractions migrating from cecum to rectum.

neoplasia 2A, congenital central hypoventilation, Bardet-Biedl, cartilage-hair hypoplasia, Riley-Day, Smith-Lemli-Opitz, and Goldberg-Shprintzen.

Known genetic variations are identified in at least 12% of cases and account for more than 50% of the observed abnormalities. Up to 11 neuro-developmental genes with high penetrance have been associated with HSCR: RET, EDNRB, GDNF, SOX10, NRTN, EDN3, ECE1, ZFHX1B, PHOX2B, KIAA1279, and TCF4 and the roles of the major susceptibility genes on chromosome 10 (RET) and chromosome 13 (EDNRB) are well established.[69]

Clinical presentation varies by age and extent of the aganglionosis. In neonates, HSCR presents with delayed passage of meconium and symptoms resembling intestinal obstruction or a more severe and potentially life-threatening presentation (HSCR associated enterocolitis [HAEC]) and rarely as bowel perforation. Infants and children with HSCR typically present with a long-standing history of medically refractory constipation or rectal therapy dependance.[70]

Abdominal radiography and contrast studies can support the diagnosis but are not sufficient to exclude it (**Fig. 6**). The presence of a transition zone or the change from a narrow rectum (aganglionic segment) to a dilated proximal colon is suggestive of HSCR. Reversal of the rectosigmoid index (ratio between the rectal and sigmoid diameters, normally >1) is suggestive of HSCR[71] but may be missed in patients with long-segment HSCR.[72] The RAIR evaluated by anorectal manometry is absent in patients with HSCR (see **Fig. 4**),[73–76] and new technology allows evaluation at an early age. Diagnostic confirmation requires a rectal biopsy demonstrating aganglionosis and submucosal nerve hypertrophy (**Fig. 7**). Calretinin and acetylcholinesterase histochemistry are ancillary techniques that improve the diagnostic accuracy. Results from a recent systematic review[77] comparing the diagnostic accuracy of tests in HSCR are summarized in **Table 1**.

Once the diagnosis of HSCR is confirmed, the goal of treatment is resecting the aganglionic segment and preserving anal sphincter function. The decision between the type of pull-through surgery or 1-stage versus 2-stage approach (diverting ostomy with later pull-through) varies between centers, but patient age, HSCR type, history of

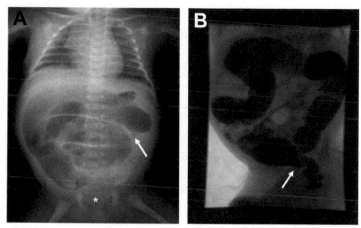

Fig. 6. Imaging studies in HSCR. (*A*) Abdominal radiography demonstrating absent gas (*asterisk*) in rectum and proximal bowel dilation (*arrow*). (*B*) Water contrast enema demonstrating transition zone (*arrow*) in rectosigmoid in a patient with HSCR.

HAEC, failure to thrive, and obstructive symptoms are key determinants. Many patients experience ongoing symptoms after surgery, and **Table 2** provides a summary of the most recent systematic review and meta-analysis describing the long-term postoperative outcomes in HSCR.[78–82] Furthermore, the American Pediatric Surgical Association HSCR Interest group has published guidelines for the management of postoperative obstructive symptoms,[83] soiling,[84] and HAEC,[85] which are summarized in **Box 1**. Anorectal manometry is useful in guiding therapy with anal *Botulinum* toxin injections.[86] CM can clarify the pathophysiology of symptoms and guide treatment postoperatively based on the motility pattern.[87] Recent studies show evidence of an association between fecal soiling and colonic hyperactivity,[88,89] so laxatives should be avoided in these cases.

Congenital Anorectal Malformations

Congenital anorectal malformations (ARMs) encompass a spectrum of anorectal disorders with variable anatomy and outcomes, with an incidence of 1 in 5000 live births

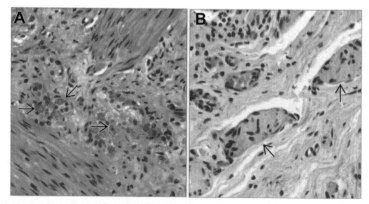

Fig. 7. (*A*) Rectal biopsy specimen (hematoxylin-eosin stain) displaying presence of submucosal ganglion cells (*arrows*) compared with (*B*) specimen from a patient with HSCR demonstrating hypertrophic nerve trunks (*arrows*) and absent ganglion cells.

Table 1
Diagnostic accuracy in Hirschsprung disease[77]

Test	Mean Sensitivity, %	Mean Specificity, %
Contrast enema	70	83
Anorectal manometry	91	94
Rectal suction biopsy		
Acetylcholinesterase stain	93	98
Hematoxylin-eosin stain	96	98

and a slight male predominance.[90] The etiology remains unclear and assumed to be multifactorial. The most frequent defect in male individuals is a rectourethral fistula and in female individuals a vestibular fistula. The Wingspread classification describes ARMs as low, intermediate, and high, and much of the literature is based on this classification, despite its lack of association with the type of surgery or outcomes. The Krickenbeck classification, which is based on the precise anatomic abnormality, has been shown to be valuable in guiding surgical management and can better define clinical outcomes.[91]

There is not a specific prenatal test to help detect ARMs. After birth, a detailed newborn examination, including careful inspection of the perineum, is key. Meconium exiting the perineum or in urine is suggestive of a fistula. In the first 24 hours of life, patients should be evaluated for associated defects especially in the presence of another syndrome, anatomic defect, or chromosomal abnormality. If there is no evidence of a fistula, a cross-table prone lateral radiograph can show air extending below the coccyx, in which case a posterior sagittal anorectoplasty (PSARP) can be performed, or gas that does not extend beyond the coccyx, in which case a 2-stage surgery should be performed.

The long-term postoperative goal is for patients to achieve bowel control through the use of medications, and dietary and behavioral modifications that are ideally individualized according to symptoms, and anorectal and colon function. The benefit of a

Table 2
Estimated prevalence of postoperative symptoms in HSCR and ARMs

Author, Year	No. of Patients	Constipation, %	Fecal Soiling, %	HAEC, %	Voiding Dysfunction, %
HSCR					
Dai et al,[78] 2020	625	14	20	N/A	0.07
Zimmer et al,[79] 2016	316	53.3	17.8	28.9	N/A
Tomuschat et al,[80] 2016	820	11.14	6.46	9.14	N/A
ARMs					
Rigueros et al,[81] 2016	455	22.2–86.7	16.7–76.7	N/A	1.7–30.5
Versteegh et al,[82] 2013	340	51	71	N/A	42

Abbreviations: ARM, anorectal malformation; HAEC, HSCR associated enterocolitis; HSCR, Hirschsprung disease; N/A, not applicable.

Box 1
Approach to patients with Hirschsprung disease with persistent postoperative symptoms

- Obstructive symptoms[83]
  - Causes:
    - Mechanical obstruction (anastomotic stricture)
    - Persistent or acquired aganglionosis, hypoganglionosis, or transition zone pull-through
    - Internal anal sphincter achalasia
    - Colon dysmotility
    - Functional megacolon (withholding behavior)
  - Approach:
    - History and physical examination including rectal examination
    - Contrast enema
    - Rectal biopsy
    - Anorectal manometry
    - Colon manometry
  - Treatment:
    - Stricture, twist, or mechanical obstruction: dilation or surgery
    - Aganglionosis, transition zone pull-through: redo pull-through
    - No neuromuscular pathology: Botulinum toxin injection, bowel management, antegrade colonic enemas, colonic resection
- Fecal soiling[84]
  - Causes:
    - Abnormal sensation
      - No sensation in neo-rectum
      - Loss of transitional epithelium
    - Inadequate sphincter control
      - Over stretch of sphincter mechanism during pull-through
      - Previous myectomy/sphincterotomy
    - Pseudo-incontinence
      - Obstruction or fecal impaction
      - Hypermotility
  - Approach:
    - History and physical examination
    - Rectal examination under anesthesia
    - Contrast enema
    - Anorectal manometry
    - Colon manometry
  - Treatment:
    - No correctable cause identified: high-fiber diet, stimulant laxatives, stool softeners as needed to maintain soft but solid stools
    - Hypermotility: constipating diet, high-fiber diet, antimotility agents
    - Persistent soiling: enema program, ostomy
- Hirschsprung disease associated enterocolitis (HAEC)[85]
  - Causes:
    - Dysbiosis of the intestinal microbiome
    - Impaired mucosal barrier function
    - Altered innate immune response
    - Bacterial translocation
  - Approach:
    - History and physical examination for grade classification
      - Grade I (possible HAEC): anorexia, diarrhea, mild abdominal distension
      - Grade II (definite HAEC): past history of HAEC, explosive diarrhea, fever, lethargy, tachycardia, abdominal distension and tenderness, explosive gas/stool on digital rectal examination
      - Grade III (severe HAEC): obstipation, obtunded, decreased peripheral perfusion, hypotension, altered mental status, marked abdominal distension, peritonitis
    - Laboratory: complete blood count with differential, chemistry, blood culture

- Abdominal radiography (mild ileus, air-fluid levels, dilated loops of bowel, rectosigmoid cutoff, pneumatosis, pneumoperitoneum)
o Treatment:
  - Grade I (outpatient): oral rehydration solution; oral metronidazole; consider rectal irrigations
  - Grade II (outpatient or inpatient): clear liquids or nothing by moth (NPO), intravenous (IV) fluid hydration; metronidazole (oral, IV), consider broad-spectrum IV coverage (ampicillin and gentamicin, or piperacillin-tazobactam); rectal irrigations
  - Grade III (inpatient, possible intensive care unit): NPO, intravenous fluids; metronidazole IV, broad-spectrum IV coverage (ampicillin and gentamicin, or piperacillin-tazobactam); rectal irrigations; proximal diversion for failure to improve with nonoperative management, exploration for pneumoperitoneum

comprehensive bowel management program is well known. Bischoff and colleagues[92] described their experience of 279 patients and reported a 95% success rate by tailoring the type of enema, medication, and diet. Stimulant laxatives are also widely used. A randomized controlled crossover design, including a washout period, that compared the effectiveness of senna and polyethylene glycol in children with corrected ARMs with fecal incontinence and constipation found a clear benefit toward senna in improving bowel movement frequency and soiling with no reported side effects.[93] The use of ACE has been reported as an effective therapy in achieving fecal continence.[55]

Postoperative anorectal and colon motility has been widely assessed. In a retrospective study of 41 patients operated on for ARMs and having defecation symptoms had total colon transit time measured by ROM and found that most had prolonged segmental transit time in the rectosigmoid.[94] A recent study aimed to describe findings in anorectal manometry among patients with different types of ARMs and found that the presence or absence of the RAIR correlated with the patient's functional outcome.[95] Anorectal manometry has also been used to describe the differences between surgical techniques, demonstrating the mean resting intra-anal resting pressure is significantly lower after PSARP compared with the laparoscopic approach but no difference was observed over the presence of the RAIR, squeeze pressures, or sensation.[96] A study using 3-dimensional high-resolution anorectal manometry demonstrated that at rest, the intra-anal resting pressures were lower both radially and longitudinally in children with a history of ARMs compared with patients with FC, but findings were not predictive of fecal continence.[97]

Regarding outcomes, a retrospective analysis by Peña and Hong[98] analyzed the long-term outcomes of 1192 patients operated for ARMs and reported that approximately 75% of their patients had voluntary bowel movements by 3 years of age and 50% of them experienced occasional soiling that improved with medical management. A systematic review reported a high prevalence of active long-term issues (constipation, fecal incontinence) in adolescents and young adults operated for ARMs, and a different study that evaluated the functional outcomes in cloaca malformations, reported similar results (see **Box 1**).[81,82] Children born with ARMs often have anomalies of the sacrum and spinal cord that impair sensory perception, sphincter control, and colon motility needed for fecal continence. Malformation type, sacral and spine involvement have been implicated in the potential for future continence in these children, and a prospective study found that the type of malformation (perineal, rectobulbar and recto-vestibular fistula, no fistula, rectal stenosis) was the only factor that predicted fecal continence, highlighting the need for long-term follow-up and bowel management programs.[99]

CLINICS CARE POINTS

- A motility disorder should be part of the differential diagnosis in infants and older children presenting with obstructive symptoms including intractable vomiting, feeding intolerance, abdominal distension, and constipation.

- The initial work up in patients with suspected CIPO should aim to identify potential causes or further explain its pathophysiology.

- Antroduodenal manometry is indicated in patients with obstructive symptoms unresponsive to medical therapy and a normal study excludes the possibility of CIPO.

- MMIHS should be suspected if a persistently distended bladder is visualized on prenatal ultrasonography.

- HSCR is typically diagnosed in the neonatal period but should be suspected in older children with medical refractory constipation.

- A normal abdominal radiography or contrast study does not rule out the possibility of HSCR.

- Anorectal manometry and CM testing is indicated in children with chronic constipation, and normal results are suggestive of a functional etiology.

- CM is useful in patients in whom surgical management is being contemplated for the treatment of medical refractory constipation.

- Defecation problems, including fecal incontinence and constipation, are common in patients with HSCR or congenital ARM after surgical repair.

- Manometry testing can help characterize anorectal and colon function and guide the postoperative medical management of HSCR and ARMs.

- A multidisciplinary approach is a well proven method in the treatment of pediatric patients with a primary or secondary motility disorder.

DISCLOSURE

The authors have nothing to disclose.

REFERENCES

1. Di Nardo G, Di Lorenzo C, Lauro A, et al. Chronic intestinal pseudo-obstruction in children and adults: diagnosis and therapeutic options. Neurogastroenterol Motil 2017;29(1). https://doi.org/10.1111/nmo.12945.
2. Thapar N, Saliakellis E, Benninga MA, et al. Paediatric intestinal pseudo-obstruction: evidence and consensus-based recommendations from an ESPGHAN-Led Expert Group. J Pediatr Gastroenterol Nutr 2018;66(6):991–1019.
3. De Giorgio R, Cogliandro RF, Barbara G, et al. Chronic intestinal pseudo-obstruction: clinical features, diagnosis, and therapy. Gastroenterol Clin North Am 2011;40(4):787–807.
4. Murr MM, Sarr MG, Camilleri M. The surgeon's role in the treatment of chronic intestinal pseudoobstruction. Am J Gastroenterol 1995;90(12):2147–51.
5. Di Lorenzo C. Pseudo-obstruction: current approaches. Gastroenterology 1999; 116(4):980–7.
6. Faure C, Goulet O, Ategbo S, et al. Chronic intestinal pseudoobstruction syndrome: clinical analysis, outcome, and prognosis in 105 children. French-Speaking Group of Pediatric Gastroenterology. Dig Dis Sci 1999;44(5):953–9.
7. Heneyke S, Smith VV, Spitz L, et al. Chronic intestinal pseudo-obstruction: treatment and long term follow up of 44 patients. Arch Dis Child 1999;81(1):21–7.

8. Muto M, Matsufuji H, Tomomasa T, et al. Pediatric chronic intestinal pseudo-obstruction is a rare, serious, and intractable disease: a report of a nationwide survey in Japan. J Pediatr Surg 2014;49(12):1799–803.

9. Vargas JH, Sachs P, Ament ME. Chronic intestinal pseudo-obstruction syndrome in pediatrics. Results of a national survey by members of the North American Society of Pediatric Gastroenterology and Nutrition. J Pediatr Gastroenterol Nutr 1988;7(3):323–32.

10. De Giorgio R, Stanghellini V, Barbara G, et al. Primary enteric neuropathies underlying gastrointestinal motor dysfunction. Scand J Gastroenterol 2000;35(2):114–22.

11. De Giorgio R, Camilleri M. Human enteric neuropathies: morphology and molecular pathology. Neurogastroenterol Motil 2004;16(5):515–31.

12. De Giorgio R, Sarnelli G, Corinaldesi R, et al. Advances in our understanding of the pathology of chronic intestinal pseudo-obstruction. Gut 2004;53(11):1549–52.

13. Isozaki K, Hirota S, Miyagawa J, et al. Deficiency of c-kit+ cells in patients with a myopathic form of chronic idiopathic intestinal pseudo-obstruction. Am J Gastroenterol 1997;92(2):332–4.

14. Stanghellini V, Corinaldesi R, Barbara L. Pseudo-obstruction syndromes. Baillieres Clin Gastroenterol 1988;2(1):225–54.

15. Mann SD, Debinski HS, Kamm MA. Clinical characteristics of chronic idiopathic intestinal pseudo-obstruction in adults. Gut 1997;41(5):675–81.

16. Stanghellini V, Cogliandro RF, De Giorgio R, et al. Natural history of chronic idiopathic intestinal pseudo-obstruction in adults: a single center study. Clin Gastroenterol Hepatol 2005;3(5):449–58.

17. Cucchiara S, Annese V, Minella R, et al. Antroduodenojejunal manometry in the diagnosis of chronic idiopathic intestinal pseudoobstruction in children. J Pediatr Gastroenterol Nutr 1994;18(3):294–305.

18. Cucchiara S, Borrelli O, Salvia G, et al. A normal gastrointestinal motility excludes chronic intestinal pseudoobstruction in children. Dig Dis Sci 2000;45(2):258–64.

19. Di Lorenzo C, Flores AF, Buie T, et al. Intestinal motility and jejunal feeding in children with chronic intestinal pseudo-obstruction. Gastroenterology 1995;108(5):1379–85.

20. Hyman PE, Di Lorenzo C, McAdams L, et al. Predicting the clinical response to cisapride in children with chronic intestinal pseudo-obstruction. Am J Gastroenterol 1993;88(6):832–6.

21. Scolapio JS, Ukleja A, Bouras EP, et al. Nutritional management of chronic intestinal pseudo-obstruction. J Clin Gastroenterol 1999;28(4):306–12.

22. Amiot A, Joly F, Alves A, et al. Long-term outcome of chronic intestinal pseudo-obstruction adult patients requiring home parenteral nutrition. Am J Gastroenterol 2009;104(5):1262–70.

23. Guarino A, De Marco G, Italian F. Natural history of intestinal failure, investigated through a national network-based approach. J Pediatr Gastroenterol Nutr 2003;37(2):136–41.

24. Hill S. Treatment and outcome of intestinal failure secondary to enteric neuromuscular disease. J Pediatr Gastroenterol Nutr 2007;45(Suppl 2):S107–9.

25. Kim HY, Kim JH, Jung SE, et al. Surgical treatment and prognosis of chronic intestinal pseudo-obstruction in children. J Pediatr Surg 2005;40(11):1753–9.

26. Navarro J, Sonsino E, Boige N, et al. Visceral neuropathies responsible for chronic intestinal pseudo-obstruction syndrome in pediatric practice: analysis of 26 cases. J Pediatr Gastroenterol Nutr 1990;11(2):179–95.

27. Emmanuel AV, Shand AG, Kamm MA. Erythromycin for the treatment of chronic intestinal pseudo-obstruction: description of six cases with a positive response. Aliment Pharmacol Ther 2004;19(6):687–94.

28. Ambartsumyan L, Flores A, Nurko S, et al. Utility of octreotide in advancing enteral feeds in children with chronic intestinal pseudo-obstruction. Paediatr Drugs 2016;18(5):387–92.

29. Emmanuel AV, Kamm MA, Roy AJ, et al. Randomised clinical trial: the efficacy of prucalopride in patients with chronic intestinal pseudo-obstruction–a double-blind, placebo-controlled, cross-over, multiple n = 1 study. Aliment Pharmacol Ther 2012;35(1):48–55.

30. Prapaitrakool S, Hollmann MW, Wartenberg HC, et al. Use of buprenorphine in children with chronic pseudoobstruction syndrome: case series and review of literature. Clin J Pain 2012;28(8):722–5.

31. Pakarinen MP, Kurvinen A, Koivusalo AI, et al. Surgical treatment and outcomes of severe pediatric intestinal motility disorders requiring parenteral nutrition. J Pediatr Surg 2013;48(2):333–8.

32. Irtan S, Bellaïche M, Brasher C, et al. Stomal prolapse in children with chronic intestinal pseudoobstruction: a frequent complication? J Pediatr Surg 2010;45(11):2234–7.

33. Lauro A, Zanfi C, Pellegrini S, et al. Isolated intestinal transplant for chronic intestinal pseudo-obstruction in adults: long-term outcome. Transplant Proc 2013;45(9):3351–5.

34. Puri P, Shinkai M. Megacystis microcolon intestinal hypoperistalsis syndrome. Semin Pediatr Surg 2005;14(1):58–63.

35. Bhagwat PK, Wangler MF. ACTG2 visceral myopathy. In: Adam MP, Ardinger HH, Pagon RA, et al, editors. GeneReviews® [Internet]. Seattle (WA): University of Washington, Seattle; 1993–2021. 2015 Jun 11 [updated 2021 May 6].

36. Gosemann JH, Puri P. Megacystis microcolon intestinal hypoperistalsis syndrome: systematic review of outcome. Pediatr Surg Int 2011;27(10):1041–6.

37. Prathapan KM, King DE, Raghu VK, et al. Megacystis microcolon intestinal hypoperistalsis syndrome: a case series with long-term follow-up and prolonged survival. J Pediatr Gastroenterol Nutr 2021;72(4):e81–5.

38. Tabbers MM, DiLorenzo C, Berger MY, et al. Evaluation and treatment of functional constipation in infants and children: evidence-based recommendations from ESPGHAN and NASPGHAN. J Pediatr Gastroenterol Nutr 2014;58(2):258–74.

39. Miller MK, Dowd MD, Friesen CA, et al. A randomized trial of enema versus polyethylene glycol 3350 for fecal disimpaction in children presenting to an emergency department. Pediatr Emerg Care 2012;28(2):115–9.

40. Bekkali NL, van den Berg MM, Dijkgraaf MG, et al. Rectal fecal impaction treatment in childhood constipation: enemas versus high doses oral PEG. Pediatrics 2009;124(6):e1108-15.

41. Bonilla S, Nurko S, Rodriguez L. Long-term use of bisacodyl in pediatric functional constipation refractory to conventional therapy. J Pediatr Gastroenterol Nutr 2020;71(3):288–91.

42. Di Lorenzo C, Nurko S, Hyams JS, et al. 1151 Linaclotide safety and efficacy in children aged 6 to 17 years with functional constipation. Am J Gastroenterol 2019;114(1):S645–6.

43. Hyman PE, Di Lorenzo C, Prestridge LL, et al. Lubiprostone for the treatment of functional constipation in children. J Pediatr Gastroenterol Nutr 2014;58(3):283–91.

44. Winter HS, Di Lorenzo C, Benninga MA, et al. Oral prucalopride in children with functional constipation. J Pediatr Gastroenterol Nutr 2013;57(2):197–203.

45. Mugie SM, Korczowski B, Bodi P, et al. Prucalopride is no more effective than placebo for children with functional constipation. Gastroenterology 2014;147(6):1285-e1.

46. Tipnis NA, El-Chammas KI, Rudolph CD, et al. Do oro-anal transit markers predict which children would benefit from colonic manometry studies? J Pediatr Gastroenterol Nutr 2012;54(2):258–62.

47. Rodriguez L, Heinz N, Colliard K, et al. Diagnostic and clinical utility of the wireless motility capsule in children: A study in patients with functional gastrointestinal disorders. Neurogastroenterol Motil 2021;33(4):e14032.

48. Rodriguez L, Sood M, Di Lorenzo C, et al. An ANMS-NASPGHAN consensus document on anorectal and colonic manometry in children. Neurogastroenterol Motil 2017;29(1). https://doi.org/10.1111/nmo.12944.

49. Siddiqui A, Rosen R, Nurko S. Anorectal manometry may identify children with spinal cord lesions. J Pediatr Gastroenterol Nutr 2011;53(5):507 11.

50. Di Lorenzo C, Flores AF, Reddy SN, et al. Use of colonic manometry to differentiate causes of intractable constipation in children. J Pediatr 1992;120(5):690–5.

51. Rodriguez L, Nurko S, Flores A. Factors associated with successful decrease and discontinuation of antegrade continence enemas (ACE) in children with defecation disorders: a study evaluating the effect of ACE on colon motility. Neurogastroenterol Motil 2013;25(2):140-e81.

52. Villarreal J, Sood M, Zangen T, et al. Colonic diversion for intractable constipation in children: colonic manometry helps guide clinical decisions. J Pediatr Gastroenterol Nutr 2001;33(5):588–91.

53. Hoekstra LT, Kuijper CF, Bakx R, et al. The Malone antegrade continence enema procedure: the Amsterdam experience. J Pediatr Surg 2011;46(8):1603–8.

54. Mugie SM, Machado RS, Mousa HM, et al. Ten-year experience using antegrade enemas in children. J Pediatr 2012;161(4):700–4.

55. Siddiqui AA, Fishman SJ, Bauer SB, et al. Long-term follow-up of patients after antegrade continence enema procedure. J Pediatr Gastroenterol Nutr 2011;52(5):574–80.

56. Badner JA, Sieber WK, Garver KL, et al. A genetic study of Hirschsprung disease. Am J Hum Genet 1990;46(3):568–80.

57. Kapur RP. Calretinin-immunoreactive mucosal innervation in very short-segment Hirschsprung disease: a potentially misleading observation. Pediatr Dev Pathol 2014;17(1):28–35.

58. O'Donnell AM, Puri P. Skip segment Hirschsprung's disease: a systematic review. Pediatr Surg Int 2010;26(11):1065–9.

59. El-Gohary Y, Skerritt C, Prasad V, et al. Case report of a skip segment Hirschsprung's disease: a real phenomenon. Int J Surg Case Rep 2021;80:105630.

60. Russell MB, Russell CA, Niebuhr E. An epidemiological study of Hirschsprung's disease and additional anomalies. Acta Paediatr 1994;83(1):68–71.

61. Goldberg EL. An epidemiological study of Hirschsprung's disease. Int J Epidemiol 1984;13(4):479–85.

62. Anderson JE, Vanover MA, Saadai P, et al. Epidemiology of Hirschsprung disease in California from 1995 to 2013. Pediatr Surg Int 2018;34(12):1299–303.

63. Bradnock TJ, Knight M, Kenny S, et al. Hirschsprung's disease in the UK and Ireland: incidence and anomalies. Arch Dis Child 2017;102(8):722–7.

64. Chia ST, Chen SC, Lu CL, et al. Epidemiology of Hirschsprung's disease in Taiwanese children: a 13-year nationwide population-based study. Pediatr Neonatol 2016;57(3):201–6.

65. Ieiri S, Suita S, Nakatsuji T, et al. Total colonic aganglionosis with or without small bowel involvement: a 30-year retrospective nationwide survey in Japan. J Pediatr Surg 2008;43(12):2226–30.

66. Amiel J, Lyonnet S. Hirschsprung disease, associated syndromes, and genetics: a review. J Med Genet 2001;38(11):729–39.

67. Moore SW, Zaahl M. Clinical and genetic differences in total colonic aganglionosis in Hirschsprung's disease. J Pediatr Surg 2009;44(10):1899–903.

68. Friedmacher F, Puri P. Hirschsprung's disease associated with Down syndrome: a meta-analysis of incidence, functional outcomes and mortality. Pediatr Surg Int 2013;29(9):937–46.

69. Moore SW. Chromosomal and related Mendelian syndromes associated with Hirschsprung's disease. Pediatr Surg Int 2012;28(11):1045–58.

70. Doodnath R, Puri P. A systematic review and meta-analysis of Hirschsprung's disease presenting after childhood. Pediatr Surg Int 2010;26(11):1107–10.

71. Garcia R, Arcement C, Hormaza L, et al. Use of the recto-sigmoid index to diagnose Hirschsprung's disease. Clin Pediatr (Phila) 2007;46(1):59–63.

72. Stranzinger E, DiPietro MA, Teitelbaum DH, et al. Imaging of total colonic Hirschsprung disease. Pediatr Radiol 2008;38(11):1162–70.

73. Emir H, Akman M, Sarimurat N, et al. Anorectal manometry during the neonatal period: its specificity in the diagnosis of Hirschsprung's disease. Eur J Pediatr Surg 1999;9(2):101–3.

74. Meinds RJ, Trzpis M, Broens PMA. Anorectal manometry may reduce the number of rectal suction biopsy procedures needed to diagnose Hirschsprung disease. J Pediatr Gastroenterol Nutr 2018;67(3):322–7.

75. Wu JF, Lu CH, Yang CH, et al. Diagnostic role of anal sphincter relaxation integral in high-resolution anorectal manometry for Hirschsprung disease in infants. J Pediatr 2018;194:136-e2.

76. Huang Y, Zheng S, Xiao X. Preliminary evaluation of anorectal manometry in diagnosing Hirschsprung's disease in neonates. Pediatr Surg Int 2009;25(1):41–5.

77. de Lorijn F, Kremer LC, Reitsma JB, et al. Diagnostic tests in Hirschsprung disease: a systematic review. J Pediatr Gastroenterol Nutr 2006;42(5):496–505.

78. Dai Y, Deng Y, Lin Y, et al. Long-term outcomes and quality of life of patients with Hirschsprung disease: a systematic review and meta-analysis. BMC Gastroenterol 2020;20(1):67.

79. Zimmer J, Tomuschat C, Puri P. Long-term results of transanal pull-through for Hirschsprung's disease: a meta-analysis. Pediatr Surg Int 2016;32(8):743–9.

80. Tomuschat C, Zimmer J, Puri P. Laparoscopic-assisted pull-through operation for Hirschsprung's disease: a systematic review and meta-analysis. Pediatr Surg Int 2016;32(8):751–7.

81. Rigueros Springford L, Connor MJ, Jones K, et al. Prevalence of active long-term problems in patients with anorectal malformations: a systematic review. Dis Colon Rectum 2016;59(6):570–80.

82. Versteegh HP, van Rooij IA, Levitt MA, et al. Long-term follow-up of functional outcome in patients with a cloacal malformation: a systematic review. J Pediatr Surg 2013;48(11):2343–50.

83. Langer JC, Rollins MD, Levitt M, et al. Guidelines for the management of postoperative obstructive symptoms in children with Hirschsprung disease. Pediatr Surg Int 2017;33(5):523–6.

84. Saadai P, Trappey AF, Goldstein AM, et al. Guidelines for the management of postoperative soiling in children with Hirschsprung disease. Pediatr Surg Int 2019;35(8):829–34.

85. Gosain A, Frykman PK, Cowles RA, et al. Guidelines for the diagnosis and management of Hirschsprung-associated enterocolitis. Pediatr Surg Int 2017;33(5):517–21.

86. Roorda D, Abeln ZA, Oosterlaan J, et al. Botulinum toxin injections after surgery for Hirschsprung disease: systematic review and meta-analysis. World J Gastroenterol 2019;25(25):3268–80.

87. Di Lorenzo C, Solzi GF, Flores AF, et al. Colonic motility after surgery for Hirschsprung's disease. Am J Gastroenterol 2000;95(7):1759–64.

88. Kaul A, Garza JM, Connor FL, et al. Colonic hyperactivity results in frequent fecal soiling in a subset of children after surgery for Hirschsprung disease. J Pediatr Gastroenterol Nutr 2011;52(4):433–6.

89. Jacobs C, Wolfson S, Di Lorenzo C, et al. Effect of colon transection on spontaneous and meal-induced high-amplitude–propagating contractions in children. J Pediatr Gastroenterol Nutr 2015;60(1):60–4.

90. Wood RJ, Levitt MA. Anorectal malformations. Clin Colon Rectal Surg 2018;31(2):61–70.

91. Holschneider A, Hutson J, Peña A, et al. Preliminary report on the International Conference for the Development of Standards for the Treatment of Anorectal Malformations. J Pediatr Surg 2005;40(10):1521–6.

92. Bischoff A, Levitt MA, Bauer C, et al. Treatment of fecal incontinence with a comprehensive bowel management program. J Pediatr Surg 2009;44(6):1278–84 [discussion: 1283–4].

93. Santos-Jasso KA, Arredondo-García JL, Maza-Vallejos J, et al. Effectiveness of senna vs polyethylene glycol as laxative therapy in children with constipation related to anorectal malformation. J Pediatr Surg 2017;52(1):84–8.

94. Demirogullari B, Ozen IO, Karabulut R, et al. Colonic motility and functional assessment of the patients with anorectal malformations according to Krickenbeck consensus. J Pediatr Surg 2008;43(10):1839–43.

95. Kyrklund K, Pakarinen MP, Rintala RJ. Manometric findings in relation to functional outcomes in different types of anorectal malformations. J Pediatr Surg 2017;52(4):563–8.

96. Chung PHY, Wong CWY, Wong KKY, et al. Assessing the long term manometric outcomes in patients with previous laparoscopic anorectoplasty (LARP) and posterior sagittal anorectoplasty (PSARP). J Pediatr Surg 2018;53(10):1933–6.

97. Ambartsumyan L, Shaffer M, Carlin K, et al. Comparison of longitudinal and radial characteristics of intra-anal pressures using 3D high-definition anorectal manometry between children with anoretal malformations and functional constipation. Neurogastroenterol Motil 2020;33:e13971.

98. Pena A, Hong A. Advances in the management of anorectal malformations. Am J Surg 2000;180(5):370–6.

99. Minneci PC, Kabre RS, Mak GZ, et al. Can fecal continence be predicted in patients born with anorectal malformations? J Pediatr Surg 2019;54(6):1159–63.

Pancreatitis in Children

Reuven Zev Cohen, MD*, A. Jay Freeman, MD

KEYWORDS

- Pediatric pancreatitis ● Acute recurrent ● Exocrine insufficiency

KEY POINTS

- Risk factors for pediatric pancreatitis are different from those for adult pancreatitis, and recognition of pediatric risk factors should guide diagnosis and management.
- Acute pancreatitis management in children should focus on fluid resuscitation, end-organ monitoring, pain management, and early nutrition.
- Acute recurrent pancreatitis in children should prompt a broader investigation into possible genetic, anatomic, and metabolic risk factors.
- Children with chronic pancreatitis require a multidisciplinary approach to manage the varied manifestations and sequelae of disease progression.

INTRODUCTIONS AND DEFINITIONS

This review of pediatric pancreatitis is organized over the spectrum of acute pancreatitis (AP), acute recurrent pancreatitis (ARP), and finally chronic pancreatitis (CP) (**Fig. 1**).[1] While each of these diagnoses requires a strict definition, there is some overlap in diagnostic approach, and management philosophies are often applicable to more than one diagnosis. Most children with AP recover with no further sequelae; however, some will develop recurrent attacks (ARP) with a subset developing irreversible pancreatic damage consistent with CP. Additionally, up to 10% of children may present with CP without prior AP or ARP.[2] Certain etiologies and interventions in particular, such as autoimmune pancreatitis (AIP) and pancreatic endotherapy, respectively, span presentations.

ACUTE PANCREATITIS SPECTRUM AND MANAGEMENT

The incidence of AP in pediatric literature is estimated to be 13 per 100,000 children[3] with rising rates of diagnosis.[4] As detailed in **Fig. 1**, the diagnosis of AP must include at least 2 of the following conditions: abdominal pain consistent with AP, serum amylase or lipase $\geq 3\times$ upper limit of normal, or imaging consistent with AP.[1] Lipase is a more

Conflicts of interest and source of funding. There are no potential conflicts of interest, real or perceived to report. No honorarium, grant, or other form of payment was given to anyone to produce the article.

Division of Pediatric Gastroenterology, Hepatology, and Nutrition, Emory University School of Medicine, Children's Healthcare of Atlanta, 1400 Tullie Road Northeast, Atlanta, GA 30329, USA

* Corresponding author.

E-mail address: Reuven.zev.cohen@emory.edu

Acute Pancreatitis (at least 2 findings)
- Abdominal pain consistent with AP
- Amylase/Lipase≥3 ULN
- Imaging consistent with AP

Acute Recurrent Pancreatitis
- ≥2 episodes AP
- Resolution of pain and/or amylase/lipse between AP episodes (1 mo)

Chronic Pancreatitis (at least 1 finding)
- Abdominal pain consistent with pancreatic origin and imaging suggestive of chronic pancreatic damage OR
- Evidence of exocrine pancreatic insufficiency and suggestive pancreatic imaging findings OR
- Evidence of endocrine pancreatic insufficiency and suggestive pancreatic imaging findings

Fig. 1. Criteria for acute, acute recurrent, and chronic pancreatitis. AP, acute pancreatitis; ULN, upper limit of normal.

accurate diagnostic marker of AP, particularly in infants.[5] Amylase and lipase can occasionally be elevated even in the absence of AP and abdominal pain, particularly in diabetic ketoacidosis (DKA),[6] and rapidly normalize after treatment for DKA.

First-line imaging for suspicion of AP is transabdominal ultrasound,[7] which has the added benefit of diagnosing biliary obstruction and identifying pancreatic fluid collections and abnormal pancreaticobiliary anatomy.

Etiology and Risk Factors for Pediatric Acute Pancreatitis Varies by Age and Differs from Adult Causes

Across all pediatric age groups, the etiology of AP is quite different than that of adults (**Fig. 2**).[8,9] Pediatric AP risk factors are more varied and most commonly the result of biliary disease, medications, or systemic disease compared to predominantly alcohol and biliary disease in adults.[10] Even within childhood, there is a shift in risk factors from infancy through toddlerhood and adolescence. In infancy and toddlerhood, AP etiologies are skewed predominantly toward trauma, systemic disease, and inborn errors of metabolism. This is in contrast to adolescence, when AP is often caused by biliary disease and medications or is idiopathic.[8]

Discrete etiologies are present within each risk category for pediatric AP as detailed in **Table 1**. In consideration of the most common risk factors for AP, a child's first presentation should include serum transaminases, bilirubin, calcium, triglycerides, and imaging with transabdominal ultrasound while reserving expanded diagnostic workups for recurrent disease or concerning history (eg, family history of pancreatic cancer or pancreatitis) or age less than 5 years at initial presentation.[1]

Medication-induced AP is potentially underreported because of difficulty linking a causative medication and lack of a clear diagnostic criteria. Temporal association and rechallenge with the medication[11,12] have been used to establish a causal link. Several high-risk medications are listed in **Table 1**, but the list is certainly not exhaustive. Genetic risk factors may predispose patients to drug-induced pancreatitis,[13] and additional risk factors, including genetic and anatomic ones, may be comorbid and must be investigated. Management of medication-induced AP is centered around cessation of possible causal medications and investigation of potential co-risk

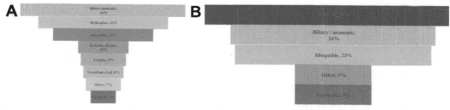

Fig. 2. Comparison of pediatric and adult risk factors for acute pancreatitis. (*Adapted from* Husain, et al and Sekimoto, et al.[8,10])

Table 1
Specific risk factors for pediatric AP

Biliary/anatomic	Medication	Systemic disease
Choledocholithiasis	Valproic acid	Autoimmune pancreatitis
Pancreas divisum	Prednisone	Sepsis
Pancreaticobiliary	Mesalamine	Lupus
maljunction	Trimethoprim/	Henoch-Schonlein purpura
Choledochal cyst	sulfamethoxazole	Kawasaki disease
Annular pancreas	Azathioprine	Inflammatory bowel disease
Intestinal duplication	Asparaginase	Hemolytic uremic syndrome
	Tetracycline	
Trauma	Other	Metabolic
Handlebar injury	Genetic	Diabetic ketoacidosis
Car accident	Inborn errors of	Hypertriglyceridemia
Nonaccidental trauma	metabolism	Hypercalcemia
Sports injury		Chronic renal failure

factors.[14] Future avenues of research must explore the mechanisms and genotype-phenotype associations of medication-induced pancreatitis.

As summarized in **Table 2**, severity of AP ranges from mild to severe.[15] Mild AP occurs in the absence of organ failure or complications and generally resolves within a week. Severity worsens with development and persistence of organ failure and local complications. Mortality for children in AP remains low and below that of adults,[16,17] potentially due to the absence of comorbidities and absence of risk factors as well as possible cellular differences that have yet to be elucidated.

Management of Acute Pancreatitis

Acute care of children with pancreatitis is focused on four domains: fluid resuscitation, end-organ monitoring and prevention of progression to severe pancreatitis, early nutrition, and pain control (**Fig. 3**).

Fluid Resuscitation in Acute Pancreatitis

Adequate intravenous (IV) crystalloid fluid is a critical front-line therapy for AP insofar as it not only treats hypovolemia but also augments pancreatic microcirculation and prevents progression to severe disease and end-organ dysfunction.[18] A preference for lactated Ringer's (LR) solution has been adopted from adult data that suggested a reduction in the incidence of systemic inflammatory response syndrome (SIRS),[19]

Table 2
Ranging severity of acute pancreatitis

Mild AP	Moderately Severe AP	Severe AP
Absence of organ failure	Transient organ failure that resolves within 48 h	Organ failure that persists for more than 48 h
Absence of local/systemic complications	Local complications	
Usual resolution within a week		

Adapted from Abu-El-Haija M, Kumar S, Szabo F, et al. Classification of Acute Pancreatitis in the Pediatric Population: Clinical Report From the NASPGHAN Pancreas Committee. Journal of pediatric gastroenterology and nutrition. 2017;64(6):984-990.

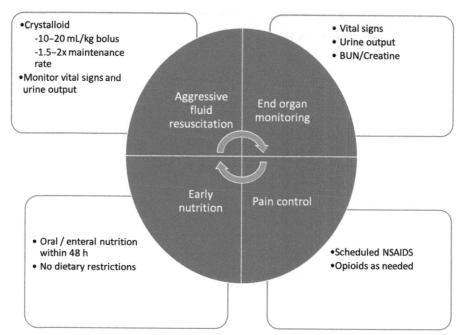

Fig. 3. Primary domains of acute pancreatitis management. BUN, blood urea nitrogen; NSAID, nonsteroidal anti-inflammatory therapy.

but a similar benefit has not been demonstrated in children with AP. Accessibility and ease of procurement of normal saline make it a suitable alternative to LR. Initial bolus of crystalloid should be 10 to 20 mL/kg followed by approximately 1.5× maintenance rate of IV fluids while monitoring urine output to assess adequate resuscitation and tolerance of oral or enteral fluids.

End-Organ Monitoring in Acute Pancreatitis

Multiorgan dysfunction including cardiac, pulmonary, and renal dysfunction are hallmarks of disease severity and increases the risk for death in AP.[20] Considering the aggressive need for IV fluid resuscitation in a milieu of increased capillary permeability, there is significant risk of third-spacing and extrapancreatic sequalae, including cardiac tamponade, acute respiratory distress syndrome, and acute kidney injury.

Pain Management in Acute Pancreatitis

There are minimal data regarding a standardized pain regimen in AP, despite the almost universal presence of abdominal pain in the diagnosis. Oral and IV nonsteroidal anti-inflammatory drugs (NSAIDs) are a mainstay of pain control.

Most children with AP will require opioids for pain control.[1] Nonetheless, children with AP who received initial pain control with an opioid ultimately received more doses of any type of analgesia than those whose initial dose was a nonopioid.[21] In comparison, patients for whom their first analgesic was a nonopioid needed fewer total doses of analgesia throughout admission. Given the risk for opioid-related adverse effects, development of opioid-sparing strategies is important. Implementation of combined opioid and NSAID, including ketorolac, is widely followed but lacks prospective efficacy data.

Nutrition Management in Acute Pancreatitis

Conventional wisdom has instructed nil per os (NPO) approach to management of AP, in an effort to presumptively suppress pancreatic enzyme production. However, NPO status has been associated with increased risk of translocation of bacterial flora from the gut causing increased morbidity in acute severe pancreatitis.[22] Furthermore, early introduction of oral or enteral nutrition is associated with decreased length of hospitalization and does not result in worsening of abdominal pain.[23-25]

The detriment of delayed nutrition is presumably due to development of a hypermetabolic state, including protein catabolism, increased energy expenditure, and increased dependence on fatty acid oxidation to provide energy that exists in the milieu of AP.[26] A full oral solid diet should be encouraged early (within 48–72 hours) of hospitalization[27] (**Fig. 4**). Fat restriction within the first 2 weeks of AP diagnosis may be considered[28] but is likely unnecessary and should not be maintained long term. For those patients unable to tolerate an oral diet, placement of a nasoenteric tube and initiation of enteral nutrition are preferred to parenteral nutrition.[29] Even in cases of severe AP in critically ill patients, there is support for early initiation of enteral nutrition and its role in improved outcomes.[30] Much of the data examining early enteral nutrition in children with AP are retrospective[5,31] but remain consistent with adult data demonstrating improved outcomes with early (<48 hours) enteral nutrition. If there is inability to reach caloric goals with enteral nutrition at 1 week, parenteral nutrition should be used for supplementation.[28]

Advanced Endoscopic Interventions in Acute Pancreatitis

Biliary obstruction is the most prevalent risk factor for pediatric AP,[8] and clues to this etiology are often in the form of elevated transaminases, bilirubin, and γ-glutamyltransferase. Ultrasound is typically an insensitive diagnostic tool for identification of a common bile duct stone,[32] and cross-sectional imaging via magnetic resonance

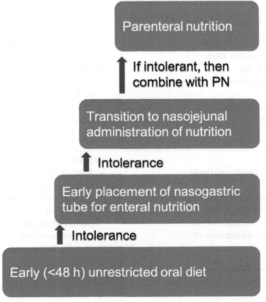

Fig. 4. Stairstep approach to nutrition in acute pancreatitis. PN, parenteral nutrition.

cholangiopancreatography (MRCP) must be obtained. In the case of biliary pancreatitis, endoscopic retrograde cholangiopancreatography (ERCP) should be pursued within 48 hours[33] if the patient has obstructive jaundice or cholangitis, and this should be followed by same-admission cholecystectomy.[34] In centers where ERCP is not readily assessable, primary cholecystectomy with intraoperative cholangiogram is a safe and effective alternative.

Management of Pancreatic Fluid Collections and Pancreatic Duct Trauma

Local complications of AP include acute pancreatic fluid collections (APFCs), acute necrotic collections (ANCs), pseudocysts, and walled-off necrosis.[35] These are characterized in the Revised Atlanta Classification[36] as adapted in **Table 3**.

The classification of these 4 types of fluid collections is mainly based on the duration, nature, and composition of the collection. APFC can develop after an episode of AP and may evolve into a pseudocyst after 4 weeks. ANC has the potential to develop after necrotizing pancreatitis and may mature into walled-off necrosis (WON) after 4 weeks. Pediatric data suggest spontaneous resolution of the overwhelming majority of APFC and pseudocysts without intervention,[35] and as such, monitoring alone generally suffices while awaiting resolution. There is no correlation between the size of the pseudocyst and the time required for resolution. The median time for pseudocyst resolution is 3 to 4 months.[37] Drainage of a pseudocyst can be considered if a child develops uncontrollable symptoms, signs of infection occur, or obstructive complications arise.

Retrospective pediatric data suggest that ANC matures to WON in approximately 68% of children, while the remainder resolve without requiring drainage.[35] Percutaneous or endoscopic ultrasound (EUS)-guided cystogastrostomy can be performed in the event of symptomatic persistence of WON (signs of gastric compression or gastric outlet obstruction) or infected fluid collections (**Table 4**). General endoscopic

Table 3	
Types of pancreatic fluid collections	
Acute pancreatic fluid collection	Acute necrotic collection
• Usually develops in the early phase of pancreatitis	• Arises from necrotizing pancreatitis
• Lack a well-defined wall	• Fluid and necrotic pancreatic parenchyma/peri-pancreatic tissue in the first 4 wk of development
• Homogenous	• May be loculated
• Confined by fascial planes	• Can become infected
• May be multiple	
• Sterile	
• Resolves spontaneously	
Pseudocyst	Walled-off necrosis
• Well-defined wall with minimal solid material	• Mature, encapsulated collection of pancreatic/peripancreatic necrosis with a well-defined inflammatory wall
• Increased amylase within the fluid	• Usually >4 wk after necrotizing pancreatitis onset
• Absence of necrotic material	• Can be infected
• Localized fluid collection >4 wk	
• Often arises from disruption of pancreatic duct	
• Rare in AP	

Adapted from Banks PA, Bollen TL, Dervenis C, et al. Classification of acute pancreatitis–2012: revision of the Atlanta classification and definitions by international consensus. Gut. 2013;62(1):102-111.[36]

Table 4
EUS utility for pediatric pancreaticobiliary disease[41]

Diagnostic	Therapeutic
Pancreatic parenchymal anatomy	Cystogastrostomy
Cystic pancreatic lesions	Celiac plexus neurolysis
Autoimmune pancreatitis	Biliary drainage if unable to access papilla.
Suspected choledocholithiasis	
Unknown etiology of obstructive jaundice	
Pancreatic mass fine needle aspiration	

principles suggest that EUS-guided drainage is preferred in mature, walled-off collections located in close proximity to the gastric wall.[38]

Blunt abdominal trauma can lead to disruption of the pancreatic duct and formation of a pancreatic pseudocyst. In these cases, ERCP can be both diagnostic to determine communication of the pseudocyst with the pancreatic duct and therapeutic with placement of a transpapillary pancreatic stent with the goal of ductal decompression through the stent given an improved pressure gradient. Early ERCP can allow for nonoperative management in cases of traumatic pancreatitis and decrease risk for development of late complications such as pancreatic duct stricture and fistula.[39] If a persistent pseudocyst cannot be drained via ERCP (discontinuous with pancreatic duct) or has complex features (infected or walled-off necrosis), EUS-guided drainage via cystogastrostomy can be used.[40] Additional indications for ERCP and EUS will be covered in more detail in discussion of CP.

Antibiotic administration in acute pancreatitis

Adult and pediatric guidelines do not recommend routine prophylactic antibiotic use in AP, even in severe cases, unless there is evidence of infected necrotizing pancreatitis or patients with necrosis who are not improving without antibiotics.[42,43]

Standardized approach

In order to improve clinical outcomes, standardized orders have been recommended for all patients admitted with isolated AP.[44] In a single-center study using a standardized order set based on the North American Society for Pediatric Gastroenterology, Hepatology, and Nutrition (NASPGHAN) AP recommendations,[43] children with AP experienced a significant reduction in opioid usage along with a clinically significant (but not statistically different) 10% reduction in hospital length of stay without increasing intensive care unit or hospital readmission rates (accepted, full ref to be added at time of proof).[45]

Children with AP should be monitored after their initial episode of AP as a single-center study reported that 70% of children developed ARP within 5 months of their initial presentation of AP.[46]

AUTOIMMUNE PANCREATITIS

Pediatric AIP is a relatively rare entity and accounts for only 4% of pediatric pancreatitis.[47] It is most prevalent in adolescence and presents with typical abdominal pain and often with direct hyperbilirubinemia and a history of weight loss. In contrast to AP, AIP often presents with normal serum amylase and lipase,[48] leading to a broader differential diagnosis that includes a host of pancreaticobiliary pathologies and

Table 5 Differentiation of AIP-1 and AIP-2		
Characterisitc	AIP-1	AIP-2
Serum IgG4	Sometimes elevated	Rarely elevated
Histology	Lymphoplasmacytic sclerosing pancreatitis and IgG4+ plasma cells	Granulocytic epithelial lesions with destruction of pancreatic duct
Other organ involvement	Sclerosing cholangitis and additional organs as a result of IgG4 disease	Ulcerative colitis
Clinical presentation	Jaundice, fatigue, abdominal pain weight loss	
Amylase/lipase	Often normal	
MRI/MRCP	• Diffuse or focal pancreatic enlargement with loss of parenchymal architecture • Peripancreatic capsular rim • T1-weighted: Decreased intensity • T2-weighted: Increased intensity • Pancreatic ductal narrowing	
Treatment	1–1.5 mg/kg/d oral prednisone (max 40–60 mg daily) for 2–4 wk followed by taper. Follow symptomatic and imaging response.	

requiring supplementary radiological and histologic information (**Table 5**). Increased serum IgG4 is a hallmark feature of type 1 AIP in adults; however, the prevalence of elevated serum IgG4 in children is lower, and there are numerous cases of seronegative type 1 AIP.[49]

First-line imaging when there is suspicion for AIP should start with transabdominal ultrasound, which may demonstrate diffuse or focal pancreatic enlargement or a mass in the context of hypoechoic pancreatic parenchyma. With suspicion for AIP, there should be a low threshold to proceed to MRCP, which, in addition to detailed parenchymal changes, can demonstrate a capsular rim on T2-weighted images and well-elucidated pancreatic or biliary ductal abnormalities consistent with AIP.[50]

Given the overlap in presentation of AIP with other biliary and neoplastic processes, a histologic diagnosis may be necessary. This is particularly true in IgG4-negative diseases. Pancreatic biopsy via EUS-guided fine needle biopsy (EUS-FNB) and ERCP-guided papillary biopsy are feasible approaches. ERCP has the added benefit of offering a therapeutic intervention for cholestasis in AIP. In diagnosing definitive AIP in adults, EUS-FNB did demonstrate marginally higher sensitivity than ERCP with papillary biopsy and was also more sensitive to differentiate type 1 and type 2 AIP histologically.[51] With wider availability of pediatric-experienced EUS providers, EUS-guided pancreatic biopsy could be the approach of choice.[48] A histologic diagnosis is additionally important in differentiating autoimmune disease from malignant processes, which, although rare in childhood, can mimic AIP presentation.

Oral corticosteroids are the first-line treatment in AIP, and therapeutic response is often helpful in clarifying the diagnosis in patients without a definitive histologic diagnosis. Both symptom resolution and imaging evidence of resolution can be used to gauge response to therapy.

Relapse of AIP in children has been reported in which case a second course of corticosteroids should be used, and for those patients who require maintenance immunomodulatory therapy, there is experience with azathioprine, mycophenolate, and 6-mercaptopurine.[47]

ACUTE RECURRENT PANCREATITIS

Approximately one-quarter of AP patients will develop ARP. Strictly defined, ARP requires at least 2 episodes of AP with either complete resolution of pain between episodes (>1 month) or complete normalization of amylase and lipase between episodes.

In addition to laboratory and imaging evaluation discussed in the evaluation of AP, children who develop ARP warrant expanded evaluation given the higher prevalence of genetic, anatomic, and metabolic risk factors.

In an effort to better understand pediatric ARP and CP, the International Study Group of Pediatric Pancreatitis: In search for a cuRE (INSPPIRE) consortium was formed.[52] Up to half of patients in the INSPPIRE cohort with ARP had at least one genetic risk factor,[53] and as such, genetic testing should be undertaken when children present with ARP. In CP, the likelihood of identifying a genetic risk factor is even higher, further supporting the need for genetic evaluation. **Table 6** details the relative frequency of the most common genetic risk factors for ARP and CP, and the role of less common mutations in genes such as *CPA1*, *CLDN2*, *CEL*, and *CEL-HYB*[53–57] is increasingly being recognized. Identification of a gain-of-function *PRSS1* mutation is particularly important in that there is high penetrance and resulting increased probability of progression to CP and possibly pancreatic cancer.[57] Additionally, there is a stronger argument for genetic counseling due to likelihood of affected relatives who will carry the *PRSS1* mutation.[58]

Imaging in Acute Recurrent Pancreatitis

In addition to the imaging investigation delineated in AP, additional aims in the evaluation of children with ARP are elucidation of treatable etiologies of ARP and delineation of signs of CP. Cross-sectional imaging with MRCP and, if available, with secretin enhancement to better delineate subtle pancreatic ductal abnormalities should be pursued in ARP. Secretin administration not only provides increased detail regarding the anatomy of the pancreatic duct but also helps to elucidate pancreatic outflow dynamics concomitantly.[59]

Anatomic Variants in Acute Recurrent Pancreatitis and Chronic Pancreatitis

The role of pancreatic anatomic variants including pancreas divisum (PD) as a causative agent in ARP and CP is controversial. While incidence of PD is higher in children with ARP and CP than that in the general population,[53,60] most patients with PD have no symptoms throughout their lifetime.[61] As the postulated pathogenic mechanism of

Table 6		
Prevalence of genetic risk factors in ARP and CP[53]		
Gene Mutation	ARP Prevalence (48%)	CP Prevalence (73%)
CFTR	34%	23%
PRSS1	17%	46%
SPINK1	13%	25%
CTRC	10%	5%

PD in pancreatitis is minor papilla obstruction, endoscopic techniques for minor papilla sphincterotomy, dilation, and stenting are often attempted in children with PD.[62] There is difficulty although in understanding whether PD is purely an association with ARP and CP or causative. Pediatric studies examining outcomes in endoscopic interventions of PD In ARP and CP are lacking, and even adult studies are generally retrospective[63] without a control arm, making assessments of pain and quality-of-life improvements difficult. From a diagnostic standpoint, while PD is presumed to be a risk factor for ARP, it is not sufficient to prevent evaluation for coexistent causes of ARP or CP. In fact, there is increasing evidence that PD could act in pathogenic concert with genetic risk factors, such as CFTR mutations, to underlie ARP or CP.[64]

Pancreatic Enzyme Supplementation in Acute Recurrent Pancreatitis

While pancreatic enzyme replacement therapy (PERT) as a treatment for pain in ARP is intuitively appealing because of theoretic negative feedback regulation of pancreatic enzymes, PERT has not shown a beneficial impact on pain[65] and should not routinely be used in children without exocrine insufficiency.[28]

CHRONIC PANCREATITIS

CP manifests with irreversible fibrosis and pathologic changes to the pancreatic parenchyma and pancreatic ductal abnormalities, which are evident radiographically with characteristic pancreatic calcifications or pancreatic duct morphologic abnormalities.[1] The diagnosis should include clinical findings of abdominal pain consistent with pancreatitis, evidence of exocrine pancreatic insufficiency (EPI), or evidence of endocrine pancreatic insufficiency. Additionally, a pancreatic biopsy demonstrating histologic evidence of CP is sufficiently diagnostic but rarely required.

Characteristic Imaging in Chronic Pancreatitis

Cross-sectional imaging in children with CP can identify calcifications, atrophy, and inflammatory changes suggestive of CP. Additionally, most children diagnosed with CP will undergo MRCP,[53] which can characteristically demonstrate morphologic abnormalities of the main pancreatic duct and side branches, intraductal calculi, stenosis and strictures, and peri-pancreatic fluid collections. ERCP can better elucidate ductal changes but is preferentially used in a therapeutic manner, as discussed later in this article. Increasingly, EUS has been used in the diagnosis of CP to try and capture early disease. Criteria for EUS diagnosis of CP in adults have been standardized with the Rosemont classification.[66] The classification is focused on parenchymal features, ductal features, and correlation of EUS findings with histology. To date, these diagnostic criteria have not been evaluated in children.

Pain Management in Chronic Pancreatitis

Chronic abdominal pain is a hallmark of CP and is a significant contributor to reduced quality of life in children with CP.[67] Identifiable organic insults often arise from pancreatic ductal hypertension, pancreatic parenchymal inflammation, ischemia, and fibrosis, in addition to extrapancreatic involvement including common bile duct pathology.[68] Over time, these insults can lead to peripheral sensitization and neural remodeling in central pain pathways and resultant autonomous pain signaling even in the absence of detectable ongoing pancreatic insult.[69] For this purpose, neuromodulating medications, including nortriptyline, duloxetine, and gabapentin, have been used.

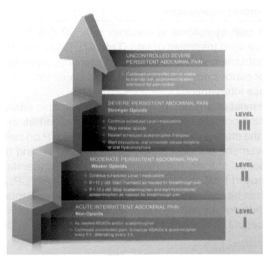

Fig. 5. NASPGHAN Pancreas Committee analgesic ladder for outpatient CP pain management.[70] (*From* Freeman AJ, Maqbool A, Bellin MD, et al. Medical Management of Chronic Pancreatitis in Children: A Position Paper by the North American Society for Pediatric Gastroenterology, Hepatology, and Nutrition Pancreas Committee. Journal of pediatric gastroenterology and nutrition. 2021;72(2):324-340.)

Multidisciplinary teams are most often used to target chronic pain in CP from multiple approaches. In addition to pediatric gastroenterologists managing children with CP, involvement of a pain clinician, therapeutic endoscopist, and physical therapist is also critical in pain intervention. Additionally, a pain psychologist with expertise in cognitive behavioral therapy is a necessary complement to medical therapy.[70]

Recent publication of CP medical management guidelines from the NASPGHAN Pancreas Committee has proposed an analgesic ladder for outpatient management of pain in children with CP[70] (**Fig. 5**). This standardized approach to analgesia consists broadly of nonopioid medications on level I, advancing to weak opioids on level II while continuing level I medications. If pain is still poorly controlled, escalation to level III is indicated which includes more potent oral opioids to replace weaker ones.

Despite attempts to study alternative nonanalgesic interventions to improve chronic pain, including low-fat diet, PERT, antioxidants, steroids, and somatostatin, none have demonstrated convincing efficacy.[65,71,72]

Table 7
Uses of ERCP for pediatric pancreaticobiliary disease

Diagnostic	Therapeutic
Pancreatic ductal hypertension	Pancreatic duct
• Stone	• Stone clearance
• Ductal stenosis/stricture	• Balloon dilation
• Leak	• Stent placement
• Papillary stenosis	Biliary stone extraction

Endotherapy for Chronic Pancreatitis

Given the hallmark pain symptoms in children with CP due to ductal hypertension, ERCP is a commonly used treatment option (**Table 7**). One goal of ERCP is to address pancreatic duct obstruction via pancreatic duct stenting, pancreatic sphincterotomy of the major and/or minor papilla, removal of main pancreatic duct stones, or some combination of these interventions.

Children with CP must often undergo repeated endoscopic interventions increasing the risk for procedural complications, including pain exacerbation, AP, infection, and bleeding. To date, the studies evaluating the effect of ERCP on pain and quality of life have shown improvement, but data consist of retrospective and nonrandomized cohorts.[73–75] Prospective studies are needed to better understand the impact of advanced endoscopy in treating chronic pain in children with CP. EUS-guided celiac plexus neurolysis has become available at several pediatric centers; however, there are no pediatric data to support its use, although adult data have demonstrated some short-term benefit.[76] Management of fluid collections is discussed earlier in this review.

Nutrition in Chronic Pancreatitis

Malnutrition manifests in up to 25% of children with CP[77] and is often multifactorial in nature[26] (**Fig. 6**).

Diagnosis of Pancreatic Exocrine Insufficiency

Approximately one-third of children with CP have EPI.[78] Manifestations of EPI generally consist of malnutrition, fat-soluble vitamin (FSV) deficiency, steatorrhea, malodorous stool, bloating, and abdominal pain. EPI can also be subclinical. Diagnosis of EPI can be performed in multiple ways, most commonly via fecal elastase-1 measurement.

Endoscopic pancreatic function testing can be performed via direct measurement of pancreatic enzymes and bicarbonate collected endoscopically after cholecystokinin or secretin stimulation.[79] This is usually not necessary if screening tests for EPI are already positive but can be useful for detecting early exocrine insufficiency or

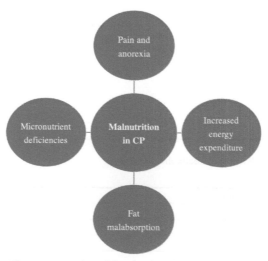

Fig. 6. Multiple contributors to malnutrition in chronic pancreatitis.

Box 1
Initiation of PERT in CP

Lipase units per kilogram body weight per meal
   500–1000 lipase units/kg/meal (half for snack). Increase by 1 capsule per meal until evidence of EPI resolved. Maximum 3000 lipase units/kg/meal.

Lipase units per gram fat in meal
   500–4000 lipase units/g fat

Enteral formula (in line cartridge)
   1 cartridge per 500 mL formula up to max 2 cartridges.

even to help make the diagnosis of CP itself. Indirect testing is most commonly obtained via fecal elastase-1. Fecal elastase is a pancreatic enzyme stable through the lower gastrointestinal tract. To accurately measure fecal elastase, the stool must be formed, as watery stool can dilute the elastase. Fecal elastase values below 100 ug/g are generally diagnostic for EPI. Administration of supplemental pancreatic enzymes, as they are porcine-derived, will not alter measurement of human fecal elastase. A 72-hour fecal fat measurement is the gold standard for indirectly detecting EPI but rarely used in clinical practice because of the cumbersome nature of collection.

Treatment of Pancreatic Enzyme Insufficiency

Generally, initiation of PERT can be initiated as detailed in **Box 1**. PERT dosing in CP is planned in a similar manner to that of cystic fibrosis–associated EPI[28] with weight-based dosing and variability based on fat content. While pancreatic enzyme insufficiency can lead to diarrhea, it should be noted that PERT does not cause constipation.

Fat-Soluble Vitamin Deficiencies in Chronic Pancreatitis

In addition to caloric insufficiency, FSV deficiencies are common in patients with CP at rates of 15%-58%.[80] FSV deficiency screening should occur every 12 to 18 months or as clinically indicated.[70] Vitamin D screening should be performed in children annually with similar interval screening for deficiencies of serum vitamin A and vitamin E. Proxy for vitamin K can be obtained with measurement of prothrombin time annually. In children with malnutrition or persistently low vitamin D levels, bone mineral density should be measured.

Additional Gastrointestinal Sequalae of Chronic Pancreatitis

Children with CP have increased risk for gastroparesis and small intestinal bacterial overgrowth (SIBO), for which symptoms of abdominal pain, early satiety, bloating, and nausea often overlap with CP symptoms. Prokinetics, including erythromycin, can be trialed for established gastroparesis, and occasionally more invasive interventions including pyloric botulinum toxin injections or postpyloric nutritional supplementation may be required.[70] Similarly, SIBO is more prevalent in patients with CP[81] and can be overlooked given the similarity in presentation with CP. Fasting glucose hydrogen breath testing can be used in establishing this diagnosis, and antibiotic treatment including rifaximin, neomycin, or metronidazole can be administered.

Endocrine Insufficiency and Pancreatogenic Diabetes Mellitus

After chronic damage to pancreatic parenchyma, it is estimated that 4% of children with CP will develop endocrine insufficiency and diabetes mellitus.[82] Children with CP should be screened annually for diabetes with fasting glucose and hemoglobin A1c.[70,83]

Surgical Management of Pancreatitis in Children

For those children with CP who do not respond to medical therapy or endoscopic therapy, there is availability of total pancreatectomy with islet autotransplantation (TPIAT). The primary aim of TPIAT is to alleviate pain from CP while preventing significant insulin dependence and endocrine insufficiency via islet autotransplantation.[84] The only indication for TPIAT is refractory pain.[85]

SUMMARY

The spectrum from acute to CP in children is unique and demands an individualized investigation and a tailored management strategy based on age, risk factors, recurrence, and complications. Evolving knowledge and broader detection of risk factors coupled with advances in therapeutic intervention in children have advanced the care of pediatric pancreatitis. Further research to better address quality of life and pharmaceutical and endoscopic interventions in children with pancreatitis is needed.

CLINICS CARE POINTS

- A child's first presentation with acute pancreatitis should include evaluation of serum transaminases, bilirubin, calcium, triglycerides, and imaging with transabdominal ultrasound while reserving expanded diagnostic workups for recurrent disease or concerning history.

- Medical management of acute pancreatitis should focus on aggressive fluid resuscitation, end organ monitoring, early oral or enteral nutrition, and pain control.

- Acute fluid collections can complicate pancreatitis. The majority of acute collection will resolve without intervention, but increasingly endoscopic retrograde cholangiopancreatography and endoscopic ultrasound-guided cystogastrostomy can be used for persistent or complicated fluid collections.

- Pediatric autoimmune pancreatitis is a rare entity and presents with typical abdominal pain and often with direct hyperbilirubinemia and a history of weight loss. Because this presentation includes a host of pancreaticobiliary pathologies, it requires supplementary radiological and histologic information.

- Genetic testing should be undertaken in children who present with recurrent pancreatitis. Cross-sectional imaging with magnetic resonance cholangiopancreatography and, if available, secretin enhancement should be obtained in recurrent cases.

- Key considerations in pediatric chronic pancreatitis that requires multidisciplinary approaches include pain management, malnutrition, and endotherapy.

REFERENCES

1. Morinville VD, Husain SZ, Bai H, et al. Definitions of pediatric pancreatitis and survey of present clinical practices. J Pediatr Gastroenterol Nutr 2012;55(3):261–5.
2. Abu-El-Haija M, Lowe M, Barth B, et al. Pediatric chronic pancreatitis without prior acute or acute recurrent pancreatitis: a report from the INSPPIRE consortium. Pancreatology 2020;20(4):781–4.
3. Morinville VD, Barmada MM, Lowe ME. Increasing incidence of acute pancreatitis at an American pediatric tertiary care center: is greater awareness among physicians responsible? Pancreas 2010;39(1):5–8.
4. Nydegger A, Heine RG, Ranuh R, et al. Changing incidence of acute pancreatitis: 10-year experience at the Royal Children's Hospital, Melbourne. J Gastroenterol Hepatol 2007;22(8):1313–6.

5. Park AJ, Latif SU, Ahmad MU, et al. A comparison of presentation and management trends in acute pancreatitis between infants/toddlers and older children. J Pediatr Gastroenterol Nutr 2010;51(2):167–70.

6. Quiros JA, Marcin JP, Kuppermann N, et al. Elevated serum amylase and lipase in pediatric diabetic ketoacidosis. Pediatr Crit Care Med 2008;9(4):418–22.

7. Trout AT, Anupindi SA, Freeman AJ, et al. North American Society for Pediatric Gastroenterology, Hepatology and Nutrition and the Society for Pediatric Radiology Joint Position Paper on noninvasive imaging of pediatric pancreatitis: literature summary and recommendations. J Pediatr Gastroenterol Nutr 2021;72(1): 151–67.

8. Husain SZ, Srinath AI. What's unique about acute pancreatitis in children: risk factors, diagnosis and management. Nat Rev Gastroenterol Hepatol 2017;14(6): 366–72.

9. Uc A, Husain SZ. Pancreatitis in children. Gastroenterology 2019;156(7): 1969–78.

10. Sekimoto M, Takada T, Kawarada Y, et al. JPN Guidelines for the management of acute pancreatitis: epidemiology, etiology, natural history, and outcome predictors in acute pancreatitis. J Hepatobiliary Pancreat Surg 2006;13(1):10–24.

11. Trivedi CD, Pitchumoni CS. Drug-induced pancreatitis: an update. J Clin Gastroenterol 2005;39(8):709–16.

12. Wolfe D, Kanji S, Yazdi F, et al. Drug induced pancreatitis: a systematic review of case reports to determine potential drug associations. PLoS One 2020;15(4): e0231883.

13. Heap GA, Weedon MN, Bewshea CM, et al. HLA-DQA1-HLA-DRB1 variants confer susceptibility to pancreatitis induced by thiopurine immunosuppressants. Nat Genet 2014;46(10):1131–4.

14. Husain SZ, Morinville V, Pohl J, et al. Toxic-metabolic risk factors in pediatric pancreatitis: recommendations for diagnosis, management, and future research. J Pediatr Gastroenterol Nutr 2016;62(4):609–17.

15. Abu-El-Haija M, Kumar S, Szabo F, et al. Classification of acute pancreatitis in the pediatric population: clinical report from the NASPGHAN pancreas committee. J Pediatr Gastroenterol Nutr 2017;64(6):984–90.

16. Bai HX, Lowe ME, Husain SZ. What have we learned about acute pancreatitis in children? J Pediatr Gastroenterol Nutr 2011;52(3):262–70.

17. Abu-El-Haija M, El-Dika S, Hinton A, et al. Acute pancreatitis admission trends: a national estimate through the kids' inpatient database. J Pediatr 2018;194: 147–51.e1.

18. Gardner TB, Vege SS, Pearson RK, et al. Fluid resuscitation in acute pancreatitis. Clin Gastroenterol Hepatol 2008;6(10):1070–6.

19. Wu BU, Hwang JQ, Gardner TH, et al. Lactated Ringer's solution reduces systemic inflammation compared with saline in patients with acute pancreatitis. Clin Gastroenterol Hepatol 2011;9(8):710–7.e1.

20. Buter A, Imrie CW, Carter CR, et al. Dynamic nature of early organ dysfunction determines outcome in acute pancreatitis. Br J Surg 2002;89(3):298–302.

21. Grover AS, Mitchell PD, Manzi SF, et al. Initial pain management in pediatric acute pancreatitis: opioid versus non-opioid. J Pediatr Gastroenterol Nutr 2018;66(2): 295–8.

22. Poropat G, Giljaca V, Hauser G, et al. Enteral nutrition formulations for acute pancreatitis. Cochrane Database Syst Rev 2015;3:Cd010605.

23. Li J, Xue GJ, Liu YL, et al. Early oral refeeding wisdom in patients with mild acute pancreatitis. Pancreas 2013;42(1):88–91.

24. Abu-El-Haija M, Wilhelm R, Heinzman C, et al. Early enteral nutrition in children with acute pancreatitis. J Pediatr Gastroenterol Nutr 2016;62(3):453–6.

25. Szabo FK, Fei L, Cruz LA, et al. Early enteral nutrition and aggressive fluid resuscitation are associated with improved clinical outcomes in acute pancreatitis. J Pediatr 2015;167(2):397–402.e1.

26. Gianotti L, Meier R, Lobo DN, et al. ESPEN guidelines on parenteral nutrition: pancreas. Clin Nutr 2009;28(4):428–35.

27. Moraes JM, Felga GE, Chebli LA, et al. A full solid diet as the initial meal in mild acute pancreatitis is safe and result in a shorter length of hospitalization: results from a prospective, randomized, controlled, double-blind clinical trial. J Clin Gastroenterol 2010;44(7):517–22.

28. Abu-El-Haija M, Uc A, Werlin SL, et al. Nutritional considerations in pediatric pancreatitis: a position paper from the NASPGHAN Pancreas Committee and ESPGHAN Cystic Fibrosis/Pancreas Working Group. J Pediatr Gastroenterol Nutr 2018;67(1):131–43.

29. Oláh A, Romics L Jr. Early enteral nutrition in acute pancreatitis-benefits and limitations. Langenbecks Arch Surg 2008;393(3):261–9.

30. Petrov MS, Pylypchuk RD, Uchugina AF. A systematic review on the timing of artificial nutrition in acute pancreatitis. Br J Nutr 2009;101(6):787–93.

31. Kumar S, Gariepy CE. Nutrition and acute pancreatitis: review of the literature and pediatric perspectives. Curr Gastroenterol Rep 2013;15(8):338.

32. Fishman DS, Chumpitazi BP, Raijman I, et al. Endoscopic retrograde cholangiography for pediatric choledocholithiasis: assessing the need for endoscopic intervention. World J Gastrointest Endosc 2016;8(11):425–32.

33. Fogel EL, Sherman S. ERCP for gallstone pancreatitis. New Engl J Med 2014; 370(2):150–7.

34. da Costa DW, Bouwense SA, Schepers NJ, et al. Same-admission versus interval cholecystectomy for mild gallstone pancreatitis (PONCHO): a multicentre randomised controlled trial. Lancet 2015;386(10000):1261–8.

35. Lal SB, Venkatesh V, Rana SS, et al. Paediatric acute pancreatitis: clinical profile and natural history of collections. Pancreatology 2020;20(4):659–64.

36. Banks PA, Bollen TL, Dervenis C, et al. Classification of acute pancreatitis–2012: revision of the Atlanta classification and definitions by international consensus. Gut 2013;62(1):102–11.

37. Bolia R, Srivastava A, Yachha SK, et al. Prevalence, natural history, and outcome of acute fluid collection and pseudocyst in children with acute pancreatitis. J Pediatr Gastroenterol Nutr 2015;61(4):451–5.

38. Dalsania R, Willingham FF. Treatment of walled-off pancreatic necrosis. Curr Opin Gastroenterol 2019;35(5):478–82.

39. Rosenfeld EH, Vogel AM, Klinkner DB, et al. The utility of ERCP in pediatric pancreatic trauma. J Pediatr Surg 2017;53(1):146–51.

40. Makin E, Harrison PM, Patel S, et al. Pancreatic pseudocysts in children: treatment by endoscopic cyst gastrostomy. J Pediatr Gastroenterol Nutr 2012;55(5): 556–8.

41. Scheers I, Ergun M, Aouattah T, et al. Diagnostic and therapeutic roles of endoscopic ultrasound in pediatric pancreaticobiliary disorders. J Pediatr Gastroenterol Nutr 2015;61(2):238–47.

42. IAP/APA evidence-based guidelines for the management of acute pancreatitis. Pancreatology 2013;13(4 Suppl 2):e1–15.

43. Abu-El-Haija M, Kumar S, Quiros JA, et al. Management of acute pancreatitis in the pediatric population: a clinical report from the north american society for

pediatric gastroenterology, hepatology and nutrition pancreas committee. J Pediatr Gastroenterol Nutr 2018;66(1):159–76.

44. Sellers ZM, Dike C, Zhang KY, et al. A unified treatment algorithm and admission order set for pediatric acute pancreatitis. J Pediatr Gastroenterol Nutr 2019;68(6): e109–11.

45. Shah M, Leong T, Freeman AJ. Order set use and education association with pediatric acute pancreatitis outcomes. Hosp Pediatr 2021;11(8):885–92.

46. Sweeny KF, Lin TK, Nathan JD, et al. Rapid progression of acute pancreatitis to acute recurrent pancreatitis in children. J Pediatr Gastroenterol Nutr 2019;68(1): 104–9.

47. Scheers I, Palermo JJ, Freedman S, et al. Recommendations for diagnosis and management of autoimmune pancreatitis in childhood: consensus from IN-SPPIRE. J Pediatr Gastroenterol Nutr 2018;67(2):232–6.

48. Scheers I, Palermo JJ, Freedman S, et al. Autoimmune pancreatitis in children: characteristic features, diagnosis, and management. Am J Gastroenterol 2017; 112(10):1604–11.

49. Pagliari D, Cianci R, Rigante D. The challenge of autoimmune pancreatitis: a portrayal from the pediatric perspective. Pancreas 2019;48(5):605–12.

50. Okazaki K, Tomiyama T, Mitsuyama T, et al. Diagnosis and classification of auto-immune pancreatitis. Autoimmun Rev 2014;13(4–5):451–8.

51. Jung JG, Lee JK, Lee KH, et al. Comparison of endoscopic retrograde cholangio-pancreatography with papillary biopsy and endoscopic ultrasound-guided pancreatic biopsy in the diagnosis of autoimmune pancreatitis. Pancreatology 2015;15(3):259–64.

52. Morinville VD, Lowe ME, Ahuja M, et al. Design and implementation of INSPPIRE. J Pediatr Gastroenterol Nutr 2014;59(3):360–4.

53. Kumar S, Ooi CY, Werlin S, et al. Risk factors associated with pediatric acute recurrent and chronic pancreatitis: lessons from INSPPIRE. JAMA Pediatr 2016; 170(6):562–9.

54. Derikx MH, Kovacs P, Scholz M, et al. Polymorphisms at PRSS1-PRSS2 and CLDN2-MORC4 loci associate with alcoholic and non-alcoholic chronic pancreatitis in a European replication study. Gut 2015;64(9):1426–33.

55. Fjeld K, Weiss FU, Lasher D, et al. A recombined allele of the lipase gene CEL and its pseudogene CELP confers susceptibility to chronic pancreatitis. Nat Genet 2015;47(5):518–22.

56. Ragvin A, Fjeld K, Weiss FU, et al. The number of tandem repeats in the carboxyl-ester lipase (CEL) gene as a risk factor in alcoholic and idiopathic chronic pancreatitis. Pancreatology 2013;13(1):29–32.

57. Whitcomb DC. Genetic risk factors for pancreatic disorders. Gastroenterology 2013;144(6):1292–302.

58. Gariepy CE, Heyman MB, Lowe ME, et al. Causal evaluation of acute recurrent and chronic pancreatitis in children: consensus from the INSPPIRE Group. J Pediatr Gastroenterol Nutr 2017;64(1):95–103.

59. Mariani A, Arcidiacono PG, Curioni S, et al. Diagnostic yield of ERCP and secretin-enhanced MRCP and EUS in patients with acute recurrent pancreatitis of unknown aetiology. Dig Liver Dis 2009;41(10):753–8.

60. Bülow R, Simon P, Thiel R, et al. Anatomic variants of the pancreatic duct and their clinical relevance: an MR-guided study in the general population. Eur Radiol 2014;24(12):3142–9.

61. Fogel EL, Toth TG, Lehman GA, et al. Does endoscopic therapy favorably affect the outcome of patients who have recurrent acute pancreatitis and pancreas divisum? Pancreas 2007;34(1):21–45.

62. Lin TK, Abu-El-Haija M, Nathan JD, et al. Pancreas divisum in pediatric acute recurrent and chronic pancreatitis: report from INSPPIRE. J Clin Gastroenterol 2019;53(6):e232–8.

63. Kanth R, Samji NS, Inaganti A, et al. Endotherapy In symptomatic pancreas divisum: a systematic review. Pancreatology 2014;14(4):244–50.

64. Bertin C, Pelletier AL, Vullierme MP, et al. Pancreas divisum is not a cause of pancreatitis by itself but acts as a partner of genetic mutations. Am J Gastroenterol 2012;107(2):311–7.

65. Yaghoobi M, McNabb-Baltar J, Bijarchi R, et al. Pancreatic enzyme supplements are not effective for relieving abdominal pain in patients with chronic pancreatitis: meta-analysis and systematic review of randomized controlled trials. Can J Gastroenterol Hepatol 2016;2016:8541839.

66. Catalano MF, Sahai A, Levy M, et al. EUS-based criteria for the diagnosis of chronic pancreatitis: the Rosemont classification. Gastrointest Endosc 2009; 69(7):1251–61.

67. Pohl JF, Limbers CA, Kay M, et al. Health-related quality of life in pediatric patients with long-standing pancreatitis. J Pediatr Gastroenterol Nutr 2012;54(5): 657–63.

68. Drewes AM, Bouwense SAW, Campbell CM, et al. Guidelines for the understanding and management of pain in chronic pancreatitis. Pancreatology 2017;17(5): 720–31.

69. Olesen SS, Krauss T, Demir IE, et al. Towards a neurobiological understanding of pain in chronic pancreatitis: mechanisms and implications for treatment. Pain Rep 2017;2(6):e625.

70. Freeman AJ, Maqbool A, Bellin MD, et al. Medical management of chronic pancreatitis in children: a position paper by the North American Society for pediatric gastroenterology, hepatology, and nutrition pancreas committee. J Pediatr Gastroenterol Nutr 2021;72(2):324–40.

71. Ahmed Ali U, Jens S, Busch OR, et al. Antioxidants for pain in chronic pancreatitis. Cochrane Database Syst Rev 2014;(8):Cd008945.

72. Dong LH, Liu ZM, Wang SJ, et al. Corticosteroid therapy for severe acute pancreatitis: a meta-analysis of randomized, controlled trials. Int J Clin Exp Pathol 2015; 8(7):7654–60.

73. Oracz G, Pertkiewicz J, Kierkus J, et al. Efficiency of pancreatic duct stenting therapy in children with chronic pancreatitis. Gastrointest Endosc 2014;80(6): 1022–9.

74. Agarwal J, Nageshwar Reddy D, Talukdar R, et al. ERCP in the management of pancreatic diseases in children. Gastrointest Endosc 2014;79(2):271–8.

75. Kohoutova D, Tringali A, Papparella G, et al. Endoscopic treatment of chronic pancreatitis in pediatric population: long-term efficacy and safety. United Eur Gastroenterol J 2019;7(2):270–7.

76. Puli SR, Reddy JB, Bechtold ML, et al. EUS-guided celiac plexus neurolysis for pain due to chronic pancreatitis or pancreatic cancer pain: a meta-analysis and systematic review. Dig Dis Sci 2009;54(11):2330–7.

77. Kolodziejczyk E, Wejnarska K, Dadalski M, et al. The nutritional status and factors contributing to malnutrition in children with chronic pancreatitis. Pancreatology 2014;14(4):275–9.

78. Schwarzenberg SJ, Bellin M, Husain SZ, et al. Pediatric chronic pancreatitis is associated with genetic risk factors and substantial disease burden. J Pediatr 2015;166(4):890–6.e1.
79. Horvath K, Mehta DI, Hill ID. Assessment of exocrine pancreatic function during endoscopy in children. J Pediatr Gastroenterol Nutr 2019;68(6):768–76.
80. Duggan SN, Smyth ND, O'Sullivan M, et al. The prevalence of malnutrition and fat-soluble vitamin deficiencies in chronic pancreatitis. Nutr Clin Pract 2014; 29(3):348–54.
81. HM NC, Bashir Y, Dobson M, et al. The prevalence of small intestinal bacterial overgrowth in non-surgical patients with chronic pancreatitis and pancreatic exocrine insufficiency (PEI). Pancreatology 2018;18(4):379–85.
82. Schwarzenberg SJ, Uc A, Zimmerman B, et al. Chronic pancreatitis: pediatric and adult cohorts show similarities in disease progress despite different risk factors. J Pediatr Gastroenterol Nutr 2019;68(4):566–73.
83. Uc A, Perito ER, Pohl JF, et al. INternational study group of pediatric pancreatitis: in search for a CuRE cohort study: design and rationale for INSPPIRE 2 from the consortium for the study of chronic pancreatitis, diabetes, and pancreatic cancer. Pancreas 2018;47(10):1222–8.
84. Abu-El-Haija M, Nathan JD. Pediatric chronic pancreatitis: updates in the 21st century. Pancreatology 2018;18(4):354–9.
85. Abu-El-Haija M, Anazawa T, Beilman GJ, et al. The role of total pancreatectomy with islet autotransplantation in the treatment of chronic pancreatitis: a report from the international consensus guidelines in chronic pancreatitis. Pancreatology 2020;20(4):762–71.

Pediatric Autoimmune Liver Diseases

Autoimmune Hepatitis and Primary Sclerosing Cholangitis

Sarah Kemme, MD*, Cara L. Mack, MD

KEYWORDS

- Autoimmune hepatitis • Chronic hepatitis • Overlap syndrome
- Pediatric liver transplantation • Primary sclerosing cholangitis

KEY POINTS

- A broad differential diagnosis should be considered in the workup of patients with chronic hepatitis.
- Autoimmune liver diseases may be asymptomatic early in the disease course; as such, a timely diagnosis requires a high index of suspicion.
- Although many medical therapies exist to achieve remission of autoimmune hepatitis, there are no effective medical therapies for primary sclerosing cholangitis or primary sclerosing cholangitis–autoimmune hepatitis overlap syndrome.
- Autoimmune liver diseases may result in the need for pediatric liver transplantation.

INTRODUCTION

Chronic hepatitis is defined as elevation of liver aminotransferases over a sustained period of time and is often associated with hepatic inflammation and fibrosis. The differential diagnosis for chronic hepatitis is broad and many etiologies can lead to the common phenotype and histologic findings. Although this article focuses on autoimmune hepatitis (AIH), primary sclerosing cholangitis (PSC), and PSC–AIH overlap syndrome (also known as autoimmune sclerosing cholangitis), the full differential diagnosis must be considered when approaching a patient with chronic hepatitis. These diagnoses may not be mutually exclusive, and a patient may have multiple etiologies for chronic hepatitis such as a concomitant diagnosis of AIH and

Section of Gastroenterology, Hepatology, and Nutrition, Digestive Health Institute, University of Colorado Denver School of Medicine and Children's Hospital Colorado, 13123 East 16th Avenue, Mailstop B290, Aurora, CO 80045, USA
* Corresponding author.
E-mail address: Sarah.Kemme@childrenscolorado.org

Pediatr Clin N Am 68 (2021) 1293–1307
https://doi.org/10.1016/j.pcl.2021.07.006
0031-3955/21/© 2021 Elsevier Inc. All rights reserved.
pediatric.theclinics.com

nonalcoholic fatty liver disease. A comprehensive list of diagnoses is outlined in **Table 1**, and **Fig. 1** provides a template for the tiered diagnostic workup of patients with chronic hepatitis. Our standard of care is to screen for hepatitis B, hepatitis C, anatomic abnormalities, nonalcoholic fatty liver disease, AIH, Wilson disease, and alpha-1-antitrypsin deficiency in all patients who present with chronic hepatitis, as illustrated in **Fig. 1**.

Table 1
Differential diagnosis for elevated aminotransferases

Infectious (acute and chronic)	Abscess (amebiasis, other)
	Adenovirus
	Coronavirus (severe acute respiratory syndrome coronavirus 2)
	Cytomegalovirus
	Enterovirus
	Epstein–Barr virus
	Hepatitis A
	Hepatitis B
	Hepatitis C
	Hepatitis E
	Herpes simplex virus
	Histoplasmosis
	HIV
	Influenza
	Parvovirus B19
	Varicella zoster
	Systemic infection (including bacterial, viral, fungal sepsis)
	Other infection
Autoimmune	AIH
	Celiac disease
	Juvenile rheumatoid arthritis
	PSC
	Systemic lupus erythematosus
Toxin mediated	Environmental
	Drug induced (prescription, herbal, and illicit)
Metabolic or genetic	Alpha-1-antitrypsin deficiency
	Cystic fibrosis
	Fatty acid oxidation disorders
	Galactosemia
	Glycogen storage disease
	Hemochromatosis (juvenile or hereditary)
	Hereditary fructose intolerance
	Niemann–Pick disease
	Other inborn errors of metabolism
	Tyrosinemia
	Wilson copper storage disease
Anatomic	Choledochal cyst
	Cholelithiasis
	Liver mass
Vascular	Budd-Chiari syndrome
	Congestive heart failure
	Shock/hypoperfusion
Infiltrative	Hemophagocytic lymphohistiocytosis
	Malignancy
	Nonalcoholic fatty liver disease

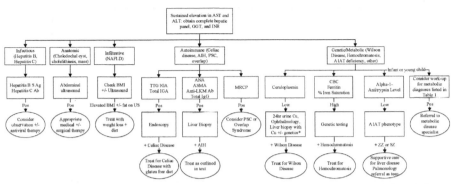

Fig. 1. Flow diagram for diagnostic workup and subsequent management of chronic hepatitis, including both standard of care and clinical scenario-specific testing that may be obtained from the initial evaluation. Ab, antibody; Ag, antigen; ALT, alanine aminotransferase; ANA, antinuclear antibody; ASMA, anti-smooth muscle actin; AST, aspartate aminotransferase; BMI, body mass index; Cu, copper; GGT, gamma glutamyl transferase; INR, international normalized ratio; MRCP, magnetic resonance cholangiopancreaticogram; NAFLD, nonalcoholic fatty liver disease.

DISCUSSION
Autoimmune Hepatitis

Definition
AIH is a chronic, immune-mediated inflammatory disease of the liver that typically presents with elevated aminotransferases, positive autoantibodies, and characteristic findings on liver biopsy. Criteria for the diagnosis of AIH include:

1. Elevated liver aminotransferases
2. One or more of the following positive autoantibodies: antinuclear antibody (ANA), anti-smooth muscle actin (ASMA)/anti-actin antibody (anti-actin), liver kidney microsomal antibody (anti-LKM), soluble liver antigen antibody, and/or liver cytosolic antigen type 1 antibody
3. AND/OR elevated IgG or globulin fraction greater than the upper limit of normal
4. AND histology with lymphocytic interface hepatitis with or without plasma cells (**Fig. 2**).

Epidemiology
The incidence of pediatric AIH ranges based on location from 0.23 (Canada) to 0.40 (United States) to 0.56 (Argentina) per 100,000 person-years.[1–3] The prevalence is similarly variable from 2.4 (non-native Canadian children) to 3.0 (United States) to 9.9 (native Canadian children) per 100,000 people.[2,4,5] It can occur at any age and within both genders, but does have a significant female predominance.[1–3,6,7] African American patients tend to present sicker, often in end-stage liver disease, and have a higher likelihood of recurrence of disease after transplantation.[8] Genetic predisposition is a factor, and most genetic associations involve the major histocompatibility complex loci.[9] Prospective studies indicate that up to 50% of all children diagnosed with AIH have a relative with a history of non–liver-related autoimmunity.[10,11]

Clinical presentation
The clinical presentation of AIH at the time of diagnosis can range from asymptomatic (approximately 10%) elevation in serum aminotransferases to acute liver failure (approximately 20%), necessitating urgent liver transplantation. The median age at

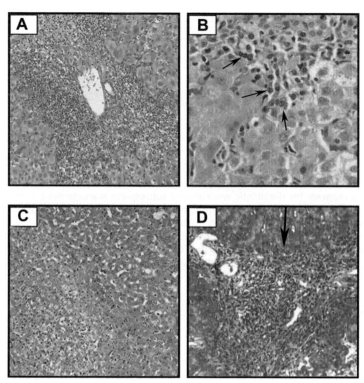

Fig. 2. Histologic findings in AIH. (*A*). Hematoxylin and eosin (H&E) staining with interface hepatitis with predominantly lymphoplasmocytic portal tract infiltrate extending beyond the limiting plate into the parenchyma. (*B*). H&E with *arrows* pointing to plasma cells. (*C*). H&E demonstrating hepatocyte necrosis (*D*). Trichrome stain demonstrating bridging fibrosis.

presentation is approximately 10 years old[1–3,6,12] and the majority of patients present with nonspecific symptoms such as fatigue (56%) and abdominal pain (44%).[3,13] Other presentations include an acute viral hepatitis-like picture with nausea, vomiting, and anorexia, or an insidious onset in approximately 30% with vague symptoms up to 2 years before diagnosis.[6,12,14] Depending on the study, cirrhosis at presentation ranges from 17% to 75% of children with AIH.[6,7,13,14] Acute, severe hepatitis, defined as hepatitis with jaundice, without encephalopathy, and with an international normalized ratio of 1.5 to 1.9, usually necessitates inpatient admission and close observation for worsening disease. Physical examination findings such as hepatomegaly and/or splenomegaly may be present in up to 50% of pediatric patients at the time of diagnosis.[6,13–15]

Diagnosis
The diagnosis of AIH is suggested by elevated liver aminotransferases, positive auto-antibodies (ANA, ASMA/anti-actin, and anti-LKM), and elevated serum IgG. Other autoantibodies are associated with AIH (see Definition), but are outside the scope of this article. Recent guidelines on AIH from the American Association for the Study of Liver Diseases describe these in more detail.[16] If autoantibodies are positive or there is suspicion for AIH despite negative autoantibodies, a liver biopsy must be performed to conclusively diagnose AIH. The hallmark histologic feature of AIH is interface hepatitis,

with portal lymphocytic and lymphoplasmacytic inflammation extending into the parenchyma.[17] The various histologic findings of AIH are shown in **Fig. 2**.

There are 2 types of pediatric AIH, categorized based on the specific positive autoantibody. Type 1 AIH is characterized by positive ANA and/or ASMA, whereas type 2 AIH has a positive anti-LKM.[18,19] Among these patients, 15% to 34% will have negative autoantibodies, but with elevated IgG and classic findings on histology and are thus classified as seronegative AIH.[13,20–22] The classification of AIH as type 1 or type 2 when applicable carries prognostic significance and may help to predict outcomes in pediatric AIH.[18,23] Patients with type 2 AIH tend to present at a younger median age (7.4–10.0 years vs 10.5–12.0 years for type 1) and have lower rates of cirrhosis at presentation (38% vs 69%), but are less likely to achieve sustained remission after drug withdrawal than patients with type 1 AIH.[3,6] Type 2 AIH also rarely presents with PSC–AIH overlap syndrome, whereas this entity is commonly seen in type 1 AIH.[16]

Special considerations
Seronegative autoimmune hepatitis. Patients who meet the histologic criteria for AIH but without positive autoantibodies are considered seronegative AIH.[13,20–22] A subset of these patients have been described to have severe aplastic anemia concomitant with or after a diagnosis of seronegative AIH.[22,24]

Drug-induced autoimmune hepatitis–like injury. Certain drugs can cause liver injury that seems to be histologically similar to AIH. Known offending drugs that are applicable to pediatric care include doxycycline, minocycline, and infliximab.[16,25,26] Minocycline, prescribed regularly for acne vulgaris, is the most common medication to cause this type of liver injury in pediatrics. Patients may have been on minocycline for 3 weeks to 2 years before development of liver injury. The majority of patients with minocycline-induced liver injury will be ANA positive (AIH type 1). The treatment is to withdraw the minocycline, induce remission with glucocorticoids, and consider treatment with azathioprine (AZA) for maintenance therapy. Approximately one-half of these patients will resolve their liver injury with no need for chronic immunosuppression.[27,28]

Conditions associated with autoimmune hepatitis
Autoimmune polyendocrinopathy–candidiasis–ectodermal dystrophy syndrome. Autoimmune polyendocrinopathy–candidiasis–ectodermal dystrophy syndrome is an autosomal recessive disease involving mutations of the autoimmune regulator gene. Fifteen percent to 20% of patients with autoimmune polyendocrinopathy–candidiasis–ectodermal dystrophy syndrome will also have AIH.[16,29,30]

Immunodysregulation polyendocrinopathy enteropathy X-linked syndrome. Immunodysregulation polyendocrinopathy enteropathy X-linked syndrome is an X-linked syndrome involving mutations of the gene encoding the forkhead box P3 transcription factor, which is necessary for normally functioning regulatory T cells. It is characterized by multisystem autoimmunity and can involve AIH.[31]

Common variable immunodeficiency. Common variable immunodeficiency is a primary immunodeficiency disorder characterized by impaired B-cell function and hypogammaglobulinemia that, in addition to its infectious complications, can cause an autoimmune phenotype. Nodular regenerative hyperplasia within the liver is frequent in patients with common variable immunodeficiency and can progress to have superimposed AIH-like features on liver biopsy.[32,33]

Hyper-IgM syndrome. Hyper-IgM syndrome is an X-linked primary immunodeficiency syndrome that is caused by mutations in the gene for CD40 ligand, which is involved in immunoglobulin class switching. It is characterized by elevated IgM with reduced IgG and IgA. Chronic infection of the biliary tract with *Cryptosporidia* can lead to a secondary sclerosing cholangitis and patients are also predisposed to both infectious hepatitis and AIH. Patients with liver disease may go on to develop cirrhosis and liver failure.[34]

Medical therapy

First-line therapies. The first-line therapy for pediatric AIH, including acute, severe AIH and acute liver failure, is glucocorticoid therapy for induction, followed by AZA for maintenance therapy (**Fig. 3**).[16] Glucocorticoid dosing should begin with prednisone 1 to 2 mg/kg/d (maximum dose of 40 mg/d) or budesonide 9 mg/d. Budesonide is preferred over prednisone when possible owing to similar efficacy and significantly fewer steroid-induced side effects, such as weight gain, mood disturbances, acne, and osteopenia.[16] One exception to the use of budesonide is in the setting of cirrhosis with portosystemic shunting. Budesonide undergoes first-pass metabolism within the liver, and in the setting of portosystemic shunting, the budesonide will not be delivered to the liver effectively or cleared from the circulation. Furthermore, prednisone or intravenous glucocorticoids should be used instead of budesonide in cases of acute, severe hepatitis or acute liver failure, because budesonide has not been trialed in these settings. Early liver transplantation must be considered for acute liver failure and glucocorticoids may have limited efficacy in this clinical scenario.[16]

Thiopurine methyltransferase (TPMT) activity should be assessed at the time of diagnosis of AIH, before starting AZA, so as to avoid severe myelosuppression in a

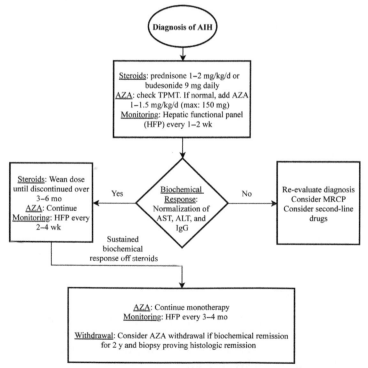

Fig. 3. First-line therapy for pediatric AIH. ALT, alanine aminotransferase; AST, aspartate aminotransferase; AZA, azathioprine; IgG, immunoglobulin G; MRCP, magnetic resonance cholangiopancreatography; TPMT, thiopurine methyltransferase.

patient with absent or near-absent TPMT activity.[16] If TPMT activity is normal and the patient has exhibited glucocorticoid responsiveness, AZA should be added to gluco-corticoid therapy to both synergistically promote the induction of remission and as maintenance therapy. AZA dosing should be tailored to achieve maximal efficacy with minimal toxicity. A 6-thioguanine level between 100 to 300 pmol/8 $\times$ 10^8 red blood cells is considered therapeutic and less toxic to bone marrow. At our center, we aim for a 6-thioguanine level between 100 and 150 pmol/8 $\times$ 10^8 red blood cells in most cases.[13] A 6-methyl-mercaptopurine level of less than 5700 pmol/8 $\times$ 10^8 red blood cells would predict lack of AZA-induced hepatotoxicity. AZA should not be used up front in acute, severe AIH or in AIH with decompensated cirrhosis. AZA can be considered after the cholestasis associated with acute, severe hepatitis has resolved.[16] Because myelosuppression is a side effect of this medication, patients may develop various cytopenias regardless of dosing and TPMT activity. If a patient has cytopenia that does not recover after 1 to 2 weeks of dose reduction, AZA should be discontinued and second-line therapies should be pursued.[16]

Second-line and salvage therapies. Mycophenolate mofetil and calcineurin inhibitors such as cyclosporin A and tacrolimus are the most prominently used second-line therapies in pediatric AIH. These are used for cases of treatment failure, partial but incomplete treatment response, and treatment intolerance.[16] Tacrolimus is preferred over cyclosporin A based on its greater efficacy and lower side effect profile, and cyclosporin A is now used infrequently. Salvage therapies such as rituximab or infliximab have been used rarely in AIH, but can be considered in refractory pediatric AIH.[16,35]

Additional management considerations and disease monitoring. An additional consideration when treating a patient with AIH is to ensure that the child has been vaccinated for hepatitis A and hepatitis B. If not, vaccination can occur after the patient has been weaned off of glucocorticoids. There is an increased risk of thyroid disease and celiac disease in the setting of AIH and, therefore, it is recommended to screen for these diseases at the time of AIH diagnosis and repeat screening thereafter if symptoms are suggestive of either diagnosis. Mental health issues such as depression or anxiety may occur, impacting medication compliance and outcomes, and thus should be monitored for and treated accordingly. While on glucocorticoids, acid suppression, vitamin D and calcium supplementation are prescribed.

The withdrawal of immunosuppression in pediatric AIH is possible in select patients, and more likely to occur without relapse in type 1 than in type 2 AIH.[36,37] After 2 years of sustained biochemical remission, defined as normal liver aminotransferases and IgG, a liver biopsy is performed to confirm histologic remission before the consideration of medication withdrawal. Approximately 30% of pediatric patients whose medications were withdrawn after confirmed histologic remission remained off of medications for the long term.[2,13]

Liver transplantation. Liver transplantation may be indicated in pediatric patients with AIH who present in acute liver failure, decompensated cirrhosis, or who are unresponsive to treatment and subsequently develop progressive decompensation. Up to 20% of pediatric patients with AIH will need liver transplantation before reaching adulthood.[2,13,14,38,39] AIH is the indication for roughly 5% of all pediatric liver transplants.[40] For chronic AIH and acute liver failure owing to AIH, the 5-year patient survival rates are 94% and 84%, respectively; the 5-year graft survival rates are 85% and 81%, respectively.[41] Graft failure after liver transplantation can occur for a variety of reasons, including transplant rejection, thrombotic complications, and recurrent

AIH. Recurrent AIH has been reported in 39% of pediatric patients with a median follow-up of 33 months.[38]

Primary Sclerosing Cholangitis

PSC is a rare, progressive autoimmune biliary disease characterized by cholestasis and fibrosis of the biliary tree. Patients with PSC may have biliary disease that affects the small, medium, and/or large bile duct branches. Approximately 80% of patients with PSC will have concurrent inflammatory bowel disease, most commonly ulcerative colitis.[42] PSC leads to biliary cirrhosis and the need for liver transplantation in the majority of patients, usually in adulthood. Furthermore, there is an increased risk for hepatobiliary and colorectal malignancies that predominantly occur in adults with PSC.[43] The pathogenesis of PSC is multifactorial and includes a genetic predisposition, an environmental or infectious trigger, and abnormal homing of gut derived T cells or proinflammatory bacterial byproducts from the intestines into the liver and biliary tree.[44] Chronic activation of innate and adaptive immune responses results in biliary injury, fibrogenesis, cirrhosis, and an increased risk for cholangiocarcinoma (approximately a 20% lifetime incidence).[45]

Definitions

Definitions of large duct PSC and small duct PSC" are provided in **Table 2**. Large duct PSC is a radiographic diagnosis and small duct PSC is a liver histologic diagnosis. Examples of magnetic resonance cholangiopancreaticogram (MRCP) findings of large duct PSC (also includes medium-sized duct abnormalities) are shown in **Fig. 4**. Liver histologic findings of small duct PSC are shown in **Fig. 5**. An important point is that the terminology used for small duct PSC implies that the cholangiographic study was normal and did not show any evidence of medium or large duct PSC. Small duct PSC is more common in children, with an incidence of approximately 20%, compared

---

Table 2
Criteria for defining large duct PSC and small duct PSC

Large Duct PSC	Small Duct PSC
1. Evidence of cholestasis on biochemistries (elevated bilirubin, GGT, and/or ALP)	1. Evidence of cholestasis on biochemistries (elevated bilirubin, GGT, and/or ALP)
2. Cholangiographic (MRCP, ERCP) findings of ≥ 1 of the following within large or medium sized bile ducts: • Focal stricturing of bile duct(s) • Dominant stricture of common bile duct[a] • Saccular dilatation of bile duct(s) • Beaded appearance of bile duct(s) • Pruning appearance of the distal bile duct branches	2. Liver histologic findings of: Definite small duct PSC • Periductal fibrosis/onion skinning around interlobular bile ducts or smaller profiles Probable small duct PSC: liver histology with ≥ 3 of 5 criteria: • Periductal edema • Periductal concentric inflammation • Bile duct epithelial injury • Ductular reaction • Neutrophils in bile ducts
3. Exclusion of secondary causes of sclerosing cholangitis (see Table 3)	3. Absence of cholangiographic abnormalities (ie, normal MRCP or ERCP)

Abbreviations: ALP, alkaline phosphatase; ERCP, endoscopic retrograde cholangiopancreaticogram; GGT, gamma glutamyl transferase; MRCP, magnetic resonance cholangiopancreaticogram.
   [a] Dominant stricture: stenosis with diameter of ≤ 1.5 mm in common bile duct or ≤ 1 mm in hepatic ducts.

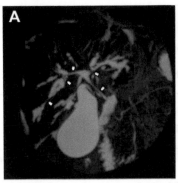
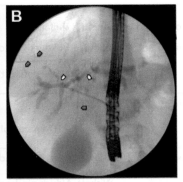

Fig. 4. Cholangiographic findings of large duct PSC. Cholangiogram images from magnetic resonance cholangiopancreaticogram (MRCP) (*A*) and endoscopic retrograde cholangiopancreaticogram (ERCP) (*B*) show multiple strictures (*yellow arrows*) with poststenotic dilations and threadlike "pruning" of the distal branches (*blue arrows*).

with less than 5% in adults with PSC.[46] It is possible that patients with large duct PSC may also have findings of small duct PSC.

Many diseases can have biliary manifestations that mimic the histologic and cholangiographic findings of PSC, suggesting that widely different insults may cause similar patterns of biliary injury. The presence of sclerosing cholangitis as a result of another underlying disorder is defined as secondary sclerosing cholangitis. It is important to consider the many causes of secondary sclerosing cholangitis (**Table 3**) to ensure that the diagnosis of PSC is correct. This process is especially important in the setting of PSC without inflammatory bowel disease.

PSC–AIH overlap syndrome (also known as ASC) is defined as the child having both PSC and AIH. PSC–AIH overlap syndrome is present in up to 33% of children with PSC[46]; therefore, autoantibodies should be obtained to screen for AIH at the time of diagnosis of PSC. If positive, then a liver biopsy should be performed to confirm the presence of interface hepatitis, which is diagnostic of AIH. AIH should be treated as detailed elsewhere in this article.

Epidemiology

The incidence of PSC in children is estimated based on a limited number of population-based studies. The incidence of PSC in children in Canada was reported

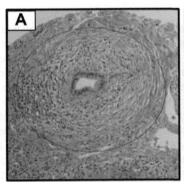
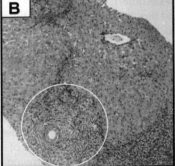

Fig. 5. Histologic findings in small duct PSC. (*A*) Hematoxylin and eosin (H&E) staining showing periductal inflammation, edema and collagen deposition (*pink*). (*B*) Trichrome stain highlighting fibrosis (*blue*).

Table 3 Causes of secondary sclerosing cholangitis	
Anatomic	Choledocholithiasis (idiopathic, sickle cell disease, other) Choledochal cyst Congenital stricture of the common bile duct Trauma
Infection	Pyogenic cholangitis Septic shock E coli 0157:H7 enterocolitis Cryptosporidium
Immunodeficiency	X-linked hyper-IgM syndrome–CD40 ligand deficiency with concurrent Cryptosporidium Wiskott–Aldrich syndrome Natural killer cell deficiency with concurrent Trichosporon infection Agammaglobulinemia with Cryptosporidium Combined variable immunodeficiency with concurrent Cryptosporidium AIDS-associated cholangiopathy with concurrent cytomegalovirus or Cryptosporidium
Neoplastic	Langerhans cell histiocytosis Hodgkin lymphoma Ductal cancer, gallbladder cancer Reticulum cell sarcoma
Congenital	Cystic fibrosis Congenital hepatic fibrosis Caroli disease Caroli syndrome (congenital hepatic fibrosis with Caroli disease) Ductal plate abnormalities

Abbreviation: MRCP, magnetic resonance cholangiopancreaticogram.

as 0.23 cases per 100,000 person-years compared with 1.11 per 100,000 person-years in adults.[47] An epidemiologic study in the United States estimated the incidence and prevalence of pediatric PSC at 0.2 and 1.5 cases per 100,000 children, respectively.[2] PSC affects all races and ethnicities. In a large cohort of pediatric patients with PSC from throughout the world, male gender was slightly more prevalent at 61%.[46]

Clinical presentation

PSC should be considered as a potential cause of liver disease in children with chronic cholestatic hepatitis (elevated aminotransferases and either elevated gamma glutamyl transferase (GGT), alkaline phosphatase or bilirubin) with or without inflammatory bowel disease, or chronic cholestatic hepatitis with the predominant symptom of pruritus. Children with inflammatory bowel disease should be screened for autoimmune liver diseases with an annual liver panel and GGT. Ninety-five percent of children with PSC will have an elevated GGT at diagnosis. There is a wide spectrum of presentations of pediatric PSC, from asymptomatic to cirrhosis with portal hypertension. The average age at diagnosis is approximately 11 to 12 years of age, although PSC has been reported as young as 2 years of age.[46,48] Daily functioning in children with PSC can be significantly altered owing to symptoms related to the disease. The most common symptoms are fatigue, pruritus, and abdominal pain. Other signs and symptoms include fever, jaundice, weight loss, delayed growth, and vitamin deficiencies.[48–50] Approximately 20% of pediatric patients with PSC have significant pruritus and in 4% it is extremely debilitating.[51,52] Intractable pruritus and fatigue can lead to sleep disturbance, depression, and impairment in school performance. An assessment of the patient's physical, psychological, and cognitive health are essential components to providing comprehensive long-term care to children with PSC.

Diagnosis

If PSC is suspected, the laboratory workup should include a liver function panel, GGT, prothrombin time/international normalized ratio, and autoantibodies (ANA, ASMA, anti-LKM) with total IgG to screen for overlap with AIH. Imaging studies should include an abdominal ultrasound examination to screen for cholelithiasis, choledocholithiasis, or bile duct dilation and an MRCP, which is the preferred modality to screen for medium and large bile duct abnormalities. Endoscopic retrograde cholangiopancreaticogram (ERCP) is an alternative to MRCP in imaging the biliary tree; however, it is more invasive, requires anesthesia, and has an added risk of post-ERCP pancreatitis. ERCP is considered when the MRCP is concerning for large duct PSC, but is inconclusive. A liver biopsy is recommended if the MRCP/ERCP is normal and there is concern for small duct PSC, or if one of the autoantibodies is positive (to confirm PSC–AIH overlap syndrome).

The majority of newly diagnosed pediatric patients with PSC will have a history of inflammatory bowel disease. If they do not have a past history of inflammatory bowel disease, it is essential to screen for inflammatory bowel disease at the time of diagnosis of PSC. Inflammatory bowel disease can manifest years before or after the diagnosis of PSC. Many children do not complain of colitic symptoms (abdominal pain, diarrhea, blood in the stool, stool urgency), but have macroscopic and microscopic evidence of inflammatory bowel disease on endoscopy evaluation. The inflammatory bowel disease that occurs in the setting of pediatric PSC has a distinct phenotype characterized by pancolitis with right-sided predominance, relative rectal sparing, backwash ileitis, and a relatively mild clinical course. Nevertheless, there is a 3- to 4-fold increased risk of colorectal cancer in adult patients with inflammatory bowel disease and PSC.[42,53]

Outcomes

Most children with PSC will have mild disease, but the rate of progression of biliary fibrosis is quite variable. The most accurate estimates of outcomes in pediatric PSC were gained through work within the Pediatric PSC Consortium, a worldwide initiative led by Mark Deneau, MD.[46] In a cohort of 781 children with PSC, 30% to 40% had evidence of portal hypertension or biliary complications (ie, biliary stricture requiring intervention) by 10 years after the diagnosis. Recent work has focused on identifying prognostic biomarkers to determine the rates of progression and complications. These biomarkers include GGT and the Sclerosing Cholangitis Outcomes in Pediatrics (SCOPE) Index. In patients with a GGT of less than 50 IU/L at 1 year after diagnosis, the 5-year event-free survival was 91%, compared with 67% for patients with a GGT of 50 IU/L or greater.[54] Events included portal hypertension, biliary stricture requiring intervention, liver transplantation, cholangiocarcinoma, or death. The SCOPE Index is calculated based on serum levels of albumin, GGT, bilirubin, and platelet count and the presence of large duct PSC. The SCOPE Index accurately prognosticates the frequency of an event on an annual basis after diagnosis.[55]

Management of primary sclerosing cholangitis

There is currently no medication that alters the progression of disease in PSC. Numerous medications have been trialed in the past without success, including immunosuppressive agents, antibiotics, and ursodeoxycholic acid. Both ursodeoxycholic acid and oral vancomycin have been reported to improve liver tests, but neither has definitively shown to slow the progression of disease.[56] Bacterial cholangitis is a complication of PSC and should be treated with broad spectrum antibiotics. Options to treat bile acid–induced pruritus include ursodeoxycholic acid, rifampin, or naltrexone. Children with PSC are at risk for deficiencies in the fat-soluble vitamins (vitamins A, D, E, and K) owing to altered bile flow. Symptomatic or dominant biliary strictures often require endoscopic therapeutic interventions, including balloon dilation of the strictures, with or without stent placement. Cholangiocarcinoma is very rare in pediatric PSC (approximately 1% of all cases); however, it is reasonable to screen for this with serum CA19-9 in the teenage years, especially if the patient has a dominant stricture.

Liver transplantation

Indications for liver transplantation in the setting of PSC or PSC–AIH overlap syndrome include cirrhosis with manifestations of end stage liver disease or debilitating pruritus that is, refractory to medical management. PSC accounts for 2% to 3% of all pediatric liver transplants. In the Pediatric PSC Consortium cohort, described elsewhere in this article, survival with the native liver was 88% at 5 years after diagnosis and 70% at 10 years.[46] The median age at transplant was 16.5 years (interquartile range, 13–19) and there was no difference between rates of transplant in patients with PSC with or without PSC–AIH overlap syndrome. Patient and graft survival is more than 90%, similar to the survival rates of patients transplanted for indications other than PSC. Patients transplanted for PSC have up to a 30% chance of recurrence of PSC disease in the allograft.

SUMMARY

In the setting of chronic hepatitis, a broad differential diagnosis should be considered to accurately identify the cause(s) of liver injury. Autoimmune liver diseases (AIH, PSC, and overlap syndrome) can occur in the absence of symptoms and, therefore, a high index of suspicion and appropriate diagnostic workup should be performed. The majority of children with AIH will achieve sustained remission with medical therapy, however there are no equivalent therapies for PSC that impact the progression of disease. Future research should include biomarker studies that will predict histologic remission in AIH and mechanistic studies that will define future treatment targets for PSC.

CLINICS CARE POINTS

- A broad differential diagnosis should be considered in the workup of patients with chronic hepatitis.

- Autoimmune liver diseases may not cause significant symptoms; as such, timely diagnosis requires a high index of suspicion.

- Although many medical therapies exist to achieve remission of AIH, there are no effective medical therapies for PSC.

- Autoimmune liver diseases may result in the need for pediatric liver transplantation.

DISCLOSURE

S. Kemme has no disclosures. C. Mack is a consultant for Albireo Pharm.

REFERENCES

1. Costaguta A, Gonzalez A, Pochettino S, et al. Incidence and clinical features of autoimmune hepatitis in the province of Santa Fe (Argentina). J Pediatr Gastroenterol Nutr 2018;67(6):e107–10.
2. Deneau M, Jensen MK, Holmen J, et al. Primary sclerosing cholangitis, autoimmune hepatitis, and overlap in Utah children: epidemiology and natural history. Hepatology 2013;58(4):1392–400.
3. Jimenez-Rivera C, Ling SC, Ahmed N, et al. Incidence and characteristics of autoimmune hepatitis. Pediatrics 2015;136(5):e1237–48.
4. Chung HV, Riley M, Ho JK, et al. Retrospective review of pediatric and adult autoimmune hepatitis in two quaternary care centres in British Columbia: increased prevalence seen in British Columbia's First Nations community. Can J Gastroenterol 2007;21(9):565–8.
5. Czaja AJ. Global disparities and their implications in the occurrence and outcome of autoimmune hepatitis. Dig Dis Sci 2017;62(9):2277–92.
6. Gregorio GV, Portmann B, Reid F, et al. Autoimmune hepatitis in childhood: a 20-year experience. Hepatology 1997;25(3):541–7.
7. Radhakrishnan KR, Alkhouri N, Worley S, et al. Autoimmune hepatitis in children–impact of cirrhosis at presentation on natural history and long-term outcome. Dig Liver Dis 2010;42(10):724–8.
8. Palle SK, Naik KB, McCracken CE, et al. Racial disparities in presentation and outcomes of paediatric autoimmune hepatitis. Liver Int 2019;39(5):976–84.
9. Oliveira LC, Porta G, Marin ML, et al. Autoimmune hepatitis, HLA and extended haplotypes. Autoimmun Rev 2011;10(4):189–93.
10. Gregorio GV, Portmann B, Karani J, et al. Autoimmune hepatitis/sclerosing cholangitis overlap syndrome in childhood: a 16-year prospective study. Hepatology 2001;33(3):544–53.
11. Wang P, Su H, Underhill J, et al. Autoantibody and human leukocyte antigen profiles in children with autoimmune liver disease and their first-degree relatives. J Pediatr Gastroenterol Nutr 2014;58(4):457–62.
12. Rodrigues AT, Liu PM, Fagundes ED, et al. Clinical characteristics and prognosis in children and adolescents with autoimmune hepatitis and overlap syndrome. J Pediatr Gastroenterol Nutr 2016;63(1):76–81.
13. Sheiko MA, Sundaram SS, Capocelli KE, et al. Outcomes in pediatric autoimmune hepatitis and significance of azathioprine metabolites. J Pediatr Gastroenterol Nutr 2017;65(1):80–5.
14. Vitfell-Pedersen J, Jorgensen MH, Muller K, et al. Autoimmune hepatitis in children in Eastern Denmark. J Pediatr Gastroenterol Nutr 2012;55(4):376–9.
15. Muratori P, Fabbri A, Lalanne C, et al. Autoimmune liver disease and concomitant extrahepatic autoimmune disease. Eur J Gastroenterol Hepatol 2015;27(10):1175–9.
16. Mack CL, Adams D, Assis DN, et al. Diagnosis and management of autoimmune hepatitis in adults and children: 2019 practice guidance and guidelines from the American Association for the Study of Liver Diseases. Hepatology 2020;72(2):671–722.
17. Balitzer D, Shafizadeh N, Peters MG, et al. Autoimmune hepatitis: review of histologic features included in the simplified criteria proposed by the international autoimmune hepatitis group and proposal for new histologic criteria. Mod Pathol 2017;30(5):773–83.

18. Czaja AJ, Manns MP. The validity and importance of subtypes in autoimmune hepatitis: a point of view. Am J Gastroenterol 1995;90(8):1206–11.

19. Maggiore G, Veber F, Bernard O, et al. Autoimmune hepatitis associated with anti-actin antibodies in children and adolescents. J Pediatr Gastroenterol Nutr 1993;17(4):376–81.

20. Heringlake S, Schutte A, Flemming P, et al. Presumed cryptogenic liver disease in Germany: high prevalence of autoantibody-negative autoimmune hepatitis, low prevalence of NASH, no evidence for occult viral etiology. Z Gastroenterol 2009;47(5):417–23.

21. Mehendiratta V, Mitroo P, Bombonati A, et al. Serologic markers do not predict histologic severity or response to treatment in patients with autoimmune hepatitis. Clin Gastroenterol Hepatol 2009;7(1):98–103.

22. Maggiore G, Socie G, Sciveres M, et al. Seronegative autoimmune hepatitis in children: spectrum of disorders. Dig Liver Dis 2016;48(7):785–91.

23. Maggiore G, Porta G, Bernard O, et al. Autoimmune hepatitis with initial presentation as acute hepatic failure in young children. J Pediatr 1990;116(2):280–2.

24. Kemme S, Stahl M, Brigham D, et al. Outcomes of severe seronegative hepatitis-associated aplastic anemia: a pediatric case series. J Pediatr Gastroenterol Nutr 2021;72(2):194–201.

25. Angulo JM, Sigal LH, Espinoza LR. Coexistent minocycline-induced systemic lupus erythematosus and autoimmune hepatitis. Semin Arthritis Rheum 1998; 28(3):187–92.

26. Elkayam O, Yaron M, Caspi D. Minocycline-induced autoimmune syndromes: an overview. Semin Arthritis Rheum 1999;28(6):392–7.

27. Bjornsson E, Talwalkar J, Treeprasertsuk S, et al. Drug-induced autoimmune hepatitis: clinical characteristics and prognosis. Hepatology 2010;51(6):2040–8.

28. Teitelbaum JE, Perez-Atayde AR, Cohen M, et al. Minocycline-related autoimmune hepatitis: case series and literature review. Arch Pediatr Adolesc Med 1998;152(11):1132–6.

29. Bruserud O, Oftedal BE, Wolff AB, et al. AIRE-mutations and autoimmune disease. Curr Opin Immunol 2016;43:8–15.

30. Lankisch TO, Jaeckel E, Strassburg CP. The autoimmune polyendocrinopathy-candidiasis-ectodermal dystrophy or autoimmune polyglandular syndrome type 1. Semin Liver Dis 2009;29(3):307–14.

31. Park JH, Lee KH, Jeon B, et al. Immune dysregulation, polyendocrinopathy, enteropathy, X-linked (IPEX) syndrome: a systematic review. Autoimmun Rev 2020;19(6):102526.

32. Crotty R, Taylor MS, Farmer JR, et al. Spectrum of hepatic manifestations of common variable immunodeficiency. Am J Surg Pathol 2020;44(5):617–25.

33. Fuss IJ, Friend J, Yang Z, et al. Nodular regenerative hyperplasia in common variable immunodeficiency. J Clin Immunol 2013;33(4):748–58.

34. Winkelstein JA, Marino MC, Ochs H, et al. The X-linked hyper-IgM syndrome: clinical and immunologic features of 79 patients. Medicine (Baltimore) 2003;82(6): 373–84.

35. Than NN, Hodson J, Schmidt-Martin D, et al. Efficacy of rituximab in difficult-to-manage autoimmune hepatitis: results from the International Autoimmune Hepatitis Group. JHEP Rep 2019;1(6):437–45.

36. Hartl J, Ehlken H, Weiler-Normann C, et al. Patient selection based on treatment duration and liver biochemistry increases success rates after treatment withdrawal in autoimmune hepatitis. J Hepatol 2015;62(3):642–6.

37. European Association for the Study of the L. EASL clinical practice guidelines: autoimmune hepatitis. J Hepatol 2015;63(4):971–1004.
38. Chai PF, Lee WS, Brown RM, et al. Childhood autoimmune liver disease: indications and outcome of liver transplantation. J Pediatr Gastroenterol Nutr 2010; 50(3):295–302.
39. Gregorio GV, McFarlane B, Bracken P, et al. Organ and non-organ specific auto-antibody titres and IgG levels as markers of disease activity: a longitudinal study in childhood autoimmune liver disease. Autoimmunity 2002;35(8):515–9.
40. Martin SR, Alvarez F, Anand R, et al. Outcomes in children who underwent transplantation for autoimmune hepatitis. Liver Transpl 2011;17(4):393–401.
41. Jossen J, Annunziato R, Kim HS, et al. Liver transplantation for children with primary sclerosing cholangitis and autoimmune hepatitis: UNOS database analysis. J Pediatr Gastroenterol Nutr 2017;64(4):e83–7.
42. Toy E, Balasubramanian S, Selmi C, et al. The prevalence, incidence and natural history of primary sclerosing cholangitis in an ethnically diverse population. BMC Gastroenterol 2011;11:83.
43. Hirschfield GM, Karlsen TH, Lindor KD, et al. Primary sclerosing cholangitis. Lancet 2013;382(9904):1587–99.
44. Karlsen TH, Folseraas T, Thorburn D, et al. Primary sclerosing cholangitis - a comprehensive review. J Hepatol 2017;67(6):1298–323.
45. Fung BM, Lindor KD, Tabibian JH. Cancer risk in primary sclerosing cholangitis: epidemiology, prevention, and surveillance strategies. World J Gastroenterol 2019;25(6):659–71.
46. Deneau MR, El-Matary W, Valentino PL, et al. The natural history of primary sclerosing cholangitis in 781 children: a multicenter, international collaboration. Hepatology 2017;66(2):518–27.
47. Kaplan GG, Laupland KB, Butzner D, et al. The burden of large and small duct primary sclerosing cholangitis in adults and children: a population-based analysis. Am J Gastroenterol 2007;102(5):1042–9.
48. Cotter JM, Browne LP, Capocelli KE, et al. Lack of correlation of liver tests with fibrosis stage at diagnosis in pediatric primary sclerosing cholangitis. J Pediatr Gastroenterol Nutr 2018;66(2):227–33.
49. Liberal R, Vergani D, Mieli-Vergani G. Paediatric autoimmune liver disease. Dig Dis 2015;33(Suppl 2):36–46.
50. Cotter JM, Mack CL. Primary sclerosing cholangitis: unique aspects of disease in children. Clin Liver Dis (Hoboken) 2017;10(5):120–3.
51. Feldstein AE, Perrault J, El-Youssif M, et al. Primary sclerosing cholangitis in children: a long-term follow-up study. Hepatology 2003;38(1):210–7.
52. Miloh T, Arnon R, Shneider B, et al. A retrospective single-center review of primary sclerosing cholangitis in children. Clin Gastroenterol Hepatol 2009;7(2): 239–45.
53. Ricciuto A, Kamath BM, Griffiths AM. The IBD and PSC phenotypes of PSC-IBD. Curr Gastroenterol Rep 2018;20(4):16.
54. Deneau MR, Mack C, Abdou R, et al. Gamma glutamyltransferase reduction is associated with favorable outcomes in pediatric primary sclerosing cholangitis. Hepatol Commun 2018;2(11):1369–78.
55. Deneau MR, Mack C, Perito ER, et al. The Sclerosing Cholangitis Outcomes in Pediatrics (SCOPE) index: a prognostic tool for children. Hepatology 2021; 73(3):1074–87.
56. Laborda TJ, Jensen MK, Kavan M, et al. Treatment of primary sclerosing cholangitis in children. World J Hepatol 2019;11(1):19–36.

Pediatric Nonalcoholic Fatty Liver Disease

Tania Mitsinikos, MD, Paula Mrowczynski-Hernandez, RD, Rohit Kohli, MBBS, MS*

KEYWORDS

• Obesity • Non-alcoholic fatty liver disease • Pediatrics • Chronic liver disease

KEY POINTS

- As the obesity epidemic worsens, pediatric nonalcoholic fatty liver disease has continued to rise.
- Screening age-appropriate children who are obese is critical to prompt evaluation and diagnosis.
- Lifestyle changes through diet modification and exercise are imperative regardless of alternative treatment modalities.
- Ongoing research is needed in pediatrics for new therapeutic interventions.

INTRODUCTION

Obesity continues to be a serious public health issue for which medical care providers have become well-versed in its associated comorbid conditions including metabolic syndrome which is characterized by specific biochemical markers as well as commonly seen conditions such as hypertension, diabetes mellitus, obstructive sleep apnea, and nonalcoholic fatty liver disease (NAFLD).

NAFLD is now a leading cause of liver disease in adults, not just in the United States but worldwide.[1] NAFLD is a chronic liver condition characterized by excess hepatic steatosis (>5%) while excluding other causes of such accumulation such as chronic viral hepatitis, steatogenic medication use, or metabolic disorders.[2] As pediatric obesity rates continue to rise, there has been a parallel increase in pediatric NAFLD prevalence such that it is now well accepted to be the most common chronic liver disease in childhood.[3,4] Furthermore, among the large number of children with NAFLD, a smaller number with nonalcoholic steatohepatitis (NASH) are the ones who will likely benefit from therapeutic interventions, including, but not limited to, liver transplantation, as they enter young adulthood.[5] With such a burden of disease, the economic burden of management will rise exponentially to care for these patients.[6] Clearly, given these alarming statistics, the need for providers to be well-versed in this condition is

---

Children's Hospital Los Angeles, 4650 Sunset Boulevard, MS #78, Los Angeles, CA 90027, USA
* Corresponding author.
E-mail address: rkohli@usc.edu

Pediatr Clin N Am 68 (2021) 1309–1320
https://doi.org/10.1016/j.pcl.2021.07.013
0031-3955/21/© 2021 Elsevier Inc. All rights reserved.

acute. From identifying at-risk populations, pursuing a focused and thoughtful workup, and finally providing necessary treatment and support for this condition, all are required for the care of these patients and, by extension, their families. The overall goals for the general pediatrician should be robust NAFLD screening protocols that help identify children with NAFLD and prompt appropriate referrals to pediatric hepatologists. Our focus of course should be to identify those with the serve form of the disease: NASH. This attention, we hope, will lead to interventions that help prevent the progression to end-stage liver disease and reverse the trend of liver transplantation in adulthood.

INCIDENCE

As mentioned previously, obesity rates in the United States continue to rise, in both the adult and pediatric populations. While the prevalence of obesity, per the Center of Disease Control, has remained rather stagnant at around 18.5% in the group younger than 18 years, when stratifying these data in different age groups, there is increasing prevalence with increasing age; 13.9% in 2 to 5 years of age, 18.4% in 6 to 11 years of age, and 20.6% in 12 to 19 years of age.[7,8] Obesity does not necessarily translate into disease; however, when Sahota and colleagues reviewed recent data on the incidence of NAFLD in the Southern California region, their results were sobering. In reviewing over 7 million patient years, in those who had been screened for NAFLD, incidence of NAFLD increased over time from 36 per 100,000 in 2009 to 58.2 per 100,000 in 2018 (P<.0001).[9] These are alarming data demonstrating the parallel increase in NAFLD to obesity rates. Given our increasing awareness of this disease in pediatrics, guidelines in the screening, diagnosis, and management of pediatric NAFLD were developed in 2017 and published by the North American Society of Gastroenterology, Hepatology, and Nutrition.[10] Vos and colleagues in this report, in accordance with other metabolic screening recommendations by the American Academic of Pediatrics, suggested screening otherwise healthy children aged 9 to 11 years with obesity as defined by a body mass index (BMI) of greater than the 95th percentile using an alanine aminotransferase (ALT) level.[10] In addition, groups with underlying high-risk conditions and comorbidities were identified for special consideration and screening for this condition; specifically those who may be overweight with a BMI greater than the 86th percentile but less than the 95th percentile, with other comorbid conditions such as central adiposity, insulin resistance, prediabetes or diabetes mellitus, dyslipidemia, sleep apnea, or family history of NAFLD/NASH.[10]

NATURAL HISTORY

The NAFLD umbrella encompasses a wide spectrum of diseases from bland steatosis to NASH with cirrhosis. The goals of screening and monitoring are to identify those at high risk for development of high grades of fibrosis and diagnosis and to treat those individuals before the onset of complications of chronic liver disease such as portal hypertension which leads to the need for liver transplantation. Pediatric care providers are in a unique position that we may identify patients early and take a more "defensive" approach than those with more advanced disease and need for "offensive" actions. Nonetheless, progression to NASH (10%–15%) and cirrhosis (5%) can and does occur with about 1% to 2% requiring liver transplantation.[11] Risk for hepatocellular carcinoma (HCC) has been described in adults with NAFLD/NASH, and thus, the risk of development of HCC in pediatric patients remains.[12–14] In those with advanced liver disease, portal hypertension, and its sequalae, liver transplantation has been described, and now NASH is increasingly recognized as one of the leading indications for liver transplantation in adults.[15]

GUIDELINES AND EVALUATION

As our awareness of this entity has heightened over the years, our frequency of screening to identify these patients has improved compared to that in prior decades.[16,17] Screening is still done based on biochemical parameters, specifically the ALT. The upper limits of this value can be quite variable and dependent on the laboratory running the test; however, established normal values have been reviewed and published where much of our guidelines rest. The SAFETY study, published in *Gastroenterology* in 2010, by Schwimmer and colleagues, examined data from a wide variety of sources that included healthy children as well as those with chronic liver diseases such as NAFLD, hepatitis B, and hepatitis C.[18] From this, they were able to determine the normal value of ALT for boys was 25.8 U/L, and for girls, 22.1 U/L.[18] These normative values have been incorporated into our clinic, and those with ALT greater than 45 U/L (about 2 times the upper limit of normal for both boys and girls) in the context of a BMI greater than the 85th percentile would be eligible for our NAFLD clinic (**Fig. 1**). This merely signals the need for ongoing workup and a close review of comorbid conditions of metabolic syndrome and does not determine the need for biopsy upon initial evaluation. Persistently elevated liver enzymes despite lifestyle changes, parental agreement, and other factors play a role in the timing of such a procedure.

Once screening has identified a patient with an elevated ALT value, many times, providers will obtain an abdominal ultrasound. The utility of such a study is less on confirming a diagnosis of NAFLD, usually outlined by increased echogenicity potentially consistent with hepatic steatosis, although overall ultrasound has a relatively poor predictive value for diagnosis or correlation of degree of hepatic steatosis.[19] Thus, we use ultrasound rather to exclude other conditions that may result in liver enzyme abnormalities such as a cholelithiasis, hepatic masses/cysts, or biliary duct abnormalities. The presence of hepatic steatosis may certainly suggest NAFLD, and based on probability along with patient anthropometrics, a likely diagnosis; however, there are many other conditions that result in such findings such as, but not limited to, hepatitis B, hepatitis C, disorders of cholesterol synthesis, Wilson's disease, medications, and alcohol use to name a few[10] that may also have hepatic steatosis as part of

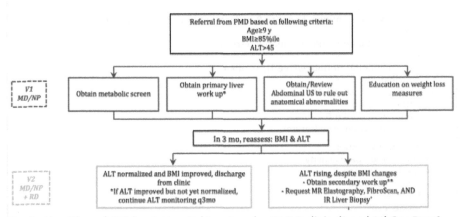

Fig. 1. Algorithm of Children's Hospital Los Angeles NAFLD clinic. (* and **) See **Box 1**.

their phenotype. Therefore, it is also important to rule out these conditions as part of the initial evaluation.

In our NAFLD clinic, our initial visit with the patient and their family focuses on many of these areas (see **Fig. 1**). First and foremost, workup to exclude other causes of asymptomatic enzyme elevation is recommended. This includes evaluation of not only many of the aforementioned disorders but also other less common metabolic and autoimmune conditions (**Box 1**). We review the ultrasound imaging that has been obtained or will request to rule out other confounding conditions. Additionally, we take a thorough history of features of other comorbid conditions such as hypertension, dyslipidemia, diabetes mellitus, obstructive sleep apnea, and polycystic ovarian syndrome in girls. Any individual screening positive to any of these conditions is recommended further workup or referred to the appropriate clinic for ongoing care. Most importantly, we take a very thorough diet and exercise history, as this is the mainstay treatment for NAFLD, as well as other obesity-related conditions previously outlined. Detailing the type and number of sugar-sweetened beverages, meal and snacking frequency, meal volumes, and food choices is important to provide realistic and tangible recommendations to families who are often overwhelmed by the lifestyle changes they know are needed. Despite our strong investment in their care and alliances made, we face challenges in follow-up and obtaining labs as this is an asymptomatic condition that makes it difficult to families to convince these often challenging and resistant teenagers for change. While we have experienced this, others have noted similar findings in obtaining the necessary follow-up labs, workup, as well as referral to gastroenterology.[20] Given this, while we may not have shown persistent elevation in liver enzymes (as defined >3 months), given the concerns for follow-up, we recommend obtaining this workup at this visit.

Box 1
Staged workup for elevated liver enzymes in the obese patient

Metabolic screen (All visits):
  Complete Blood Count with differential
  Chemistry panel
  Gamma Glutamyl Transpeptidase
  Fasting lipid panel
  Hemoglobin A1c

Primary liver workup:
  Hepatitis B surface Antigen, Hepatitis B surface Antibody (Ab), Hepatitis C Ab
  Celiac Ab screen
  Serum iron, Total Iron Binding Capacity ferritin
  Ceruloplasmin
  Thyroid Stimulating Hormone/Free Thyroxine4
  Anti Nuclear Ab
  Liver kidney microsomal Ab
  Smooth muscle Ab
  Total Immunoglobulin G
  Alpha 1 Anti-trypsin level (serum)

Secondary liver workup:
  Lysosomal acid lipase activity
  Soluble liver antigen
  Liver pancreas-1 Ab
  Insulin level
  C-peptide level

Our current approach requires follow-up with our multidisciplinary team every 3 months. After their initial assessment and workup, subsequent processes include evaluation and recommendation by a registered dietician with specific expertise in those with conditions associated with obesity such as NAFLD and diabetes mellitus. Additionally, our team includes a psychologist to assist patients and families with psychosocial stressors and mental health issues that may be contributing to behaviors leading to poor lifestyle choices. Frequent follow-up was recommended as prior studies showed that not only frequent follow-up but also multidisciplinary approaches help improve anthropometric and biochemical parameters of disease. Specifically, the study published in 2013 by DeVore and colleagues was able to demonstrate in children adherent to follow-up that they have improved BMI Z scores, Aspartate Amino transferase (AST), ALT, total cholesterol, and low-density lipoprotein cholesterol that were statistically significant.[21]

At this juncture, if ALT remains elevated despite lifestyle change efforts, liver biopsy is typically recommended. This not only helps formal diagnosis of diseases, for NAFLD, this is the established gold standard method, but also helps stratify risk based on NAFLD activity score and prognosticate based on fibrosis scores. While generally a safe procedure, the cost and procedural risk of repeated biopsies are not to be ignored, and surrogate measures of fibrosis and advancement of disease have been developed for disease monitoring and progression. Specifically, transient elastography (FibroScan) as well as magnetic resonance (MR) elastography are the two modalities shown to be able to differentiate higher grades of fibrosis in this disease and have shown good correlation of fibrosis in adults.[22,23] Currently, our clinic uses both modalities to establish baseline at the time of liver biopsy and then periodic monitoring over time during the course of treatment. The ALT, however, is the primary biochemical marker followed to assess progression of disease as well as treatment.[24]

IMAGING

FibroScan is an inexpensive, portable, bedside study that can provide rapid results on liver fibrosis and even hepatic steatosis. It uses an ultrasound probe to transmit vibrations inducing a shear wave that propagates through the tissue of interest. Ultrasound then measures the shear wave velocity which corresponds into stiffness and, in the case of the liver, fibrosis, a representative image of which is provided in **Fig. 2**.[25] The faster the shear wave propagates through the tissue, the stiffer it is, and thus, higher grade of fibrosis. Currently, established cutoffs for kilopascal (kPa) measurements are outlined in **Table 1**. Other pediatric studies have established slightly different cutoffs in pediatrics, specifically F3-F4 greater than 8.6 kPA and F4 greater than 11.5 kPa with 81% and 84% accuracy, respectively.[26] Controlled attenuation parameter provides fat quantification that correlates closely to liver histology.[27] There are some limitations to this study, particularly abdominal adiposity, which increases the distances between the probe and liver, BMI greater than 30 kg/m^2, and operator experience.[28] Castera demonstrated a failure rate of about 3.1% as defined by zero measurements obtained and unreliable results when fewer than ten measures were obtained, which was as high as 15.8%.[25] Nonetheless, this study proves to be a highly useful one and is now being integrated into other noninvasive biomarker scoring systems which help providers to stratify patients' risk for progressive disease without the need for continued liver biopsy.[29,30]

MR elastography provides results similar to those of the FibroScan and mitigates many of the failures or unreliable measures that can occur with transient elastography. The principles of this study are the same as those of the FibroScan; however, MR

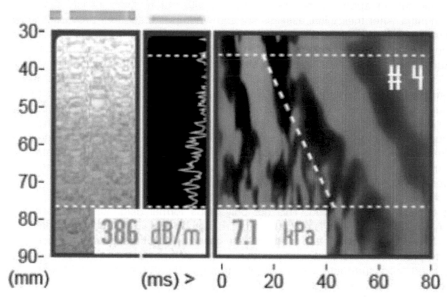

Fig. 2. Image of FibroScan measurement. (*Courtesy of* Debra Browne, NP, GI Division, CHLA.)

elastography may provide a more comprehensive assessment of the liver given its broader range of tissue under elasticity for measurement.[31] Representative photos of MR elastography in **Fig. 3** highlight this study's ability to capture data of the entire liver. After demonstrating reliable and accurate results in adults, pediatric studies have demonstrated similar success. Normal values in children without the underlying liver disease were found to have a kPa of 2.1 independent of age, sex, or BMI.[32] In chronic liver disease, MR elastography in a pediatric cohort demonstrated a cutoff value of 2.71 kPa to identify significant fibrosis as compared to histopathology with 88% sensitivity and 85% specificity.[33] Additionally, hepatic steatosis measures can also be obtained and trended over time.[34,35] However, it does have some important limitations including the need for breath holds, cost, and time.

TREATMENT
Nutritional Counseling

The mainstay of pediatric NAFLD/NASH treatment remains lifestyle-mediated weight loss. Targeting lifestyle changes, such as increased physical activity, and modifying the affected child's diet using a multidisciplinary team including dietitians are key to achieving this goal. Increasing physical activity is important; however, greater

Table 1 Established cutoff values for various grades of fibrosis using FibroScan	
Liver Stiffness Cutoff (kPa)	**Fibrosis Score (Metavir)**
2.5–7.0	F0-F1
7.0–9.5	F2
9.5–12.5	F3
>12.5	F4

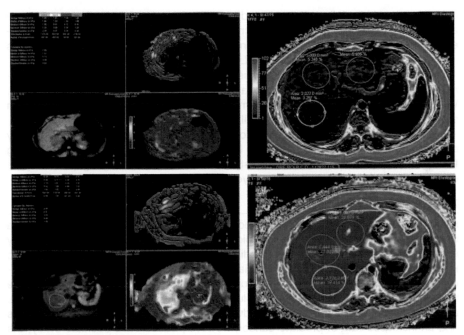

Fig. 3. Image of MR elastography. (*Courtesy of* Dr. Skorn Pontarana, Radiology Department, CHLA.)

emphasis is placed on dietary modifications. No specific diet or program is recommended for the treatment of NAFLD.

Studies have shown that reducing excessive energy intake from added sugars in the diet, such as sugar-sweetened beverages, may reduce biomarkers for NAFLD activity. In our clinic, the first intervention of treatment is counseling patients to eliminate all sugar-sweetened beverages and juices while promoting water as the preferred fluid for hydration. This is emphasized in all follow-up visits. The second intervention may be identifying areas of excessive energy or sugar intake. A diet recall may be reviewed, and goals are discussed to help reduce the intake of excessive sugar while including balanced meals with protein, fat, and fiber-rich carbohydrate sources such as fruits, vegetables, and whole grains. Balanced meal examples are demonstrated using the foods the families report, including those often consumed at home, while being mindful of portions and eating behaviors that may contribute to a child's excessive energy intake.

Establishing lifestyle approaches to having regular meals, snacks, and staying hydrated with unsweetened fluids is discussed. Lifestyle approaches may also include participation in daily physical activities that the child enjoys and body movement that brings them joy. Sleep hygiene and stress management are also discussed in relation to the quantity and quality of foods the child may be eating. The dietitian works with families to help identity behaviors that may be contributing to excessive energy intake. It is also important to note that the dietitian aims to communicate the nutrition recommendations with children and families in a manner that promotes self-care and compassion rather than restrictive dieting or dangerous weight loss methods. The goal is to encourage healthy habits that embrace balance and nutrition education for long-term health.

The mainstay of pediatric NAFLD/NASH treatment remains lifestyle-mediated weight loss. Targeting lifestyle changes by appropriately modifying the affected child's diet using a multidisciplinary team including dieticians as well as increasing physical activity are key to achieving this goal. Increasing physical activity is important; however, most emphasis is placed on dietary modifications. No specific diet or program is recommended for the treatment of NAFLD.

In our clinic, the approach is stepwise. The most important intervention is eliminating all sugar-sweetened beverages, and this is emphasized in all follow-up visits. We discuss establishing limits on the number of meals per day and minimizing portion size. Food choices are reviewed in detail.

We have developed an educational video targeted to our preteen patients so they may gain better understanding of what NAFLD is but more importantly highlighting these points to promote a healthier lifestyle in a medium and language that may be easier for them to comprehend (https://youtu.be/4CFYMAx5-7E).

Therapeutic Interventions

In addition to lifestyle changes, we also recommend the use of vitamin E (400 IU twice a day of the natural form) in children with biopsy-proven NASH. This is currently the only effective and approved treatment for pediatric NAFLD. The Treatment of Nonalcoholic Fatty Liver Disease in Children (TONIC) trial, a double-blinded, placebo-controlled, randomized trial, demonstrated that at this dose and frequency, it is possible to improve hepatic histology and have greater resolution of NASH.[36] There are safety concerns associated with the use of vitamin E in adult studies, particularly cardiovascular events and an increased rate of prostate cancer; however, based on a pediatric study, the TONIC study, there were no reported adverse events over the 2-year study period.[36,37] We advise children with biopsy-confirmed NASH to be trialed on vitamin E for 2 years, with the goal of significant biochemical response defined as improved ALT levels.[37]

FUTURE DIRECTION

Emphasis should be placed not only on ways to improve diagnostic accuracy and noninvasive testing but also more importantly on treatment. While there are nearly 200 clinical trials ongoing for NAFLD, only 20 of them target pediatric disease, highlighting the need for more data in this area with its ever-rising incidence.[38] Various drug targets as well as supplements have been investigated with varying results.

Obeticholic Acid

Obeticholic acid (OCA) derives from chenodeoxycholic acid and an agonist of the farnesoid X receptor and has been identified as a promising target for chronic liver diseases, including NASH by improving histologic features of NASH.[39–41] Younossi and colleagues recently published phase 3 trial data from a study of over 900 adult patients with NASH, with fibrosis, without cirrhosis.[42] After an 18-month intervention, a primary end-point analysis found fibrosis improvement of greater than or equal to 1 stage with no worsening of NASH or NASH resolution with no worsening of fibrosis, and those with higher dose OCA showed significant improvement in fibrosis, with 23% reaching the primary endpoint; however, the study is ongoing to assess longer term outcomes.[42] Generally, the medication was well tolerated with pruritus being the most common side effect.

Cysteamine Bitartrate — Delayed Release

As many therapeutic options target different pathophysiologic mechanisms, oxidative stress is an area that can have benefit, similar to vitamin E.[43] Cysteamine is known to support glutathione synthesis, which is an intracellular oxidant and when depleted leads to hepatocellular injury.[44] In a small open-label pilot study, 13 patients were treated with cysteamine bitartrate-delayed release, which improved liver enzymes; however, despite the improvement in ALT and lobular inflammation on histology, there was no significant different in fibrosis.[45]

Rebaudioside

Xi and colleagues published promising data for the use of noncaloric sweeteners in a NAFLD-induced mouse model, demonstrating that rebaudioside in drinking water improved liver enzymes and liver fibrosis.[46] This has now been extended to a clinical trial in patients with biopsy-proven NASH, examining the effects of commercially available rebaudioside drinks, currently in active recruitment.

Microbiome

Other investigations examining microbiome and fecal microbial transplant in an NAFLD mice model have been conducted but have not demonstrated protection or disease reversal in such instances.[47] Fecal contents from an NAFLD-induced mouse model fed diets that demonstrated improvement of NAFLD histologically were isolated and gavaged to mice who were maintained on an NAFLD-induced diet. This did not demonstrate any protective effects or disease reversal in those mice. It is worth nothing, in that same study, the shift in macronutrient distribution of the diet of NAFLD-induced mice with improved histologic disease both in degree of steatosis as well as fibrosis.[47,48] Others have explored the use of synbiotics, and while shifts in the microbiome were identified, this did not change disease characteristics or fibrosis.[49] Further work needs to be conducted to better understand the interplay of diet, microbiome, and its effects on NAFLD.

SUMMARY

In conclusion, we advocate for a multidisciplinary approach to care in children with NAFLD/NASH. This should include specific support involving nutritional services to provide counseling and guidance for successful weight loss and improvement in hepatic steatosis as well as appropriate psychosocial support when appropriate. The utility of noninvasive markers and assessment of liver disease is ever evolving, but currently FibroScan and MR elastography are helpful tools in stratifying those with advanced grades of fibrosis and help reduce the need for invasive procedures such as repeated liver biopsies. In the interim, we in pediatrics have a unique opportunity to help identify the children most at risk from the worst manifestations of this epidemic and to provide interventions at an early age to help prevent serious life-altering consequences from chronic liver disease in adulthood such as HCC and liver transplantation.

CLINICS CARE POINTS

- Fatty liver disease (NAFLD/NASH) is a diagnosis of exclusion needing other causes of hepatic steatosis to be ruled out, and the gold standard for its diagnosis is a liver biopsy.

- Abdominal ultrasound is a useful tool for ruling out hepatobiliary structural abnormalities; however, it should not be used in establishing a diagnosis of NAFLD/NASH.

- Lifestyle modification, especially diet changes, should be strongly emphasized at frequent follow-up encounters to patients/families as it remains the mainstay of treatment for pediatric NAFLD.

- Noninvasive imaging for monitoring disease progression such as vibration-controlled transient elastography or magnetic resonance elastography may help decrease need for follow-up liver biopsies.

DISCLOSURE

Dr R. Kohli declares Data Safety Monitoring Board/research agreements with Albireo Pharma, Takeda Pharmaceutical Company, Mirum Pharmaceuticals, Vision Pharma, and Epigen Pharma. Dr R. Kohli is a consultant for/received speaking compensation from Intercept Pharmaceuticals, Alexion Pharmaceuticals, and Sanofi-Genzyme. Other authors have nothing to disclose.

REFERENCES

1. Younossi ZM, Koenig AB, Abdelatif D, et al. Global epidemiology of nonalcoholic fatty liver disease-meta-analytic assessment of prevalence, incidence, and outcomes. Hepatology 2016;64(1):73–84.
2. Chalasani N, Younossi Z, Lavine JE, et al. The diagnosis and management of nonalcoholic fatty liver disease: practice guidance from the American Association for the Study of Liver Diseases. Hepatology 2018;67(1):328–57.
3. Loomba R, Sanyal AJ. The global NAFLD epidemic. Nat Rev Gastroenterol Hepatol 2013;10(11):686–90.
4. Yu EL, Golshan S, Harlow KE, et al. Prevalence of nonalcoholic fatty liver disease in children with obesity. J Pediatr 2019;207:64–70.
5. Younossi ZM, Stepanova M, Afendy M, et al. Changes in the prevalence of the most common causes of chronic liver diseases in the United States from 1988 to 2008. Clin Gastroenterol Hepatol 2011;9(6):524–30.e1 [quiz e60].
6. Younossi ZM, Henry L, Bush H, et al. Clinical and economic burden of nonalcoholic fatty liver disease and nonalcoholic steatohepatitis. Clin Liver Dis 2018; 22(1):1–10.
7. Hales CM, Carroll MD, Fryar CD, et al. Prevalence of obesity among adults and youth: United States, 2015-2016. NCHS Data Brief 2017;10(288):1–8.
8. Ogden CL, Carroll MD, Lawman HG, et al. Trends in obesity prevalence among children and adolescents in the United States, 1988-1994 Through 2013-2014. JAMA 2016;315(21):2292–9.
9. Sahota AK, Shapiro WL, Newton KP, et al. Incidence of nonalcoholic fatty liver disease in children: 2009-2018. Pediatrics 2020;146(6). https://doi.org/10.1542/peds.2020-0771.
10. Vos MB, Abrams SH, Barlow SE, et al. NASPGHAN clinical practice guideline for the diagnosis and treatment of nonalcoholic fatty liver disease in children: recommendations from the expert committee on NAFLD (ECON) and the North American Society of Pediatric Gastroenterology, Hepatology and Nutrition (NASPGHAN). J Pediatr Gastroenterol Nutr 2017;64(2):319–34.
11. Rinella M, Charlton M. The globalization of nonalcoholic fatty liver disease: prevalence and impact on world health. Hepatology 2016;64(1):19–22.
12. Oliveira S, Samba AK, Towbin AJ, et al. Incidental inflammatory adenoma with β-catenin activation in the setting of paediatric NASH. Pediatr Obes 2018; 13(1):70–3.
13. Kanwal F, Kramer JR, Mapakshi S, et al. Risk of hepatocellular cancer in patients with non-alcoholic fatty liver disease. Gastroenterology 2018;155(6):1828–37.e2.
14. Natarajan Y, Kramer JR, Yu X, et al. Risk of cirrhosis and hepatocellular cancer in patients with non-alcoholic fatty liver disease and normal liver enzymes. Hepatology 2020. https://doi.org/10.1002/hep.31157.
15. Younossi ZM. Nonalcoholic fatty liver disease and nonalcoholic steatohepatitis: implications for liver transplantation. Liver Transpl 2018;24(2):166–70.

16. Riley MR, Bass NM, Rosenthal P, et al. Underdiagnosis of pediatric obesity and underscreening for fatty liver disease and metabolic syndrome by pediatricians and pediatric subspecialists. J Pediatr 2005;147(6):839–42.
17. Schwimmer JB, Newton KP, Awai HI, et al. Paediatric gastroenterology evaluation of overweight and obese children referred from primary care for suspected non-alcoholic fatty liver disease. Aliment Pharmacol Ther 2013;38(10):1267–77.
18. Schwimmer JB, Dunn W, Norman GJ, et al. SAFETY study: alanine aminotransferase cutoff values are set too high for reliable detection of pediatric chronic liver disease. Gastroenterology 2010;138(4):1357–64, 1364.e1–2.
19. Awai HI, Newton KP, Sirlin CB, et al. Evidence and recommendations for imaging liver fat in children, based on systematic review. Clin Gastroenterol Hepatol 2014; 12(5):765–73.
20. Ferguson AE, Xanthakos SA, Siegel RM. Challenges in screening for pediatric nonalcoholic fatty liver disease. Clin Pediatr (Phila) 2018;57(5):558–62.
21. DeVore S, Kohli R, Lake K, et al. A multidisciplinary clinical program is effective in stabilizing BMI and reducing transaminase levels in pediatric patients with NAFLD. J Pediatr Gastroenterol Nutr 2013;57(1):119–23.
22. Garcovich M, Veraldi S, Di Stasio E, et al. Liver stiffness in pediatric patients with fatty liver disease: diagnostic accuracy and reproducibility of shear-wave elastography. Radiology 2017;283(3):820–7.
23. Singh S, Venkatesh SK, Loomba R, et al. Magnetic resonance elastography for staging liver fibrosis in non-alcoholic fatty liver disease: a diagnostic accuracy systematic review and individual participant data pooled analysis. Eur Radiol 2016;26(5):1431–40.
24. Newton KP, Lavine JE, Wilson L, et al. Alanine aminotransferase and gamma-glutamyl transpeptidase predict histologic improvement in pediatric nonalcoholic steatohepatitis. Hepatology 2021;73(3):937–51.
25. Castera L. Non-invasive diagnosis of steatosis and fibrosis. Diabetes Metab 2008;34(6 Pt 2):674–9.
26. Lee CK, Mitchell PD, Raza R, et al. Validation of transient elastography cut points to assess advanced liver fibrosis in children and young adults: the boston children's hospital experience. J Pediatr 2018;198:84–9.e2.
27. Desai NK, Harney S, Raza R, et al. Comparison of controlled attenuation parameter and liver biopsy to assess hepatic steatosis in pediatric patients. J Pediatr 2016;173:160–4.e1.
28. Castéra L, Foucher J, Bernard PH, et al. Pitfalls of liver stiffness measurement: a 5-year prospective study of 13,369 examinations. Hepatology 2010;51(3): 828–35.
29. Newsome PN, Sasso M, Deeks JJ, et al. FibroScan-AST (FAST) score for the non-invasive identification of patients with non-alcoholic steatohepatitis with significant activity and fibrosis: a prospective derivation and global validation study. Lancet Gastroenterol Hepatol 2020;5(4):362–73.
30. Boursier J, Vergniol J, Guillet A, et al. Diagnostic accuracy and prognostic significance of blood fibrosis tests and liver stiffness measurement by FibroScan in non-alcoholic fatty liver disease. J Hepatol 2016;65(3):570–8.
31. Kennedy P, Wagner M, Castéra L, et al. Quantitative elastography methods in liver disease: current evidence and future directions. Radiology 2018;286(3): 738–63.
32. Trout AT, Anupindi SA, Gee MS, et al. Normal liver stiffness measured with MR elastography in children. Radiology 2020;297(3):663–9.

33. Xanthakos SA, Podberesky DJ, Serai SD, et al. Use of magnetic resonance elastography to assess hepatic fibrosis in children with chronic liver disease. J Pediatr 2014;164(1):186–8.

34. Reeder SB, Cruite I, Hamilton G, et al. Quantitative assessment of liver fat with magnetic resonance imaging and spectroscopy. J Magn Reson Imaging 2011; 34(4):729–49.

35. Ma J. Dixon techniques for water and fat imaging. J Magn Reson Imaging 2008; 28(3):543–58.

36. Lavine JE, Schwimmer JB, Van Natta ML, et al. Effect of vitamin E or metformin for treatment of nonalcoholic fatty liver disease in children and adolescents: the TONIC randomized controlled trial. JAMA 2011;305(16):1659–68.

37. Bjelakovic G, Nikolova D, Gluud LL, et al. Antioxidant supplements for prevention of mortality in healthy participants and patients with various diseases. Cochrane Database Syst Rev 2012;(3):CD007176.

38. Pediatric NAFLD. Available at: ClinicalTrials.gov. Accessed May 13, 2021.

39. Lin CH, Kohli R. Bile acid metabolism and signaling: potential therapeutic target for nonalcoholic fatty liver disease. Clin Transl Gastroenterol 2018;9(6):164.

40. Mudaliar S, Henry RR, Sanyal AJ, et al. Efficacy and safety of the farnesoid X receptor agonist obeticholic acid in patients with type 2 diabetes and nonalcoholic fatty liver disease. Gastroenterology 2013;145(3):574–82.e1.

41. Neuschwander-Tetri BA, Loomba R, Sanyal AJ, et al. Farnesoid X nuclear receptor ligand obeticholic acid for non-cirrhotic, non-alcoholic steatohepatitis (FLINT): a multicentre, randomised, placebo-controlled trial. Lancet 2015;385(9972): 956–65.

42. Younossi ZM, Ratziu V, Loomba R, et al. Obeticholic acid for the treatment of nonalcoholic steatohepatitis: interim analysis from a multicentre, randomised, placebo-controlled phase 3 trial. Lancet 2019;394(10215):2184–96.

43. Sanyal AJ, Campbell-Sargent C, Mirshahi F, et al. Nonalcoholic steatohepatitis: association of insulin resistance and mitochondrial abnormalities. Gastroenterology 2001;120(5):1183–92.

44. Dohil R, Schmeltzer S, Cabrera BL, et al. Enteric-coated cysteamine for the treatment of paediatric non-alcoholic fatty liver disease. Aliment Pharmacol Ther 2011; 33(9):1036–44.

45. Schwimmer JB, Lavine JE, Wilson LA, et al. In children with nonalcoholic fatty liver disease, cysteamine bitartrate delayed release improves liver enzymes but does not reduce disease activity scores. Gastroenterology 2016;151(6):1141–54.e9.

46. Xi D, Bhattacharjee J, Salazar-Gonzalez RM, et al. Rebaudioside affords hepatoprotection ameliorating sugar sweetened beverage- induced nonalcoholic steatohepatitis. Sci Rep 2020;10(1):6689.

47. Mitsinikos FT, Chac D, Schillingford N, et al. Modifying macronutrients is superior to microbiome transplantation in treating nonalcoholic fatty liver disease. Gut Microbes 2020;12(1):1–16.

48. Mitsinikos FT, Chac D, Shillingford N, et al. Microbiome and histologic changes in non-alcoholic fatty liver disease following shifts in macronutrient distribution. Abstract, Digestive disease week (DDW). Gastroenterology 2017;152(5):S1118–9.

49. Scorletti E, Afolabi PR, Miles EA, et al. Synbiotic alters fecal microbiomes, but not liver fat or fibrosis, in a randomized trial of patients with non-alcoholic fatty liver disease. Gastroenterology 2020. https://doi.org/10.1053/j.gastro.2020.01.031.

Hepatitis C: Current State of Treatment in Children

Sanu R. Yadav, MD[a], Deborah A. Goldman, MD[a], Karen F. Murray, MD[b],*

KEYWORDS

- Hepatitis C • HCV • Direct-acting antivirals • Screening • Diagnosis • Treatment

KEY POINTS

- Pediatric hepatitis C infections are rising due to increasing infections in adolescents and women of reproductive age, driven largely by the opioid epidemic.
- All children at high risk should be tested with anti–hepatitis C virus (HCV) antibody at least once. All children born to positive mothers should be tested for anti-HCV antibody at 18 months of age or RNA detection by polymerase chain reaction in the first year of life.
- Oral direct-acting antivirals (DAAs) interfere with viral replication and have high cure rates. They have good tolerance and safety profile in children.
- All children older than 3 years chronically infected with HCV should be considered for treatment with DAAs irrespective of genotype and disease severity.
- A strong public health and awareness strategy is needed for early identification of chronic infections in children and easy access to affordable DAAs.

INTRODUCTION

Within 30 years of discovery of the virus, a cure for hepatitis C is now possible. The story behind this herculean scientific feat dates back to the 1970s when scientists were perplexed by a presumed viral agent causing post blood transfusion hepatitis, that was neither hepatitis A nor hepatitis B. Termed at the time non-A non-B hepatitis, it was not until 1979 when in *Science* was published the description of a clone of the genome of a non-A non-B hepatitis virus,[1] a single-stranded RNA virus of the Flaviviridae family; the name hepatitis C (HCV) was applied. The discovery of HCV enabled scientists to characterize the exact details of this viral particles' genome, develop HCV screening tests, including antibody tests, and later apply polymerase chain reaction (PCR) to identify and quantitate presence of the viral genome. Eventually this foundational discovery resulted in decreased incidence of transfusion-associated HCV through donor-blood screening, identification of populations at increased risk for

a Department of Pediatric Gastroenterology, Hepatology, and Nutrition, Cleveland Clinic Children's Hospital, 8950 Euclid Avenue, R3, Cleveland, OH 44195, USA; b Cleveland Clinic Children's Hospital, 8950 Euclid Avenue, R3, Cleveland, OH 44195, USA
* Corresponding author.
E-mail address: murrayk5@ccf.org

Pediatr Clin N Am 68 (2021) 1321–1331
https://doi.org/10.1016/j.pcl.2021.07.008
0031-3955/21/© 2021 Elsevier Inc. All rights reserved.

pediatric.theclinics.com

HCV infection, and spawned the development of antiviral treatments, culminating in the direct-acting antiviral agents (DAA), that can now cure most chronic hepatitis C infections. Characterization of the hepatitis C viral genome was so noteworthy that the 2020 Nobel Prize in Medicine and Physiology was awarded to the researchers, Houghton, Rice, and Alter, who were instrumental in the story behind HCV discovery.[2] The focus of the next decade for HCV is ensuring that DAAs are available to the millions of people worldwide infected with the virus, with the World Health Organization (WHO) setting a goal of eliminating HCV by 2030.[3]

In this review, the epidemiology of pediatric HCV infection, its natural history, and the treatments approved by the Food and Drug Administration (FDA) available for children, adolescents, and adults with chronic HCV infection are reviewed. Understanding which patients are at risk for infection allows for the implementation of preventive education to halt viral spread, and effective screening strategies for early identification of people who need access to the best available treatments, before sequela of chronic liver disease can occur.

VIROLOGY

Hepatitis C is a single-stranded positive RNA virus within the Flaviviridae family. Genetic variation evolving via mutation in geographically distinct regions has resulted in 6 distinct genotypes, along with several subtypes. The genotypes vary worldwide, with genotype 1 being the most common ($\sim$70%) in North America and in Europe, and genotypes 2 and 3 contributing the next most common variants at $\sim$20%. Genotypes 4, 5, and 6 predominate in the Middle East, Asia, and Africa, respectively. The viral genome is composed of 5' and 3' nontranslated regions, along with genes encoding a large polyprotein of 3011 amino acids that consists of the structural and nonstructural proteins (**Fig. 1**). E1 and E2 structural proteins allow for viral entry into host cells, and the nonstructural proteins are involved with viral replication, and are the target sites for the DAA agents. The primitive viral RNA polymerase, which replicates the viral genome, is "error" prone, resulting in at least 100 genetic variations daily, offering survival advantage to the virus but also thwarting efforts to develop a vaccine against HCV thus far.[4]

EPIDEMIOLOGY AND TRANSMISSION OF HEPATITIS C VIRUS

The virus is transmitted via parenteral spread. Before the introduction of screening measures in 1992, HCV was the major blood-borne viral pathogen. With mandated screening of blood products, the risk of transfusion-related infection significantly declined, now being less than 1 in a million units transfused in countries that adhere to the most rigorous screening recommendations.[5] Parenteral exposure underlies transmission, with intravenous (IVDU) and intranasal drug use, and high-risk sexual practices, being the most common mechanisms in adults. With the recent opioid epidemic in the United States, there have been increasing cases of HCV in both adult and adolescent populations, with the incidence tripling from 2011 to 2016, and a four-fold increase in young adults aged 20 to 30 years.[6]

In 2015, WHO estimated that there were 71 million people with chronic HCV worldwide.[7] Of these, the calculated incidence in children was reported to be approximately 5 million, with the prevalence in developing countries higher than in the United States and Europe. Despite slow progression of the disease, the possibility of eventual development of cirrhosis and hepatocellular carcinoma exist in both children and adults. The infection has had a global impact on both morbidity and mortality, with almost 400,000 deaths from complications related to chronic liver disease or cancer

Hepatitis C Targeted Therapies

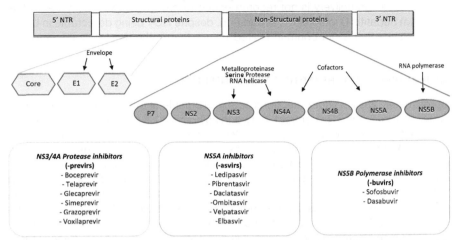

Fig. 1. Hepatitis C viral genome with targets of various DAAs. The viral genome is a positive single-stranded RNA encoding a single polyprotein (consisting of 3011 amino acids) that undergoes proteolysis to generate 3 structural proteins (Core, E1, and E2) and 7 nonstructural proteins (p7, NS2, NS3, NS4A, NS4B, NS5A, and NS5B). The DAAs are grouped according to their target of action: the NS3/4A protease inhibitors ("-previrs") interfere with HCV RNA unwinding and polyprotein cleavage; NS5A inhibitors ("-asvirs") prevent multiple functions of proteins involved in virion assembly; and the NS5B polymerase inhibitors ("-buvirs") target RNA-dependent RNA polymerase.

associated with HCV. This, coupled with an increased public health awareness of the infection, prompted the WHO goal to eliminate HCV by 2030. Specifically, the goal is to achieve a 90% reduction in chronic HCV and a 65% reduction in the mortality associated with the virus.[3] Feasibility of this scheme is largely driven by major advances in the development of the DAA agents, which have truly revolutionized treatment of HCV with simple and highly effective regimens.

It is estimated that there are at least 2.7 million individuals with active HCV infection in the United States, of whom at least 50% are unaware that they harbor the virus. In addition, approximately 135,000 children and adolescents in the United States reportedly have active HCV infection.[8] Further, populations at highest risk often have not been screened, and when identified as having chronic HCV, may currently have limited access to DAA regimens.

In children, vertical or perinatal transmission is responsible for most pediatric HCV infections (~60%).[9] Other modes of transmission mirror those in adults, with IVDU and high-risk sexual practices spreading infection, and rarely intrafamilial spread through blood exposure with shared household items such as razors or toothbrushes. One percent to 2.5% of pregnant women in the United States are estimated to be positive for HCV, with numbers steadily increasing over the past decade in the setting of increasing opioid use. Perinatal mother-to-child (vertical) transmission occurs in approximately 2% to 7% of pregnancies in women who are HCV infected. Transmission rates are higher in women who are coinfected with human immunodeficiency virus (HIV) and in those who have high levels of circulating HCV. Other associations with higher rates of vertical transmission are seen with neonates who have had internal scalp monitoring devices, with prolonged rupture of membranes (>6 hours), and with prolonged neonatal exposure to maternal blood such as can occur with a large episiotomy. The route of delivery does not seem to influence vertical transmission rates, so cesarean delivery is not recommended to prevent transmission if a mother has known hepatitis C infection.[10] In addition, despite HCV being detectable in breast milk, breastfeeding is not contraindicated unless the mother is also coinfected with HIV.

NATURAL HISTORY OF HEPATITIS C VIRUS INFECTION

Approximately 75% of acute infections acquired outside of the perinatal period lead to chronic viral infection.[11] In contrast, between 25% and 40% of infants infected perinatally clear the virus spontaneously by age 2 years; another 10% of young children may clear the infection in early childhood.[12] The exact mechanism of spontaneous clearance is not known, but may relate to viral genotype, host, and immune factors. Infection with genotype 3 HCV, presence of single nucleotide polymorphisms in IFN3/IL28b, and variations in the immunogenetic profile (such as HLA, Killer-cell immunoglobulinlike receptor and its ligand-binding domains) of the mother and child, have been linked to the development of chronicity versus spontaneous clearance in children.[13,14] Once cleared of the infection, it is considered a "cure," as recurrences rarely occur without repeat exposure.

The natural history of the virus is a slow and indolent infection, typically with minimal to no symptoms. Symptomatic acute HCV infection is rare, but when present it is characterized by nonspecific viral symptoms such as fever, myalgia, and fatigue. Even more rarely does an acute infection with HCV lead to acute liver failure. In those who fail to clear the virus, fluctuating levels of serum aminotransferase levels are typical, and over several decades it can result in gradual progression of liver disease with a risk of cirrhosis as high as ~20% after 20 years of disease. Risk factors and comorbidities that are associated with increased severity of disease include older age at onset, longer duration of disease, obesity, homelessness or incarceration, history of childhood cancer, anemias requiring chronic transfusions, concomitant alcohol use, IVDU, and coinfections with HIV or hepatitis B virus (HBV).[12] Because most HCV infections are asymptomatic, it is critical to have a high index of suspicion for screening to identify those individuals who are infected and at higher risk of severe disease, and provide timely effective treatment. In addition, although not contributing to severe advancement of chronic HCV, coinfection with hepatitis A (HAV) can result in more significant acute HAV impact, underscoring the importance of vaccination for HAV in those chronically infected with HCV.

SCREENING AND DIAGNOSIS OF HEPATITIS C VIRUS INFECTION

Because of rising prevalence, and silent transmission of infection, the prevention of HCV infection heavily depends on identification of people living with chronic HCV through easy, reliable, and universal screening strategies. Screening for hepatitis C infection should occur in patients with risk factors as noted in **Box 1**. These include patients with unexplained chronic elevations of liver enzymes, a history of IVDU, high-risk sexual behaviors, incarcerated teenagers, and children born to HCV-positive mothers. Screening is done via the anti-HCV antibody test and, if positive, infection is confirmed by a positive HCV RNA test by PCR amplification. Further, the US Preventive Services Task Force expanded these guidelines in March 2020 to recommend a one-time universal screening of all asymptomatic (including pregnant) adults aged 18 to 79 years.[8] Children suspected of HCV exposure or those in any high-risk category (**Box 1**) also should be screened. The American Academy of Pediatrics further recommends screening children born to HCV-positive mothers with anti-

---

Box 1
Considerations for hepatitis C virus (HCV) screening in children

Children born to HCV-positive mothers
- American Academy of Pediatrics recommendation: anti-HCV antibody screening at 18 months of age, confirmation of positive children with polymerase chain reaction (PCR) testing after 3 years of age.
- American Association for the Study of Liver Disease guidance: consider HCV RNA detection by PCR during first year of life (optimal time unknown, earliest at 2 months of age).
- Siblings of children with vertically acquired HCV infection, born through same mother, also should be tested.

Young children and adolescents with high risk for HCV infection (at least 1-time screening with anti-HCV antibody testing, periodic screening if continued risk)
- Injection/intranasal drug use
- High-risk sexual practices: multiple partners, unprotected sex, men having sex with men
- Children with human immunodeficiency virus or hepatitis B virus infection
- Children requiring hemodialysis
- Children in correctional facilities or homeless environment
- International adoptees
- Unexplained chronic liver disease or enzyme elevations
- Children who received tattoos and piercings from unregulated places

Adults and pregnant women:
- US Preventive Services Task Force recommendation: universal 1-time anti-HCV antibody testing for all adults (including pregnant women).
- Strong consideration for testing all pregnant women for HCV infection.

HCV antibody at or after 18 months of age, to allow for passively transferred maternal antibodies to wane. Any child with a positive antibody against HCV should have infection confirmed by HCV RNA testing by 3 years of age.[15] To prevent the need to wait 18 months after a child's birth to screen for HCV, an American Association for the Study of Liver Disease-Infectious Disease Society of America (AASLD-IDSA) panel recommends consideration of HCV RNA detection by PCR during the first year of life, which can be done as early as 2 months.[16] The optimal strategy for maximizing timely detection of HCV in children who will develop chronic HCV infection after exposure, to allow for optimally early treatment, remains unknown.

Children and adolescents confirmed to have HCV infection (with quantitative HCV RNA by PCR) should be further evaluated with serum aminotransferases, γ-glutamyl transferase, fractionated bilirubin, albumin, prothrombin time/international normalized ratio, α-fetoprotein, a complete blood count, and a liver and spleen ultrasound. Children younger than 3 years, or those older who are not treated, should be followed annually with these laboratory tests.[17] Repeat quantitative HCV RNA should be performed in anticipation of anti-HCV treatment. Pediatric hepatology consultation should be sought for any child with a positive HCV RNA.

TREATMENT

The treatment of hepatitis C has seen a paradigm shift over the past 3 decades with the advent of DAAs. Before DAAs, the best available treatment was a combination of pegylated-interferon with ribavirin, requiring 24 to 48 weeks of therapy, subcutaneous administration, intense monitoring because of numerous potential side effects, and with suboptimal sustained virological response rates. As our understanding of the

HCV viral genome and the replication cycle of the virus improved, identification of potential targets for direct viral interference resulted in a class of antiviral agents, the DAAs. DAA drugs are now considered standard of care for chronic HCV treatment, and have replaced the interferon-based regimens, with improved ease of administration, tolerance, and viral clearance.

The DAAs are grouped according to their target of action: the NS3/4A protease inhibitors ("-previrs") that interfere with HCV polyprotein cleavage; NS5A inhibitors ("-asvirs") that prevent formation of membranous web and virion assembly; and the NS5B polymerase inhibitors ("-buvirs") that inhibit the RNA-dependent RNA polymerase, key to viral replication. Hepatitis C RNA clearance rates in adults, later shown to also represent cure rates in most subjects, saw dramatic rise with the approval of boceprevir and telaprevir in 2011. A decade later, there are now multiple DAA agents available for treatment of chronic HCV in adults (**Table 1**).

The safety and efficacy of DAAs in children was established in 2016 via a phase 2 multicenter open-label trial of 100 adolescents (12–18 years) with genotype 1 HCV infection, treated with ledipasvir-sofosbuvir for 12 weeks.[18] Findings demonstrated a sustained viral suppression response at 12 weeks posttreatment (SVR12) in 98% of the participants, with no virological failure or serious adverse events reported. The relative short duration of treatment, with a quantifiably high HCV RNA clearance rate, acceptable safety profile, and ease of oral administration, have resulted in the FDA approval of 4 different DAA combination regimens in children and adolescents to date (**Table 2**). There are now FDA-approved options available to treat children as young as 3 years of age covering all genotypes of HCV. Pan-genotypic DAA combinations (effective for treatment of any HCV genotype), well established in adults, are also now available to treat children as young as 3 years.[19] This exponential growth in therapeutics for chronic HCV infection has brought the eradication of HCV virus within the realm of achievable goals. The challenge globally has now shifted from finding effective therapy to identifying cases efficiently and linking them to the treatments with affordability and accessibility.

Current guidelines, established by the AASLD-IDSA, recommend treatment of chronic HCV infection with DAA combination regimens for all children aged 3 years and older, regardless of disease severity.[16] This recommendation is based on the longevity of children who have a lifetime risk for development of complications of chronic HCV, such as cirrhosis and hepatocellular carcinoma, along with the potential for viral transmission to others. Multiple studies have proven that HCV treatment in children is cost-effective.[20] One study compared the cost-utility of early treatment at 6 years of age versus deferral of treatment until 18 years, and found that treating 10,000 children early would prevent 330 cases of cirrhosis, 18 cases of hepatocellular carcinoma, and 48 liver-related deaths over a period of 20 years.[21] Hence, treatment should be initiated in all children with chronic HCV aged 3 years or older.

Viral genotyping is currently recommended in children to aid selection of the most effective DAA regimen because the ones available for children are still HCV genotype-specific; the need for viral genotyping is expected to soon be obsolete, however, as highly effective pan-genotypic regimens become increasingly available for children. Similarly, the need to perform a liver biopsy for histologic evaluation, which was once considered part of the pretreatment strategy, is no longer required to initiate treatment in children.[22]

Treatment should be deferred in children younger than 3 years because of high rates of spontaneous viral clearance in very young children, and lack of approved treatments. However, there are case reports of successful use of DAAs in early infancy, including sofosbuvir-ledipasvir use in a 5-month-old infant with genotype 4a infection

Table 1
Direct-acting antivirals (DAAs) approved by the Food and Drug Administration (FDA) for use in adults

Drug	FDA Approval	Comments
Boceprevir (Victrelis) Telaprevir (Incivek)	2011	*Discontinued due to availability of newer DAAs with better safety profile*
Simeprevir (Olysio)	2013	*Discontinued in the United States*
Sofosbuvir (Sovaldi)	2013	Used in combination regimen with ledipasvir or velpatasvir, covers all genotypes when used in combination regimens
Sofosbuvir/Ledipasvir (Harvoni)	2014	Currently in use for genotype 1
Ombitasvir/Paritaprevir/Ritonavir with Dasabuvir (Viekira Pak) or without Dasabuvir (Technivie)	2014, 2015	*Discontinued in the United States*
Daclatasvir (Daklinza)	2016	Used in combination with sofosbuvir, ribavirin for genotypes 1 and 3
Grazoprevir/Elbasvir (Zepatier)	2016	Genotype 1 and 4
Sofosbuvir/Velpatasvir (Epclusa)	2016	Pan-genotypic regimen
Sofosbuvir/Velpatasvir/Voxilaprevir (Vosevi)	2017	Pan-genotypic, useful in treatment failures with other DAA regimens
Glecaprevir/Pibrentasvir (Mavyret)	2017	Pan-genotypic regimen

before gene therapy for adenosine deaminase–deficient severe combined immunodeficiency[23]; and daclatasvir-sofosbuvir-ribavirin therapy in an 8-month-old infant with genotype 3 infection before liver transplantation for carbamoyl phosphate synthetase I deficiency.[24]

In children aged 3 to 17 years, there are currently 4 different DAA combinations approved by the FDA (see **Table 2**). Sofosbuvir-ledipasvir combination with weight-based dosing for 12 weeks, is available for treatment of genotype 1, 4, 5, and 6 HCV infections in children ≥3 years of age,[25] whereas sofosbuvir-ribavirin combination regimen is available for children ≥3 years of age with genotype 2 and 3 HCV infection (treatment durations of 12 and 24 weeks, respectively).[26] The pan-genotypic DAA combination of glecaprevir-pibrentasvir for 8 weeks' duration in adolescents older than 12 years was approved in April 2019,[27] and sofosbuvir-velpatasvir for 12 weeks' duration in children older than 6 years was approved in March 2020 and more recently for age 3 years and above in June 2021.[28] Ongoing trials are evaluating the safety and efficacy of DAAs in expanded age groups, genotypes, with prior treatment failure, and with chronic coinfections (see **Table 2**).

All DAA therapies that are currently approved for use in children have demonstrated remarkable efficacy and safety profile. Pediatric trials for the DAA combination regimens have all had sustained virological response at 12 weeks of more than 95%, with only minor adverse effects noted commonly, including headache (18%–29%), nausea (~27%), vomiting (24%–36%), fatigue (13%–18%), diarrhea (14%–39%), drug-related fever (17%–21%), and upper respiratory infection–like symptoms (13%–19%).[22] There were no serious adverse events noted in any of the pediatric DAA combination trials. However, cases of reactivation of HBV in patients with HCV/HBV coinfection, occasionally in fulminant forms, have been associated with HCV clearance when targeted DAA therapies are initiated.[29,30] It is recommended to

Table 2
Current Direct-acting antivirals available for treatment or ongoing trials in children

Drug Regimen	Genotypes	Approval Status	Dosing
Ledipasvir + sofosbuvir Duration of treatment: 12 wk	1, 4, 5, 6	FDA approved for ages 3–11 (Sept 2019), ages 12–17 (April 2017)	Fixed dose combo (ledipasvir/sofosbuvir) <17 kg: 33.75 mg/150 mg 17 to <35 kg: 45 mg/200 mg ≥35 kg: 90 mg/400 mg
Sofosbuvir + ribavirin Duration of treatment: 12 wk	2, 3	FDA approved for ages 3–17 (Aug 2019)	Sofosbuvir <17 kg: 150 mg 17 to <35 kg: 200 mg ≥35 kg: 400 mg Ribavirin <47 kg: 15 mg/kg 47–49 kg: 600 mg 50–65 kg: 800 mg 66–80 kg:1000 mg >80 kg: 1200 mg
Glecaprevir + pibrentasvir Duration of treatment: 8 wk	Pangeno-typic	FDA approved for ages 12–17 (April 2019), Ongoing trials for age 3–11 (estimated completion Nov 2022)	Fixed dose combo (glecaprevir/pibrentasvir) >12 y: 300 mg/120 mg
Sofosbuvir + velpatasvir Duration of treatment: 12 wk	Pangeno-typic	FDA approved for ages 6–17 (March 2020), approved for ages 3–6 years (June 2021)	Sofosbuvir/Velpatasvir <17 kg: 150 mg/37.5 mg 17 to <30 kg: 200 mg/50 mg >30 kg: 400 mg/100 mg
Elbasvir + grazoprevir	1, 4	Ongoing trials for age 3–17	To be determined
Daclatasvir + sofosbuvir	Pangeno-typic	Ongoing trials for age 3–17	To be determined
Sofosbuvir + velpatasvir + voxilaprevir	Pangeno-typic	Ongoing trials for age 3–17 Received European Medicines Agency waiver for use in children age <12 y in Europe	To be determined

screen all patients for HBV infection before initiating HCV-targeted DAA regimens, and either concurrent treatment for active HBV infection or close monitoring at regular intervals for HBV reactivation (depending on HBV viral DNA levels) should be pursued in these patients. Timely HBV vaccination is recommended for all susceptible individuals.

CHALLENGES AND FUTURE DIRECTIONS

Although there is a paucity of data on prevalence and treatment of HCV infection in children, the evidence base is steadily growing and newer, safer, and broader DAA coverage for pediatric HCV infections are being developed. This advancement in drug development, however, has not translated into improved access and utilization in this unique population. Children often have minor symptoms and usually do not develop severe disease or complications, whereas DAA therapies have often been restricted to advanced disease by many insurance providers. It needs to be emphasized that providing timely treatment to children who do not clear the virus spontaneously will be crucial in reducing the long-term burden of chronic disease as well as in the eventual global elimination of HCV. Universal screening at the population level is still lacking, and especially so in children with perinatal exposure and in high-risk adolescents. Identification of children who are chronically infected, and linking them to an accessible care system that facilitates treatment adherence, will require a strong public health strategy.

CLINICS CARE POINTS

- All children at high risk should be tested with anti-HCV antibody. Positive antibody tests should be confirmed with HCV RNA detection by PCR.
- Infants born to an HCV-positive mother should be tested with anti-HCV antibody at or after 18 months. Early HCV RNA detection by PCR can be considered as early as 2 months of age.
- All children ≥3 years of age with HCV infection should receive treatment with DAAs regardless of the genotype or disease severity. Early treatment is cost-effective and reduces lifetime risk of complications.
- Children with chronic HCV should be vaccinated for HBV and HAV infections. Screening for chronic HBV infection should be routinely done before initiating targeted DAA therapy.
- Pediatric hepatology consultation should be sought for any child with positive HCV RNA.

DISCLOSURE

S.R. Yadav: nothing to disclose. D.A. Goldman: nothing to disclose. K.F. Murray: consultant to Gilead and Albireo.

REFERENCES

1. Choo QL, Kuo G, Weiner AJ, et al. Isolation of a cDNA clone derived from a blood-borne non-A, non-B viral hepatitis genome. Science 1989;244(4902): 359–62.
2. Burki T. Nobel Prize for hepatitis C virus discoverers. Lancet 2020;396(10257): 1058.
3. WHO | Global health sector strategy on viral hepatitis 2016-2021. Available at: https://www.who.int/hepatitis/strategy2016-2021/ghss-hep/en/. Accessed April 2, 2021.

4. Rabaan AA, Al-Ahmed SH, Bazzi AM, et al. Overview of hepatitis C infection, molecular biology, and new treatment. J Infect Public Health 2020;13(5):773–83.

5. Fong IW, Fong IW. Blood Transfusion-Associated Infections in the Twenty-First Century: New Challenges. Current Trends and Concerns in Infectious Diseases 2020;191-215. Available at: https://www.ncbi.nlm.nih.gov/pmc/articles/PMC7120358/.

6. 2016 surveillance data for viral hepatitis in U.S. | CDC. Available at: https://www.cdc.gov/hepatitis/statistics/2016surveillance/commentary.htm. Accessed April 4, 2021.

7. WHO | Global hepatitis report. 2017. Available at: https://www.who.int/hepatitis/publications/global-hepatitis-report2017/en/. Accessed April 4, 2021.

8. Chou R, Dana T, Fu R, et al. Screening for hepatitis C virus infection in adolescents and adults: updated evidence report and systematic review for the US Preventive Services Task Force. JAMA 2020;323(10):976–91.

9. Ragusa R, Simone Corsaro L, Frazzetto E, et al. Hepatitis C virus infection in children and pregnant women: an updated review of the literature on screening and treatments. Am J Perinatol Rep 2020;10:121–7.

10. Hughes BL, Page CM, Kuller JA. Hepatitis C in pregnancy: screening, treatment, and management. Am J Obstet Gynecol 2017;217(5):B2–12.

11. Thomas DL, Astemborski J, Rai RM, et al. The natural history of Hepatitis C virus infection: host, viral, and environmental factors. J Am Med Assoc 2000;284(4):450–6.

12. Mack CL, Gonzalez-Peralta RP, Gupta N, et al. NASPGHAN Practice guidelines: diagnosis and management of hepatitis c infection in infants, children, and adolescents. J Pediatr Gastroenterol Nutr 2012;54(6):838–55.

13. Indolfi G, Azzari C, Resti M. Polymorphisms in the IFNL3/IL28B gene and hepatitis C: from adults to children. World J Gastroenterol 2014;20(28):9245–52.

14. Ruiz-Extremera A, Pavó N-Castillero EJ, Florido M, et al. Influence of HLA class I, HLA class II and KIRs on vertical transmission and chronicity of hepatitis C virus in children. PLoS One 2017. https://doi.org/10.1371/journal.pone.0172527.

15. Hepatitis C | Red Book® 2018 | Red Book Online | AAP Point-of-Care-Solutions. Available at: https://redbook.solutions.aap.org/chapter.aspx?sectionid=189640105&bookid=2205#192299167. Accessed April 5, 2021.

16. HCV in children | HCV guidance. Available at: https://www.hcvguidelines.org/unique-populations/children. Accessed April 5, 2021.

17. Squires JE, Balistreri WF. Treatment of Hepatitis C: a new paradigm toward viral eradication. J Pediatr 2020. https://doi.org/10.1016/j.jpeds.2020.02.082.

18. Balistreri WF, Murray KF, Rosenthal P, et al. The safety and effectiveness of ledipasvir–sofosbuvir in adolescents 12-17 years old with hepatitis C virus genotype 1 infection. Hepatology 2017;66(2):371–8.

19. Available at: https://www.gilead.com/news-and-press/press-room/press-releases/2021/6/us-food-and-drug-administration-approves-new-formulation-of-epclusa-expanding-pediatric-indication-to-treat-children-ages-3-and-older-with-chronic.

20. Nguyen J, Barritt AS, Jhaveri R. Cost effectiveness of early treatment with direct-acting antiviral therapy in adolescent patients with hepatitis C virus infection. J Pediatr 2019;207:90–6.

21. Greenaway E, Haines A, Ling SC, et al. Treatment of chronic hepatitis C in young children reduces adverse outcomes and is cost-effective compared with deferring treatment to adulthood. J Pediatr 2020. https://doi.org/10.1016/j.jpeds.2020.08.088.

22. Leung DH, Squires JE, Jhaveri R, et al. Hepatitis C in 2020: A North American Society for Pediatric Gastroenterology, Hepatology, and Nutrition Position Paper. J Pediatr Gastroenterol Nutr 2020;71(3):407–17.

23. Tucci F, Calbi V, Barzaghi F, et al. Successful treatment with ledipasvir/sofosbuvir in an infant with severe combined immunodeficiency caused by adenosine deaminase deficiency with HCV allowed gene therapy with Strimvelis. Hepatology 2018;68(6):2434–7.

24. Huang AC, Beadles A, Romero D, et al. Sustained virologic remission in an 8-month-old pediatric patient with carbamoyl phosphate synthetase i deficiency and hepatitis c infection using direct-acting antivirals prior to liver transplant. J Pediatr Gastroenterol Nutr 2021;72(3):e79–80.

25. Schwarz KB, Rosenthal P, Murray KF, et al. Ledipasvir-sofosbuvir for 12 weeks in children 3 to <6 years old with chronic hepatitis C. Hepatology 2020;71(2): 422–30.

26. Rosenthal P, Schwarz KB, Gonzalez-Peralta RP, et al. Sofosbuvir and ribavirin therapy for children aged 3 to <12 years with hepatitis c virus genotype 2 or 3 infection. Hepatology 2020;71(1):31–43.

27. Jonas MM, Squires RH, Rhee SM, et al. Pharmacokinetics, safety, and efficacy of glecaprevir/pibrentasvir in adolescents with chronic hepatitis C virus: part 1 of the DORA study. Hepatology 2020;71(2):456–62.

28. A Phase 2, Open-Label, Multicenter, Multi-cohort Study to Investigate the Safety and Efficacy of Sofosbuvir/Velpatasvir in Adolescents and Children With Chronic HCV Infection. ClinicalTrials.gov Identifier: NCT03022981. Updated October 8, 2020. Available at: https://clinicaltrials.gov/ct2/show/study/NCT03022981 Accessed August 19, 2021.

29. Chen G, Wang C, Chen J. Hepatitis B reactivation in hepatitis B and C coinfected patients treated with antiviral agents: a systematic review and meta-analysis. Hepatology 2017;66(1):13–26.

30. Mücke MM, Backus LI, Mücke VT. Hepatitis B virus reactivation during direct-acting antiviral therapy for hepatitis C: a systematic review and meta-analysis. Lancet Gastroenterol Hepatol 2018;3(3):172–80.

Biliary Atresia/Neonatal Cholestasis

What is in the Horizon?

Sara E. Yerina, BSN, RN[a], Udeme D. Ekong, MD, MPH[a,b],*

KEYWORDS

- Cystic BA • Kasai portoenterostomy • Adjuvant therapy • BA outcome
- Native liver survival

KEY POINTS

- Biliary atresia (BA) is a global disease seen across all ethnic groups with important distinctions.
- Scientific advances in adjuvant therapies are on the horizon.
- There are important considerations for young people surviving with their native liver and BA.

INTRODUCTION

Biliary atresia (BA) is a progressive fibroinflammatory, obliterative disorder of the extrahepatic and intrahepatic biliary tree, occurring in infants, that leads to cirrhosis and liver failure.[1–4] The reported incidence varies across different countries, ranging from 0.52 to 0.71 per 10,000 live births in Western countries,[5–8] 1.06 per 10,000 live births in Korea,[9] to 1.1 to 1.48 per 10,000 live births in Japan and Taiwan.[10–12] In spite of the low incidence, it remains the commonest cause of neonatal cholestasis,[3] end-stage liver disease in children, and the leading indication of pediatric liver transplantation worldwide.[13,14] BA can be classified into 4 major groups,[1] namely isolated BA accounting for 70% to 80% of all BA cases; syndromic BA accounting for 10% to 20% of BA cases in Western countries and Korea[9] and less than 2%, 6%, and 4.9% of BA cases in Japan, Taiwan, and Mainland China, respectively[15–17]; cystic BA characterized as a cystic change in an otherwise obliterated biliary tract accounting for 5% to 10% of BA cases[18] (**Fig. 1**A–B); and cytomegalovirus (CMV)-associated BA, which is reported in up to 50% of BA cases in China[19] based on a liver biopsy

[a] Medstar Georgetown Transplant Institute, Medstar Georgetown University Hospital, 3800 Reservoir Road, NW, Washington, DC, USA; [b] Department of Pediatrics, Georgetown University School of Medicine, Washington, DC, USA
* Corresponding author. Medstar Georgetown Transplant Institute, Medstar Georgetown University Hospital, 3800 Reservoir Road, NW, Washington, DC.
E-mail address: Udeme.D.Ekong@gunet.georgetown.edu

Pediatr Clin N Am 68 (2021) 1333–1341
https://doi.org/10.1016/j.pcl.2021.08.002
0031-3955/21/© 2021 Elsevier Inc. All rights reserved.

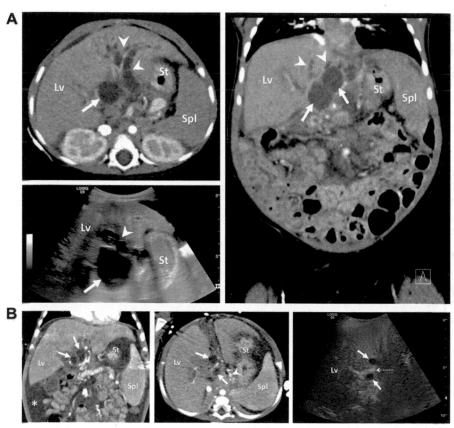

Fig. 1. Radiologic images of cystic form of biliary atresia. (*A*) A 7-month-old infant with cystic biliary atresia. Contrast-enhanced axial CT (*left, top panel*) shows tubular, dilated biliary radicles (*arrowheads*) and round cystic focus (*solid arrow*) in the central liver and porta hepatis, respectively. Transverse grayscale ultrasound (*left, bottom panel*) shows corresponding anechoic cystic and tubular structures along the central liver and porta hepatis. Coronal CT reconstruction (*right panel*) demonstrates mixed cystic and tubular biliary radicle dilatation. (*B*) A 5-month-old infant with advanced liver disease and cystic biliary atresia. Contrast-enhanced coronal CT (*left panel*) demonstrates morphologically cirrhotic liver, splenomegaly, ascites (*asterisk*), and absence of the gallbladder. Two small rounded cystic structures (*solid arrows*) at the porta hepatis were noted. Axial CT (*middle panel*) also demonstrates the small cystic foci (*solid arrows*), absent gallbladder, and mild perigastric varices (*arrowhead*). Transverse B-mode sonography of the right upper quadrant (*right panel*) demonstrates the cystic structures (*solid arrows*) at the porta hepatis, distinct from nearby portal vein (*dashed arrow*). CT, computed tomography; Lv, liver; St, stomach; Spl, spleen. *Courtesy of* Arash R. Zandieh MD, Department of Radiology, Medstar Georgetown University Hospital, Washington, DC.

study and 10% of patients with BA (mostly non-Caucasian) in another series.[2] Congenital anomalies reported in syndromic BA include biliary atresia splenic malformation syndrome (BASM), intestinal atresia, cleft palate, and polycystic kidney, coloboma, anorectal atresia, and congenital heart disease.[20] The Japanese Association of Pediatric Surgeons has an abbreviated classification that uses the most proximal level of extrahepatic biliary obstruction: type 1: level of the common bile duct; type 2: level of the common hepatic duct; type 3: level of the portal hepatis.

ETIOPATHOGENESIS
Developmental/Genetic

Development of the biliary system begins in the fourth week of gestation,[21] and because the key components of BASM develop between the second and eighth week of gestation, BASM is thought to arise due to failure of development of the extrahepatic duct.[22] Recently, biallelic and heterozygous *PKD1L1* variants were identified in children with BASM. *PKD1L1* has dual roles in determination of laterality and ciliary function; moreover, it is expressed by cholangiocytes, suggesting that *PKD1L1* is a biologically plausible candidate gene for the BASM syndrome.[23] Liu and colleagues[24] similarly report on *PDGFA* gene rs9690350 polymorphism, increasing the risk for development of BA in Southern Chinese children. *PDGFA* is a mitogen for hepatic stellate cells and an important fibrogenic factor in chronic liver disease. Vascular remodeling of hepatic artery branches, in addition to hypoxia-ischemia in livers, may be associated with disappearance of interlobular bile ducts, progressing over time to a decreased cholangiocyte mass with resultant development of BA.[25,26]

Infection/Inflammation/Innate Immunity

Several viruses have been posited to be initiators of inflammation,[27,28] and several groups have suggested that an immune-mediated liver injury and inflammation underlie development of BA.[29–34] The presence of antibodies (immunoglobulin M [IgM]) against CMV has been linked to the poorest HPE outcome and highest mortality[27] and an exaggerated proinflammatory response observed in liver biopsies. In contradistinction, a Th2 response is reported in the subgroup of patients with cystic BA and associated with improved drainage following Kasai portoenterostomy.[34] Increasing evidence also suggests involvement of the innate immune system from disease onset.[34]

EVALUATION OF THE CHOLESTATIC INFANT

Suffice to say, early diagnosis of BA is important, as the prognosis has been shown to correlate with the timing of surgery, and the treatment window is narrow. The approach to the evaluation of a cholestatic infant is elegantly illustrated in the 2017 NASPGHAN/ESPGHAN guidelines[35]; however, there are a few important points that will be emphasized here as pertains to screening and early diagnosis of BA.

Harpavat and colleagues[36–38] show that conjugated bilirubin is elevated on the day of birth and effectively discriminates between infants with BA and controls suggesting that these infants already have an obstructed biliary tree at birth. Of 124,385 newborns, screening identified infants with BA with a sensitivity of 100% (95% confidence interval [CI], 56.1%–100%), specificity of 99.9% (05% CI, 99.9%–99.9%), a positive predictive value of 5.9% (95% CI, 2.6%-12.2%), and a negative predictive value of 100% (95% CI, 100%–100%). Importantly, the age at which infants underwent the Kasai portoenterostomy was significantly younger after screening was implemented (mean age, 56 $\pm$ 19 days before screening implementation vs 36 $\pm$ 22 days after screening implementation; [95% CI, 7–32 days]; P = .004).[38] In Asia, the universal stool color chart screening has been adopted in Mainland China, Taiwan, and Japan and has resulted in a significant reduction in delayed diagnosis of BA in Japan[39]; similarly, both age at portoenterostomy and native liver survival improved compared with the era that predated screening in Taiwan (portoenterostomy at <60 days of age: 66% vs 49%; 3-year jaundice-free survival: 57% vs 31.5%),[40] and in Shenzen, the age at diagnosis decreased from 81 $\pm$ 12 days to 56 $\pm$ 15 days, jaundice clearance rate improved from 47.1% to 54.4%, and 2-year native liver survival increased from

44.4% to 52.6%.[41] Lastly, serum matrix metalloproteinase-7 has been reported to potentially improve the accuracy of diagnosis of BA with a sensitivity of 98.67% and specificity of 95%,[42] however, it has not been validated outside China.

Hepatobiliary scintigraphy using 99m Tc-mebrofenin (hepatobiliary iminodiacetic acid [HIDA] scan) is used in some centers to assess patency of the biliary system, with the assumption that the presence of tracer in the bowel constitutes patency and excludes BA; however, there are published reports of infants with biliary patency reported on HIDA scans who were ultimately diagnosed with BA,[43] suggesting that biliary excretion noted on a HIDA scan does not exclude a diagnosis of BA. Infants with BA may have pigmented stools initially but over the first weeks or months of life develop progressive jaundice with acholic stools, which indicates biliary obstruction. Thus, given the progressive nature of BA, it is probably not surprising to find variation in tracer excretion depending on the timing of the scan with respect to complete occlusion of the extrahepatic biliary tree.[43] Liver biopsy, with features of biliary obstruction, has been demonstrated to have a higher diagnostic accuracy for the diagnosis of BA than HIDA scan.[44]

MANAGEMENT: SURGICAL TREATMENT AND ADJUVANT THERAPIES

The primary surgical treatment of BA remains the Kasai portoenterostomy, and excision of the fibrous cord at a precise level at the porta and portoenterostomy introduced by Kasai is regarded as the best method when attempting to salvage the native liver and restore bile flow.[45] Reports out of England and Wales and Finland suggest that centralizing resources improves the outcomes of patients with BA[46,47] (Table 1). Even with clearance of jaundice, most of these children go unto liver transplantation[48,49] raising a clear unmet medical need to improve outcomes and reduce the need for liver transplantation and its attendant complications. Given that inflammation is a key component of the pathogenesis of BA, the antiinflammatory properties of steroids has been harnessed to promote bile drainage following portoenterostomy. Its usefulness as adjunctive therapy following portoenterostomy has been studied quite extensively.[50–52] Clearance of jaundice has been reported to be related to the age at portoenterostomy in infants who receive high-dose steroids with resultant improvement in native liver survival.[53] The subgroup of infants with CMV IgM + BA have been reported to have a very poor response to portoenterostomy,[27] and adjunctive antiviral therapy has been reported to improve clearance of jaundice and native liver survival.[28,54,55]

Other agents under study include N-acetylcysteine, a precursor to glutathione, a known choleretic, as adjunctive therapy following portoenterostomy[56]; this is presently undergoing phase II clinical trials. Intravenous immunoglobulin (IVIG) was studied as adjuvant therapy in BA, in a multicenter, phase I/IIA clinical trial; however, it

Table 1 Reported outcomes following hepatoportoenterostomy				
	Japan[10,11]	Korea[9]	Taiwan[10,12]	England & Wales[46]
HPE drainage rate	1 y: 60%	5 y: 75%	3 mo: 58%	6 mo: 55%
Short-term native liver survival	1 y: 70%	-	2 y: 52%	-
Long-term native liver survival	20 y: 49%	5 y: 63%	5 y: 64%	5 y: 46% 10 y: 40%

Abbreviation: HPE, hepatoportoenterostomy.

failed to demonstrate any trend to lower bilirubin levels or improved 360-day native liver survival.[57] Lastly, a phase II clinical trial of an inhibitor of the apical sodium-dependent bile acid transporter/ileal bile acid transporter (ASBT), as a potential therapeutic agent for the treatment of BA is underway. The rationale being elevated serum bile acid levels are associated with increased morbidity and mortality in several cholestatic liver diseases; specifically, large increases in serum bile acid levels are a well-known feature of BA,[58] thus, high bile acid levels are understood to be an important driver of liver disease in patients with BA after portoenterostomy.[59] A consistent body of literature has demonstrated that bile drainage, as measured by bilirubin levels at 3 and 6 months after portoenterostomy is a prognostic indicator of long-term native liver survival in BA.[49,60] A reduction in serum and hepatic bile acid levels in patients with BA is hypothesized to slow or prevent liver injury, thereby improving long-term native liver survival. By virtue of its ability to inhibit bile acid absorption and lower circulating bile acid levels, iASBTs have the potential to reduce the long-term sequelae of BA.

BILIARY ATRESIA IN YOUNG ADULTS: TRANSITION TO ADULT HEPATOLOGY CARE

Native liver survival greater than 20 years in young adults with BA ranges between 14% and 44%.[61] About 60.5% of long-term survivors alive with their native liver have progressive liver-related complications namely cholangitis in 100%, portal hypertension in 80%, gastrointestinal bleeding in 45%, and hepatocellular carcinoma in 1.3%. About 7.6% received liver transplantation after the age of 20 years.[62] Recurrent episodes of cholangitis in the absence of significant chronic liver disease should prompt investigation into roux loop obstruction from adhesions and/or progressive shortening of the roux loop length over time. A radionuclide scan can assess hepatic excretion and function, whereas a liver ultrasound may demonstrate dilated biliary radicals.[63] Large liver nodules are more likely regenerative nodules than malignant transformation. Hepatopulmonary syndrome and portopulmonary syndrome are complications of cirrhosis; although less frequently reported in children with BA, Karrer and colleagues[64] report 2 cases of each over a 44-year period, in 320 children with BA at their institution, and Ueno and colleagues[65–67] report a frequency of 6.8% and 3.4%, respectively, in their cohort of 88 children with BA followed over a median of 11.6 years. As the phenotype of young adults with BA is different from the usual adult liver diseases, specialist multidisciplinary care is essential in the transition of these patients to adult hepatology care.

SUMMARY

BA remains a challenging disease with less than perfect outcomes. Postoperative serum bilirubin level measured after Kasai portoenterostomy remains the most accurate clinical predictor of native liver survival.[49] With more patients living into adulthood with their native liver, awareness of the long-term complications in this patient population is important for health professionals.

CLINIC CARE POINTS

Diagnosis
- Obtain direct or conjugated bilirubin levels in addition to total bilirubin in newborn infants evaluated for jaundice, as patients with a diagnosis of BA may have elevated direct or conjugated bilirubin levels at 24 to 48 hours after birth.

Interventions of care

- Total bilirubin greater than or equal to 2.0 mg/dL by 3 months after hepatoportoenterostomy identifies most of the children who will die or require liver transplant by 2 years of age. Moreover, it is a predictor of adverse clinical outcomes related to advancing liver disease such as growth failure, ascites, or hypoalbuminemia.

- Infants whose total bilirubin does not become less than 2 mg/dL within 3 months of hepatoportoenterostomy are at high risk for early disease progression, and consideration should be given to referral for liver transplant evaluation.

- Intensive nutritional monitoring and interventions may be warranted, most especially considering growth failure and fat-soluble vitamin deficiencies in infants with poor bile flow following hepatoportoenterostomy.

DISCLOSURE

The author has no financial disclosures.

BIBLIOGRAPHY

1. Davenport M. Biliary atresia: from Australia to the zebrafish. J Pediatr Surg 2016; 51(2):200–5.
2. Lakshminarayanan B, Davenport M. Biliary atresia: a comprehensive review. J Autoimmun 2016;73:1–9.
3. Nizery L, Chardot C, Sissaoui S, et al. Biliary atresia: clinical advances and perspectives. Clin Res Hepatol Gastroenterol 2016;40(3):281–7.
4. Verkade HJ, Bezerra JA, Davenport M, et al. Biliary atresia and other cholestatic childhood diseases: advances and future challenges. J Hepatol 2016;65(3): 631–42.
5. Hopkins PC, Yazigi N, Nylund CM. Incidence of biliary atresia and timing of hepatoportoenterostomy in the United States. J Pediatr 2017;187:253–7.
6. Wildhaber BE, Majno P, Mayr J, et al. Biliary atresia: swiss national study, 1994-2004. J Pediatr Gastroenterol Nutr 2008;46(3):299–307.
7. Schreiber RA, Barker CC, Roberts EA, et al. Biliary atresia: the Canadian experience. J Pediatr 2007;151(6):659–65, 665.e1.
8. Chardot C, Buet C, Serinet MO, et al. Improving outcomes of biliary atresia: French national series 1986-2009. J Hepatol 2013;58(6):1209–17.
9. Lee KJ, Kim JW, Moon JS, et al. Epidemiology of biliary atresia in Korea. J Korean Med Sci 2017;32(4):656–60.
10. Jimenez-Rivera C, Jolin-Dahel KS, Fortinsky KJ, et al. International incidence and outcomes of biliary atresia. J Pediatr Gastroenterol Nutr 2013;56(4):344–54.
11. Nio M, Ohi R, Miyano T, et al. Five- and 10-year survival rates after surgery for biliary atresia: a report from the Japanese Biliary Atresia Registry. J Pediatr Surg 2003;38(7):997–1000.
12. Hsiao CH, Chang MH, Chen HL, et al. Universal screening for biliary atresia using an infant stool color card in Taiwan. Hepatology 2008;47(4):1233–40.
13. Suchy FJ, Burdelski M, Tomar BS, et al. Cholestatic liver disease: working group report of the first world congress of pediatric gastroenterology, hepatology, and nutrition. J Pediatr Gastroenterol Nutr 2002;35(Suppl 2):S89–97.
14. Lampela H, Kosola S, Heikkila P, et al. Native liver histology after successful portoenterostomy in biliary atresia. J Clin Gastroenterol 2014;48(8):721–8.
15. Nio M. Japanese biliary atresia registry. Pediatr Surg Int 2017;33(12):1319–25.

16. Zhan J, Feng J, Chen Y, et al. Incidence of biliary atresia associated congenital malformations: a retrospective multicenter study in China. Asian J Surg 2017; 40(6):429–33.
17. Chiu CY, Chen PH, Chan CF, et al, Taiwan Infant Stool Color Card Study G. Biliary atresia in preterm infants in Taiwan: a nationwide survey. J Pediatr 2013;163(1): 100–103 e1.
18. Caponcelli E, Knisely AS, Davenport M. Cystic biliary atresia: an etiologic and prognostic subgroup. J Pediatr Surg 2008;43(9):1619–24.
19. Xu YY J, Zhang R, Yin Y, et al. The perinatal infection of cytomegalovirus is an important etiology for biliary atresia in China 2012. p. 109–13.
20. Allotey J, Lacaille F, Lees MM, et al. Congenital bile duct anomalies (biliary atresia) and chromosome 22 aneuploidy. J Pediatr Surg 2008;43(9):1736–40.
21. Crawford JM. Development of the intrahepatic biliary tree. Semin Liver Dis 2002; 22(3):213–26.
22. Davenport M, Savage M, Mowat AP, et al. Biliary atresia splenic malformation syndrome: an etiologic and prognostic subgroup. Surgery 1993;113(6):662–8.
23. Berauer JP, Mezina AI, Okou DT, et al. Identification of polycystic kidney disease 1 like 1 gene variants in children with biliary atresia splenic malformation syndrome. Hepatology 2019;70(3):899–910.
24. Liu F, Zeng J, Zhu D, et al. PDGFA gene rs9690350 polymorphism increases biliary atresia risk in Chinese children. Biosci Rep 2020;40(7). BSR20200068.
25. dos Santos JL, da Silveira TR, da Silva VD, et al. Medial thickening of hepatic artery branches in biliary atresia. A morphometric study. J Pediatr Surg 2005;40(4): 637–42.
26. Fratta LX, Hoss GR, Longo L, et al. Hypoxic-ischemic gene expression profile in the isolated variant of biliary atresia. J Hepatobiliary Pancreat Sci 2015;22(12): 846–54.
27. Zani A, Quaglia A, Hadzic N, et al. Cytomegalovirus-associated biliary atresia: an aetiological and prognostic subgroup. J Pediatr Surg 2015;50(10):1739–45.
28. Parolini F, Hadzic N, Davenport M. Adjuvant therapy of cytomegalovirus IgM+ve associated biliary atresia: prima facie evidence of effect. J Pediatr Surg 2019; 54(9):1941–5.
29. Davenport M, Gonde C, Redkar R, et al. Immunohistochemistry of the liver and biliary tree in extrahepatic biliary atresia. J Pediatr Surg 2001;36(7):1017–25.
30. Mack CL, Tucker RM, Sokol RJ, et al. Biliary atresia is associated with CD4+ Th1 cell-mediated portal tract inflammation. Pediatr Res 2004;56(1):79–87.
31. Narayanaswamy B, Gonde C, Tredger JM, et al. Serial circulating markers of inflammation in biliary atresia–evolution of the post-operative inflammatory process. Hepatology 2007;46(1):180–7.
32. Hill R, Quaglia A, Hussain M, et al. Th-17 cells infiltrate the liver in human biliary atresia and are related to surgical outcome. J Pediatr Surg 2015;50(8):1297–303.
33. Lages CS, Simmons J, Maddox A, et al. The dendritic cell-T helper 17-macrophage axis controls cholangiocyte injury and disease progression in murine and human biliary atresia. Hepatology 2017;65(1):174–88.
34. Ortiz-Perez A, Donnelly B, Temple H, et al. Innate immunity and pathogenesis of biliary atresia. Front Immunol 2020;11:329.
35. Fawaz R, Baumann U, Ekong U, et al. Guideline for the evaluation of cholestatic Jaundice in infants: joint recommendations of the North American Society for Pediatric Gastroenterology, Hepatology, and Nutrition and the European Society for Pediatric Gastroenterology, Hepatology, and Nutrition. J Pediatr Gastroenterol Nutr 2017;64(1):154–68.

36. Harpavat S, Finegold MJ, Karpen SJ. Patients with biliary atresia have elevated direct/conjugated bilirubin levels shortly after birth. Pediatrics 2011;128(6): e1428–33.

37. Mysore KR, Shneider BL, Harpavat S. Biliary atresia as a disease starting in utero: implications for treatment, diagnosis, and pathogenesis. J Pediatr Gastroenterol Nutr 2019;69(4):396–403.

38. Harpavat S, Garcia-Prats JA, Anaya C, et al. Diagnostic yield of newborn screening for biliary atresia using direct or conjugated bilirubin measurements. JAMA 2020;323(12):1141–50.

39. Matsui A. Screening for biliary atresia. Pediatr Surg Int 2017;33(12):1305–13.

40. Lien TH, Chang MH, Wu JF, et al. Effects of the infant stool color card screening program on 5-year outcome of biliary atresia in Taiwan. Hepatology 2011;53(1): 202–8.

41. Zheng J, Ye Y, Wang B, et al. Biliary atresia screening in Shenzhen: implementation and achievements. Arch Dis Child 2020;105(8):720–3.

42. Yang L, Zhou Y, Xu PP, et al. Diagnostic accuracy of serum matrix metalloproteinase-7 for biliary atresia. Hepatology 2018;68(6):2069–77.

43. Adeyemi A, States L, Wann L, et al. Biliary excretion noted on hepatobiliary iminodiacetic acid scan does not exclude diagnosis of biliary atresia. J Pediatr 2020;220:245–8.

44. Lee JY, Sullivan K, El Demellawy D, et al. The value of preoperative liver biopsy in the diagnosis of extrahepatic biliary atresia: a systematic review and meta-analysis. J Pediatr Surg 2016;51(5):753–61.

45. Tam PKH, Chung PHY, St Peter SD, et al. Advances in paediatric gastroenterology. Lancet 2017;390(10099):1072–82.

46. Davenport M, Ong E, Sharif K, et al. Biliary atresia in England and Wales: results of centralization and new benchmark. J Pediatr Surg 2011;46(9):1689–94.

47. Lampela H, Ritvanen A, Kosola S, et al. National centralization of biliary atresia care to an assigned multidisciplinary team provides high-quality outcomes. Scand J Gastroenterol 2012;47(1):99–107.

48. Shneider BL, Brown MB, Haber B, et al. A multicenter study of the outcome of biliary atresia in the United States, 1997 to 2000. J Pediatr 2006;148(4):467–74.

49. Shneider BL, Magee JC, Karpen SJ, et al. Total serum bilirubin within 3 months of hepatoportoenterostomy predicts short-term outcomes in biliary atresia. J Pediatr 2016;170:211–7, e1–2.

50. Davenport M, Parsons C, Tizzard S, et al. Steroids in biliary atresia: single surgeon, single centre, prospective study. J Hepatol 2013;59(5):1054–8.

51. Bezerra JA, Spino C, Magee JC, et al. Use of corticosteroids after hepatoportoenterostomy for bile drainage in infants with biliary atresia: the START randomized clinical trial. JAMA 2014;311(17):1750–9.

52. Dong R, Song Z, Chen G, et al. Improved outcome of biliary atresia with postoperative high-dose steroid. Gastroenterol Res Pract 2013;2013:902431.

53. Tyraskis A, Davenport M. Steroids after the Kasai procedure for biliary atresia: the effect of age at Kasai portoenterostomy. Pediatr Surg Int 2016;32(3):193–200.

54. Fischler B, Casswall TH, Malmborg P, et al. Ganciclovir treatment in infants with cytomegalovirus infection and cholestasis. J Pediatr Gastroenterol Nutr 2002; 34(2):154–7.

55. Shah I, Bhatnagar S. Biliary atresia with cytomegalovirus infection and its response to ganciclovir. Trop Gastroenterol 2014;35(1):56–8.

56. Tessier MEM, Shneider BL, Brandt ML, et al. A phase 2 trial of N-Acetylcysteine in Biliary atresia after Kasai portoenterostomy. Contemp Clin Trials Commun 2019; 15:100370.
57. Mack CL, Spino C, Alonso EM, et al. A Phase I/IIa trial of intravenous immuno-globulin following portoenterostomy in biliary atresia. J Pediatr Gastroenterol Nutr 2019;68(4):495–501.
58. Chen HL, Liu YJ, Chen HL, et al. Expression of hepatocyte transporters and nuclear receptors in children with early and late-stage biliary atresia. Pediatr Res 2008;63(6):667–73.
59. Harpavat SHJ, Karpen SJ. Prognostic value of serum bile acids after Kasai portoenterostomy in biliary atresia 2019. p. 137.
60. Chusilp S, Sookpotarom P, Tepmalai K, et al. Prognostic values of serum bilirubin at 7th day post-Kasai for survival with native livers in patients with biliary atresia. Pediatr Surg Int 2016;32(10):927–31.
61. Jain V, Burford C, Alexander EC, et al. Prognostic markers at adolescence in patients requiring liver transplantation for biliary atresia in adulthood. J Hepatol 2019;71(1):71–7.
62. Bijl EJ, Bharwani KD, Houwen RH, et al. The long-term outcome of the Kasai operation in patients with biliary atresia: a systematic review. Neth J Med 2013;71(4): 170–3.
63. Samyn M. Transitional care of biliary atresia. Semin Pediatr Surg 2020;29(4): 150948.
64. Karrer FM, Wallace BJ, Estrada AE. Late complications of biliary atresia: hepatopulmonary syndrome and portopulmonary hypertension. Pediatr Surg Int 2017; 33(12):1335–40.
65. Ueno T, Saka R, Takama Y, et al. Onset ages of hepatopulmonary syndrome and pulmonary hypertension in patients with biliary atresia. Pediatr Surg Int 2017; 33(10):1053–7.
66. Nightingale S, Stormon MO, O'Loughlin EV, et al. Early posthepatoportoenterostomy predictors of native liver survival in biliary atresia. J Pediatr Gastroenterol Nutr 2017;64(2):203–9.
67. Tyraskis A, Parsons C, Davenport M. Glucocorticosteroids for infants with biliary atresia following Kasai portoenterostomy. Cochrane Database Syst Rev 2018; 5(5):CD008735.

UNITED STATES POSTAL SERVICE® Statement of Ownership, Management, and Circulation (All Periodicals Publications Except Requester Publications)

1. Publication Title	2. Publication Number	3. Filing Date
PEDIATRIC CLINICS OF NORTH AMERICA	424 – 66	9/18/2021

4. Issue Frequency	5. Number of Issues Published Annually	6. Annual Subscription Price
FEB, APR, JUN, AUG, OCT, DEC	6	$250.00

7. Complete Mailing Address of Known Office of Publication (Not printer) (Street, city, county, state, and ZIP+4®)

ELSEVIER INC.
230 Park Avenue, Suite 800
New York, NY 10169

Contact Person
Malathi Samayan

Telephone (Include area code)
91-44-4299-4507

8. Complete Mailing Address of Headquarters or General Business Office of Publisher (Not printer)

ELSEVIER INC.
230 Park Avenue, Suite 800
New York, NY 10169

9. Full Names and Complete Mailing Addresses of Publisher, Editor, and Managing Editor (Do not leave blank)

Publisher (Name and complete mailing address)

DOLORES MELONI, ELSEVIER INC.
1600 JOHN F KENNEDY BLVD. SUITE 1800
PHILADELPHIA, PA 19103-2899

Editor (Name and complete mailing address)

KERRY HOLLAND, ELSEVIER INC.
1600 JOHN F KENNEDY BLVD. SUITE 1800
PHILADELPHIA, PA 19103-2899

Managing Editor (Name and complete mailing address)

PATRICK MANLEY, ELSEVIER INC.
1600 JOHN F KENNEDY BLVD. SUITE 1800
PHILADELPHIA, PA 19103-2899

10. Owner (Do not leave blank. If the publication is owned by a corporation, give the name and address of the corporation immediately followed by the names and addresses of all stockholders owning or holding 1 percent or more of the total amount of stock. If not owned by a corporation, give the names and addresses of the individual owners. If owned by a partnership or other unincorporated firm, give its name and address as well as those of each individual owner. If the publication is published by a nonprofit organization, give its name and address.)

Full Name	Complete Mailing Address
WHOLLY OWNED SUBSIDIARY OF REED/ELSEVIER, US HOLDINGS	1600 JOHN F KENNEDY BLVD. SUITE 1800 PHILADELPHIA, PA 19103-2899

11. Known Bondholders, Mortgagees, and Other Security Holders Owning or Holding 1 Percent or More of Total Amount of Bonds, Mortgages, or Other Securities. If none, check box ▶ ☐ None

Full Name	Complete Mailing Address
N/A	

12. Tax Status (For completion by nonprofit organizations authorized to mail at nonprofit rates) (Check one)
The purpose, function, and nonprofit status of this organization and the exempt status for federal income tax purposes:
☒ Has Not Changed During Preceding 12 Months
☐ Has Changed During Preceding 12 Months (Publisher must submit explanation of change with this statement)

PS Form 3526, July 2014 [Page 1 of 4 (see instructions page 4)] PSN: 7530-01-000-9931 PRIVACY NOTICE: See our privacy policy on www.usps.com.

13. Publication Title	14. Issue Date for Circulation Data Below
PEDIATRIC CLINICS OF NORTH AMERICA	JUNE 2021

15. Extent and Nature of Circulation			Average No. Copies Each Issue During Preceding 12 Months	No. Copies of Single Issue Published Nearest to Filing Date
a. Total Number of Copies (Net press run)			568	483
b. Paid Circulation (By Mail and Outside the Mail)	(1)	Mailed Outside-County Paid Subscriptions Stated on PS Form 3541 (Include paid distribution above nominal rate, advertiser's proof copies, and exchange copies)	276	264
	(2)	Mailed In-County Paid Subscriptions Stated on PS Form 3541 (Include paid distribution above nominal rate, advertiser's proof copies, and exchange copies)	0	0
	(3)	Paid Distribution Outside the Mails Including Sales Through Dealers and Carriers, Street Vendors, Counter Sales, and Other Paid Distribution Outside USPS®	220	180
	(4)	Paid Distribution by Other Classes of Mail Through the USPS (e.g., First-Class Mail®)	0	0
c. Total Paid Distribution (Sum of 15b (1), (2), (3), and (4))		▶	496	444
d. Free or Nominal Rate Distribution (By Mail and Outside the Mail)	(1)	Free or Nominal Rate Outside-County Copies Included on PS Form 3541	51	22
	(2)	Free or Nominal Rate In-County Copies Included on PS Form 3541	0	0
	(3)	Free or Nominal Rate Copies Mailed at Other Classes Through the USPS (e.g., First-Class Mail)	0	0
	(4)	Free or Nominal Rate Distribution Outside the Mail (Carriers or other means)	0	0
e. Total Free or Nominal Rate Distribution (Sum of 15d (1), (2), (3) and (4))		▶	51	22
f. Total Distribution (Sum of 15c and 15e)		▶	547	466
g. Copies not Distributed (See Instructions to Publishers #4 (page #3))		▶	21	17
h. Total (Sum of 15f and g)		▶	568	483
i. Percent Paid (15c divided by 15f times 100)		▶	90.67%	95.27%

* If you are claiming electronic copies, go to line 16 on page 3. If you are not claiming electronic copies, skip to line 17 on page 3.

16. Electronic Copy Circulation		Average No. Copies Each Issue During Preceding 12 Months	No. Copies of Single Issue Published Nearest to Filing Date
a. Paid Electronic Copies	▶		
b. Total Paid Print Copies (Line 15c) + Paid Electronic Copies (Line 16a)	▶		
c. Total Print Distribution (Line 15f) + Paid Electronic Copies (Line 16a)	▶		
d. Percent Paid (Both Print & Electronic Copies) (16b divided by 16c × 100)	▶		

☒ I certify that 50% of all my distributed copies (electronic and print) are paid above a nominal price.

17. Publication of Statement of Ownership

☒ If the publication is a general publication, publication of this statement is required. Will be printed in the OCTOBER 2021 issue of this publication. ☐ Publication not required.

18. Signature and Title of Editor, Publisher, Business Manager, or Owner

Malathi Samayan

Malathi Samayan - Distribution Controller

Date 9/18/2021

I certify that all information furnished on this form is true and complete. I understand that anyone who furnishes false or misleading information on this form or who omits material or information requested on the form may be subject to criminal sanctions (including fines and imprisonment) and/or civil sanctions (including civil penalties).

PS Form 3526, July 2014 (Page 3 of 4)   PRIVACY NOTICE: See our privacy policy on www.usps.com.

Moving?

Make sure your subscription moves with you!

To notify us of your new address, find your **Clinics Account Number** (located on your mailing label above your name), and contact customer service at:

Email: journalscustomerservice-usa@elsevier.com

800-654-2452 (subscribers in the U.S. & Canada)
314-447-8871 (subscribers outside of the U.S. & Canada)

Fax number: 314-447-8029

Elsevier Health Sciences Division
Subscription Customer Service
3251 Riverport Lane
Maryland Heights, MO 63043

*To ensure uninterrupted delivery of your subscription, please notify us at least 4 weeks in advance of move.

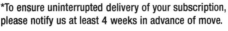